STEVE SOLOMON

Growing NUTRIENT-DENSE vegetables

A COOL-CLIMATE GUIDE

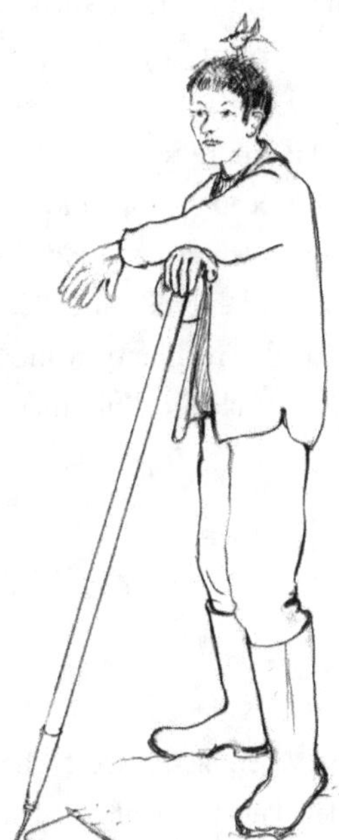

MELLIODORA PUBLISHING

A Note from the Publisher

Growing Nutrient-Dense Vegetables was originally self-published by the author as *Growing Vegetables South of Australia*. In an "apology" note to the reader, Steve explains, "I produced this book without help from a copy editor—someone who knows how to dot eyes and cross teas, make sure that subordinate clauses are not dangling in front of an adverb, and makes sure that when the author refers to something in another chapter it actually is in that chapter...." Rather than smooth away these quirks with our publishing wand, we have also chosen to forego professional copyediting, leaving Steve's idiosyncrasies, and charm, intact.

You'll also find references to Tasmanian suppliers, products and places. Steve's view, and ours, is that they offer a useful framework for what to look for in your own region – as well as a practical directory for those growing "south of Australia".

If you're reading this with a copy of Steve's original self-published edition on your bookshelf, you'll find no surprises here, just the comfort of a classic with a fresh coat of paint. If you're on a Steve-Solomon-spree after discovering *The Intelligent Gardener*, this nutrient-dense growing guide will not disappoint. And if you're coming to Steve's work for the first time, you're in good hands. He's been growing most of his own food for over fifty years — first in Oregon, where he founded Territorial Seed Company, and then in Tasmania, where he settled in 1998. As he explains in his own preface to this edition, roughly half his growing life was spent in each place, and the cool-temperate climate links them more than the distance separates them.

— *The Publishers*

Growing Nutrient-Dense Vegetables: A Cool-Climate Guide by Steve Solomon

Published by Melliodora Publishing July 2026 • ISBN 978-0-6456065-7-7

Originally self-published as *Growing Vegetables South of Australia* by Steve Solomon (2002-2025).

First Melliodora Publishing edition, 2026. **melliodora.com**

Illustrations by Muriel Brown. Additional text and cover artwork: Catie Payne.

Project management, layout and cover design: Richard Telford.

Table of Contents

Vegetables by Family

An alphabetical guide to the vegetables in Chapter 9, How to Grow It — grouped by botanical family. These groupings double as a crop rotation guide: after harvesting one family from a garden bed, plant something from a different family in its place.

Preface

Dear Reader,

In 1979 I paid for printing the first 6,000 copies of what eventually became the book you're reading right now. Back then this book was called *Growing Vegetables West of the Cascades*, which are a line of tall volcanic mountains in both Oregon and Washington states. The Cascades create a temperate maritime climate on their western side that is different than the rest of the United States. In respect to climate, Cascadia is similar to Tasmania, where I live now. My message was crammed into 64 pages because that was all I could afford. The first edition sold out in a few months; then I gave my book to a regional publishing company and expanded the second edition to its current size. The third edition was entirely rewritten in 1984, and so was the fourth edition in 1987. The main reason for all those revisions was that I had learned so much.

Then life brought me to settle in Tasmania. The home gardening situation I found upon arrival in 1998 was highly reminiscent of how Oregon was in 1978 when I homesteaded there. Oregon has a unique maritime climate featuring mild rainy/frosty winters and mostly cool, dry, sunny summer days. The garden books used by Cascadians prior to my arrival there came from the eastern United States, where summers can be scorching and winters freeze the soil one metre deep. The seeds offered to Cascadians then also came from the East, and many of them did not thrive so well in cool summer weather, whilst the crops designed to be harvested in autumn before the soil froze solid all finished too quickly and usually did not withstand Cascadia's humid, frosty winters. So after two years in Oregon I wrote a local gardening guide.

Tasmania was similar. The vegetable gardening books and most vegetable seeds came from mainland Australia, where the climates are entirely different. So I wrote *Growing Vegetables South of Australia*. I did not seek a mainland Australian publisher because the population of Tasmania is only half a million. Instead I purchased a minimum-sized office copy centre and started printing the insides of my book at home. It took me about five days to print 400 copies, feeding the machine 500 sheets of paper at a time, starting after breakfast and continuing until dinner time. A local printer made the covers and did the binding of batches of 400 books. From the very get-go, annual sales amounted to around 600 copies. So I estimate that from 2002 until the end of 2025 I sold 14,000 copies. Only a few were purchased by tourists; the rest went to Tasmanians. I'm not bragging about selling that many books into such a small population. The important thing is that doing one or two print runs every year offered me many opportunities to tweak the text. Which I did. In fact, I learned so much during those years that I completely rewrote the book twice.

I am 83 now. So far I'm experiencing ageing as reduced endurance. I need to nap almost every day. As fast as my body declines, I enjoy a corresponding increase in spiritual awareness. My interests are changing. It seems time for me to stop improving the book I started in 1979 and spend more time reading the Holy Scriptures and walking the paddock with my dog. I conclude that this must be the right action for me because within months of deciding to quit writing *Growing Vegetables South of Australia*, God sent me Melliodora, a proper publisher who recognized that *South of Australia* could help others in similar climates worldwide if the book had a different title. I hope this *Cool Climate Guide* will inspire similar local books for other climate regions.

Blessings,

Winter Solstice, June 2026

Introduction

Son, the cheapest experience you can get comes second hand . . . if you'll only buy it.

Sidney Solomon, my father, in private conversation

I divide food gardeners into two main groups. I name the largest group *casual gardeners*—these folks grow a few small backyard beds or a community garden plot. Much of what they know about vegie gardening came from TV presenters and magazines. Their gardens produce only a tiny part of what their family eats all year. I call the other group *serious gardeners.* I am one of them. We are few. We believe that the quality of our family's food supply is so important that we'll devote a lot of time and effort to growing a large part of it ourselves.

My own gardening career skipped the casual stage. Our first house was small, old and unattractive on a dusty unsealed street in the western edge of Los Angeles. We bought the place because it was on a one acre block where I could grow a big food garden. The soil there was naturally well mineralized but I was not yet smart enough to appreciate how that particular soil made our vegies taste so delicious—so delicious that I became a vegetableatarian. The word doesn't mean that I reject animal-sourced foods. It means I'm an omnivore that mostly eats vegetables most of the time.

After five years of gardening in Babylon we sold our home and small business in order to homestead in Oregon, much like mainland Australians settle in Tasmania as a lifestyle choice. All we could afford without debt was five acres of grassy hillside that (we didn't yet know) had lost all its topsoil from decades of growing winter wheat. When that eroded hillside could no longer produce a profitable wheat crop its fertility had been further depleted by selling hay off the property until the amount of grass it produced did not cover the cost of cutting and baling it. And then that totally mined-out land it was subdivided into five acre lifestyle blocks for fools from the city. Like us.

I soon discovered that organically grown vegetables produced on heavily leached, mined-out subsubsoil are not nutritious. In fact, the longer I ate from that land the poorer my health became. Seven years of health decline strongly motivated me. I learnt how to build soil fertility in a manner that more or less complies with organic certification requirements *and* also produces highly nutrient-dense vegetables. And from that point my health improved rapidly. Another garden writer who appreciated what I have achieved described my method as "beyond organic."

•

I believe that human bodies were Designed to prefer nutrient dense food because it tastes better. However, these days no matter how much you are prepared to pay, no matter how diligently you search the Saturday market, truly nutrient-dense vegetables and fruit are rarely on offer. Fresh?, usually. Attractive?, yes. Nutrient dense? not particularly. And that's why I grow most of my family's food.

I've been shown a great many backyards. When I've inquired about why there was so little (or none) food being grown I heard all the usual justifications. Most of them come down to lack of time and energy after using it to earn enough money to buy the illusion of happiness. This lifestyle makes no sense to me. I won't bore you with a money not buying happiness sermon but this entire book is really about how time and energy *can* buy health. Although maybe less time and energy than you imagine now. This book also teaches efficient methods that make growing the family's food more remunerative than working for wages.

Tasmanians need their own gardening book. Our circumstances are quite different than they are across the Bass Strait. Tasmania's soils have been strongly depleted of nutrients by winter rains; the rocks forming our agricultural soils differ from mainland geology. Tassie's climate is dominated by the surrounding ocean, whose temperature is far more stable than a continental land mass. So Tasmania's climate is more like southern England than like Victoria. Our climate is much like western Oregon; that is where I once made my living by selling regionally-appropriate vegetable garden seeds and writing regionally-focused how-to-garden books.

At age 55 it was time to relocate. I chose Tasmania because I feel completely at home here, because Tassie culture and economy now are similar to what Oregon was like when I was young. I took possession of a seven acre bush property in Upper Rosevears on November 1, 1998. There wasn't time to raise my own seedlings. Whatever I found at the local garden centre would have to do. Consequently I discovered that our garden centre tomato seedlings were not nearly as early to ripen nor as productive nor as tasty as the varieties I had provided to Oregonians when I ran Territorial Seed Company. The eggplant seedlings turned out to be a heat loving variety that probably did fine on the mainland but for me it grew a fruitless bush because Tasmanian nights were too cool. The capsicums produced only a few fruits of medium size that ripened late. Mainland lettuce varieties proved insufficiently winter hardy. I observed that wintertime vegie gardens near me didn't have much growing in them.

Clearly my new neighbours needed help. After accumulating a few years of experience I self-published the first edition of this book. I called it "South of Australia" because Tassie, like other small countries, depends upon imports—including gardening books originating from that big island to the north of us. Tasmanians bought seeds from mainland catalogue sellers and from mainland picture packet distributors providing varieties that often were not suited to Tasmanian conditions. And we repeated the state's unofficial mantra—near enough is good enough.

Since 2002 I have sold over 10,000 copies of this book—all but a handful of them to Tasmanians. My book has had an effect. These days many gardeners take fuller advantage of Tasmania's year-round growing possibilities and have learnt what nutrient density means when you bite into it.

I feel blessed to have helped this happen.

I grow most of my own food

I've been a homesteader since my early 30s. The word *homesteading* means creating products or services from your own home that earn income or that are personal survival necessities, like food or firewood. I encourage others to practice this lifestyle because people develop confidence when they create any part of their necessities. Then they're less concerned with pleasing the Authority paying their salary; they're less dependent on government. I think life would be better for everyone if more people produce much of their own basic survival requirements instead of working a joyless job to earn money with which to buy them.

Independence-mindedness greatly increases when a person enjoys a high degree of physical well-being but these days the majority of Australians are trapped in a diminishing spiral of worsening health that actually began before birth with their mother's inadequate nutrition and continued into childhood when they established unfortunate eating habits that led to dependency on medicines that further lower overall health. The way out is not found by finding a smarter doctor. The way out requires (1) overcoming unhealthy eating habits by switching to nutrient-dense foods, and (2) eliminating otherwise decent foods that happen to be inappropriate for your body's genetic makeup or foods it reacts badly to. In my opinion that's all it takes for most people to enjoy a sense of well being most of the time, make them energetic and optimistic, make the overall tone of my neighbourhood become more positive, make people enjoyably live longer—and thereby get wiser. For those whose bodies haven't yet degenerated too far, eating right completely heals diseases caused by years of wrong feeding.

Overcoming harmful food habits can be difficult. I assert that dietary repentance has been made even more difficult because the nutritional content of all foods has declined by more than half over the last century. Consequently the basic foods like wheat and meat as well as fruits and vegetables—whether conventionally or organically grown—are not nearly as nutrient dense as they should be. They do not taste as good as they could. *They do not satisfy.* Consequently, eating mostly nutrient-undense foods creates irresistible urges to eat over-seasoned junk.

Certified organic is more nutritious than most "conventionally grown" but most organic foods are not even close to what food could be. One proof of my assertion are people who have largely replaced conventional foods with certified organic but still crave junk food—such as starch fried in vegetable oil—but obtain it from the health-food shop. I believe there is a more effective way to reform eating habits and improve health—simply enjoy the wonderful flavours of fresh home-garden vegetables that were grown in such a way as to make them nutrient dense. Give that a few years to work on you and a big vegie garden can effortlessly uplift your food preferences.

Foods produced on fully remineralized soil taste enormously better *because* they contain much more nutrition. I don't mean the insignificant 25 percent increase over conventionally grown that the organic farming industry propaganda claims about its fruits and vegetables. I'm talking about packing 200 to 300 percent more nutrition into food. Imagine eating a carrot that tastes twice as carroty with complex undertones of raspberry and ginger, a barely sensed aroma of carnations, a lingering pleasant aftertaste and so sweet that any sweeter would be disgusting. That's the sort of thing I mean. I mean steamed French beans that don't *need* butter, salt or pepper. That sort of thing.

If the majority of Australian farms grew nutrient-dense crops then the overall health and intelligence of Australians would improve enormously. But remineralizing exhausted soils is not affordable when the only way most farmers can find to make a profit is by minimizing the cost of inputs.

I think the full social cost of industrial food includes at least two-thirds the current burden of medical care, 90 plus percent of all dental care (there still would be sports injuries and car wrecks), plus the huge social costs arising from people self-medicating with legal- and illegal mood altering substances. Ethical social accounting would show that soil remineralization is the low cost solution to a great many ills. However, remineralization is never-never-never mentioned in mainstream conversation because, in my opinion, restoration of our farmlands would soon bankrupt the AMA and the medical schools controlled by the AMA, and bankrupt the drugs businesses—both medical and illegal—and pretty much end the mental health industry, the agricultural poison industry, etc.

•

Have you seen those huge tables in the appendices of 1960s how-to-be-healthy books, informing us that 100 grams of broccoli contain exactly so many milligrams of vitamin B_6 and so forth? These numbers are not The Truth. They act, in fact, like a powerful statistical deception because those numbers are *averages* of a great many samples grown on different soils at different times of year. Had you been shown the range instead of the average then you would realize that one sample contains five times more B_6 than the average, another sample might provide next to none.

Do these differences really matter? Doesn't it all average out? Sorry! No matter how correct a person's food choices seem, intaking average nutrient density no longer produces vibrant health because the overall nutrition in *all* foods, be they organically grown or conventional, has decreased steadily over the last 100 years. This decline has been indisputably documented regarding American conventionally grown foods. Comparing the most recent USDA report (1990s) with a similar report from the early 1960s shows a 40 to 60 percent decline in almost all nutritional elements in all types of fruits and vegetables. (All amounts following are in milligrams/100 grams.) Between 1963 and 2000 the average vitamin C content of capsicum dropped from 128 mg to 89 mg. The vitamin A content of apples dropped from 90 mg to 53 mg. Nearly half the calcium and vitamin A once found in broccoli has disappeared. The potassium content of collards has fallen from 400 mg to 170 mg and magnesium from 57 mg to 9 mg. Cauliflower has lost half its vitamin C, thiamine and riboflavin. Calcium in pineapple has dropped from 17 mg to 7 mg. Etc. (Source: "Vegetables Without Vitamins," *Life Extension Foundation Magazine*, www.Lef.org, March 2001, available online at soilandhealth.org.)

The Americans have a huge organic farming industry that proudly declares that OG food contains 25 percent more nutrition than conventional. But if roughly half the nutrient content of all conventionally grown foods has been lost then organically grown food these days provides a bit under two-thirds of the nutrition that conventionally grown foods provided in 1963. It's much worse than that: foods in 1963 contained much less nutrition on average than they did before the First World War because after WWI chemicals replaced crop rotations, green- and animal manures.

To yield nutrient-dense food the soil has to contain adequate organic matter and *abundantly* provide plants with 11 chemical elements in concentrations that must be proportionate to each other, as well as provide many other plant nutrient elements in very small quantities. Farmers can't fertilize soil to that extent and also make a profit. Instead, the soil is only fed enough to produce the highest-possible bulk yield at the lowest-possible cost. And this is a typical result: potatoes grown on balanced remineralized soil can contain about 11 percent protein; however, the usual industrial farming supermarket sort, the frozen French fries by the 50-pound-bag processor sort—about 8 percent protein. The 11 percent protein spud also provides far higher concentrations of minerals, vitamins and other nutritional factors. But 8 percent protein potatoes yield more bushels per acre. The grower of calorie-dense food spends much less on fertilizer—and stays in business.

Suppose that you are a potato farmer with a mortgage and business debts; which sort of spud are you going to grow? A certified organic potato farmer might agonize over the choice, but could they choose differently? It's a rare farmer practicing any agricultural religion that could choose to harvest fewer bushels per acre while incurring higher production costs.

Suppose Tasmanians had to depend on potatoes as their staff of life, much like Irish cottagers did around 1,800—spuds making up much of every meal. We *could* satisfy our appetites with simply prepared nutrient dense potatoes or else we surely would artfully season relatively tasteless demineralized devitaminized potatoes. If we lived on 8 percent protein potatoes, then over a few generations we'd become shorter in height; our average lifespan would decrease; we'd be less intelligent. And collectively, socially, we would have to spend far more than any amount of money we saved by not perfecting soil fertility . . . on hospitals, on doctors, on mental therapists, on disability care, on prisons . . . not considering the cost of all that pain and suffering. I think my previous sentence accurately describes what actually is happening right now.

There is a simple mathematical equation that expresses this concept:

$$\text{HEALTH} = \text{NUTRITION} \div \text{CALORIES}$$

The average health of a broad population equals the nutrition in their total dietary intake divided by the total number of calories accompanying these nutrients.

If we receive 2,000 units of nutrition from our daily 2,000 calories, then our health equals "one," but if only 1,000 units of nutrition are in our 2,000 daily calories, then our health equals "one-half" while most peoples' body size increases quite a bit. Perhaps this idea seems too simple to explain such a complex subject but the truth actually is that simple. If people ate so that their nutritional intake was high compared to the number of calories they were consuming then they would be slender, far healthier, more intelligent and longer-lived compared to what is normal these days.

In 1939 an American research dentist named Weston Price published *Nutrition and Physical Degeneration.* * The book should have become and still should be required reading in high school but it still is widely ignored. Price documented many extremely remote communities where everyone had perfect teeth, legendary good health and very long lives. Everybody. The cause was extreme isolation. There was no shop in the village. There were no tins of jam or Spam or condensed milk, no sugar, no white flour. These people grew, gathered, fished or hunted everything they ate. They had no choice but to raise food naturally and prepare it simply. The community was so healthy because over time it had learned which foods healed illness and which local foods developed health—and concentrated on those. I consider Price's book one of the most important works of the twentieth century because without this information we would be entirely lost in a stormy sea of illness without the slightest idea of how healthy and long-lived properly nourished humans could be.

Weston Price and his wife made three globe-spanning journeys between 1933 and 1936. Their first trip was to Europe where they visited healthy communities in extremely remote Swiss highland valleys and the Outer Hebrides islands off Scotland. They subsequently visited Africa, Peru, Australia (very remote aboriginals), Melanesia, Polynesia and far north Canada. In every isolated community almost everyone lived past age 80 and often much longer; they possessed all their teeth in old age with not a sign of tooth decay, gum disease or loose teeth from loss of jawbone. Price provides many photos showing bright toothy smiles without there being a toothbrush in the community. He also found no sign of the degenerative diseases we consider normal these days—cancer, heart disease, diabetes, etc. Childbirth was rarely difficult; almost all mothers and children survived it. Infant mortality was very low and the birth rate usually was in balance with that. Death arrived from misadventure or old age. Price also commented on the high moral standards in these well-nourished communities. The people seemed more intelligent than the usual, poised and spiritually aware (without religious formalities). Price also analysed their foods as best he could using the limited (portable) chemistry of his era. He found that people in these healthy communities received about five times the average mineral nutrition (calcium, magnesium, potassium) of working class Americans of that time. The American dietary of that era consisted of very few vegetables, much devitalized white flour, pork fat, denatured white corn, potatoes, overcooked and often processed/preserved red meat and sugar. Milk products were degraded by pasteurization.

One lesson I take from Price's book is that no one dietary is optimum for all humans. The highland Swiss thrived on rye bread and dairy products; the Scots in the Outer Hebrides ate seafood, kale and oats. The isolated Native Americans

* *The best books about improving human (and animal) health with better farming methods were written between 1930 and 1960. Often not even one used copy of these titles is for sale on the internet. I have made many of these books available as free downloads from www.soilandhealth.org. Complete bibliographic information on every book I will mention can be found in the Additional Reading section at the end. You are invited to study the contents of Soil and Health Library; it will substantiate everything I have asserted in this Introduction.*

of northern Canada ate mostly animal foods (but not only muscle tissue). Healthy highland Africans ate mostly cereals; isolated tropical Africans ate starchy roots. Long-lived remote Pacific Islanders mostly ate tree fruit, garden vegetables and seafoods. And especially of interest to us, remote Australian aboriginals eating bush tucker had long lives, perfect teeth and excellent health. It seems obvious to me that after a group of wandering humans settled in a new region, their children with genetics that didn't suit the local food possibilities failed to run the gauntlet of childhood disease. That is how a community's genes came to match the available foods. People, considered as a group, can thrive on almost any reasonable assortment of foods except for one possibility—to be really healthy our foods *must* be nutrient dense.

No community now on this planet except perhaps in the most inaccessible parts of the Amazon rainforest remained free of industrial foods after the Second World War. People in these no-longer-remote-enough places still share pretty much the same genetics their ancestors had but their extraordinary health and longevity has disappeared. Price's book provides the best documentation we have about the human potential for health and longevity. His research proves to me that a long, healthy life is the entitlement of almost every body but we have sold our God-given birthright for cheap industrial food.

I'm not quite done ranting about 'health equals nutrition divided by calories.' Please examine a few foods through this lens. Take refined white sugar. It is all calories and no nutrition. None! Every calorie we eat as sugar reduces our total nutritional intake because taking in empty calories *prevents* us from eating foods that do contain nutrition. Worse, we now know that eating more than a few teaspoons of table sugar per day causes deadly metabolic diseases; high fructose corn syrup is worse than table sugar in this respect.

Fats are more calorie dense than sugar is. Most fats contain very little nutrition. Every calorie of low quality fat we intake reduces our ability to consume foods that do contain the nutrients we need. Ask yourself please: what proportion of most peoples' total caloric intake these days comes in the forms of cheap vegetable oil and sugar? Half? More than half? When I was a young man it would have been way less than 25 percent. In the remote communities Price described these kinds of non-foods were not available.

So if sugar and most fats are the worst, what's at the extreme healthy end of the food spectrum? The best single food I know of, the one that offers the most nutrition for the amount of calories it provides is an uncooked dark green leaf that was grown on balanced remineralized soil. A person would have to spend half their entire day chewing in order to take in enough calories from a diet of only raw leaf lettuce, kale, spinach, endive, silverbeet, etc. Their jaw muscles would become very strong; they would be slender (and very healthy) no matter how much they ate.

To live long in good health people must mostly eat nutrient-dense foods. Our foods must not have been devitalised or denatured (some nutritional elements removed) like white wheat flour is. Our foods must not be adulterated with slightly toxic preservatives or other artificial ingredients. And most important, our foods must be grown on soils we have intentionally made as fertile and balanced as they possibly can be.

To learn more I suggest starting with *The Wheel of Health** by G. T. Wrench. It is a brief and easy-to-comprehend book about the human potential for health and longevity. Dr. Wrench explains that your current state of health was strongly influenced by your maternal grandmother's nutrition and that a mother's poor nutrition permanently lessens their own children's health and longevity. A person whose body got a good nutritional start and then mostly eats whole unadulterated nutrient-dense foods can enjoy perfect teeth for their lifetime without ever seeing a dentist, will not experience degenerative disease and can look forward to a long and physically pleasant life. Our God-given birthright includes the possibility of a gentle death after a long life—if we are healthy. Alternatively, we may experience a lot of disease but with medical intervention suffer on for almost as many years, with suboptimum health all the way. Which way it goes could most often be our choice.

I rarely find highly nutrient-dense vegies on offer. The local growers I chat with at weekend markets sell vegetables that look as good as anything in the supermarket. Often they are certified organically grown. But most of these growers have not specifically added trace elements to their soil. Their soil's major nutrients—nitrogen, calcium, magnesium potassium, phosphorus and sulfur—have been increased but not brought into balance. Their food is better, but not nearly better enough. That's most of why I grow most of my own. That's why Annie and I mostly eat whatever comes fresh from the garden. There have been moments when I wished to travel, to adventure, to not be responsible for my nutrition beyond making reasonably healthy choices the majority of the time. And I have tried that route more than once. But my health suffered each time I depended on industrial foods for more than a few months.

I believe serving others is God's purpose for me. So you are welcome to write to me. I maintain a contact page at www.soilandhealth.org.

Chapter 1
Basics

The agriculturalist is the servant of the plant.
Louise Howard, second wife of Sir Albert Howard.

Before the Second World War the majority of Tasmanians lived on farms or else in small towns where most residential building blocks were a half-acre. Growing backyard vegies was the usual thing. Children learned how to by helping. People these days understand smart phones, mass market entertainment, recreational drugs and fast-food restaurants; they know little or nothing about growing plants. So this chapter tries to compensate.

Competition

The best way I know to understand another being is to imagine their boots and then try to walk in them. So let's consider the awareness of a wild plant and then assume the viewpoint of a garden vegetable.

Sure, plants are aware! We don't notice this because plants aren't concerned about the same things humans are. And unlike humans, plants do not possess individuality. A plant is like a skin cell, part of a broad protective layer—skin. Kill a few cells and the skin grows back. I wonder: does each skin cell consider itself to be the whole skin? I believe that plants similarly participate in a shared consciousness involving all the plants of their species in the region. Their collective interest is survival that is usually accomplished by domination.

The spiritual nature of plants is best grasped by direct observation; it can't be easily communicated with words. What I hope these words will achieve is to suggest there is an insight to be had. One way to entice that understanding is spending time leaning on a hoe.

Here's how-to. When your muscles become a bit tired from hoeing weeds or digging beds, rest the working end of the tool on the soil, hold the handle near the top and take some weight off your feet. Then stare into the distance or at some part of your garden and just *look,* don't think. When you inevitably do think, don't give yourself a problem about thinking when you're supposed to not think—which is a mistake that people who practice meditation often make—just resume working. And don't let anyone call hoe-leaning laziness! Hoe-leaning is every bit as vital a gardening task as hoe sharpening is.

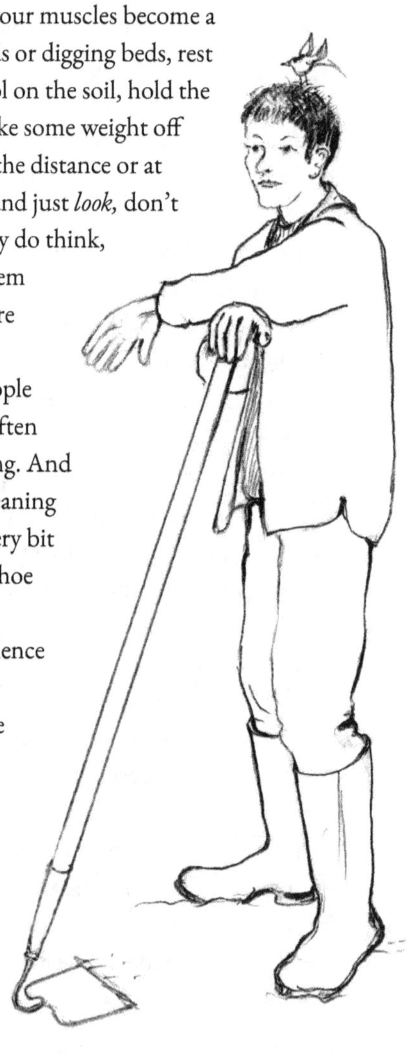

Hoe-leaning helps to silence mental chatter and brings forth insight; to paraphrase The Book on this, 'be still and ye shall Know.' My observations revealed that plants are focused on a life-or-death struggle to access light and soil resources and to dominate space. And that plants are not kind. They steal the other guy's light and poison the other guy's soil.

Each species has its own cunning strategy. Young trees put no energy into making seeds for their first years but instead grow taller faster. Once they secure some space they then make jillions of seeds that can travel long distances because of the height they're released.

Wild lettuce rapidly spreads broad leaves over its neighbours as its juicy taproot patiently stores up food and moisture against the day that its seed stalk will rapidly overtop them. Tasmania's mild winters support many biennial species using a similar strategy. Biennials mature seeds in summer while conditions are dry and then they die. These seeds sprout with the autumn rains and proceed to grow slowly through winter, storing up food. In spring biennials consume their reserves to outgrow their competitors.

Wild plants withstand intense competition; many species thrive in compact infertile soil. They survive drought. They cope with strong wind. When edible wild plants became garden vegetables they received a protected environment, richer moister looser soil, far less competition and assisted reproduction. In exchange they make tender leaves without bitterness, extra-large juicy seedpods; unnecessarily huge flowers; bigger, sweeter fruit; fatter tastier seeds. Vegetables have become grotesque weaklings in order to please us but they only thrive in rich garden soil. Weeds, still being wild plants, always outdo them. New gardeners soon realize that weeds crowd vegetables out. What many do not realize is that overcrowded vegetables do nearly as poorly as if they were competing with weeds.

Gardeners have been misled about plant spacing ever since the intensive method was made politically correct in the mid-1970s. Intensive supposedly achieves a much higher yield from the area involved. Intensive requires deeply digging a great deal of compost into wide raised beds and then packing plants as close together as they can seem to withstand each other's competition. Intensive supposedly yields more from the amount of irrigation supplied. (I will discredit that assertion when I discuss dry gardening.) The driving force behind intensive appears to be John Jeavons—but maybe not. John first appeared on the national scene a few months before I started food gardening. His method must have appealed to the Powers That Be because within seven years every mainstream garden book, national garden magazine and government garden publication promoted intensive. I practiced the intensive method for ten years until I learned better. I still think intensive makes sense for a casual gardener with only a few square metres to play in.

After six years of gardening intensively I went into the vegetable garden seed business. To do that ethically I grew variety trials in order to discover the best ones for home gardening in my climate. A trial requires careful observation of many varieties, all given the same opportunity. A trial shows if almost every plant from that packet of seed is similar to the others and productive or if the packet makes plants of little value. Every plant under trial must be given enough growing room to fully express itself so I organized the trials ground in long rows with a walkway between each row so that I could closely observe every plant. Most of my trial rows were 1,200 mm apart centre to centre. Cauliflower and broccoli plants were positioned 600 mm apart in the row. Each variety of a small-sized vegetable like carrot or beetroot was allowed two row metres but to be able to inspect enough plants of each variety I put them in two lines that were 300 mm apart, one line along each side of the row centre. Vining species like cucumbers had to be separated enough that there was no doubt about which fruit belonged to which plant—which meant one plant per position, each position 1,200 apart in the row, the rows 1,200 apart. Pumpkin vines were positioned 3 metres apart, in rows 2,400 apart.

I soon discovered that the amount of work required to grow a half-acre of variety trials was little more than what it took to grow an intensive garden that was one-eighth acre. I discovered that the trials ground needed watering far less often, that most species grew much larger, seemed healthier and some kinds of vegetables produced for more weeks. My biggest surprise was discovering that the spread out vegetables in the trials ground produced nearly as much food per square metre per growing week as my intensive kitchen garden did. The bottom line: intensive only makes sense when a person has more time than they have space.

Weeds

The more often I weed the garden the less time and effort it takes. In spring I thoroughly weed the entire garden *once a week*. That way the weeds are always small and easily eliminated. But if I were to weed every two weeks it would require three or four times as much work. Attention ladies: weekly weeding with a sharp hoe takes little more effort than sweeping or vacuuming floors.

Extensive layouts save time and reduce effort because they can be weeded efficiently with a lightweight *sharp* hoe. Plants on intensive beds are packed so tightly that they must be weeded bent over with dull fingers. Pulling out some weed species can be nearly impossible if the weed got very large—the top snaps off when you tug, leaving the growing point intact. Then the weed grows a new top. Hoeing just below the surface efficiently slices off the growing point; hoeing almost inevitably kills weeds. Occasionally a hoed weed is badly damaged but not killed; it is sure not to survive when I hoe it again one week later. And hoeing is not hard on the back or knees although doing it does develop strong wrists.

These days my vegetable beds total about 150 square metres, not including the paths between them. That much garden amply provides two oldies year-round. Weeds that appear at summer's end I allow to grow unmolested (*and very slowly*) through winter. Weeds start growing fast in September; these will make seeds. So during this month, nearly every afternoon that the weather is pleasant I spend an hour hoeing paths and cleaning beds. Weeding takes much less time from October through March and very little from April through August.

My vegie garden consists of *slightly* raised beds with narrow footpaths between them. The beds do not have retaining walls. Starting about mid-August I clean paths; I am especially focused on grasses. If I didn't do this grasses would form a tough sod that spreads into the beds. (You gardeners who mow grass paths between your beds are making a lot of unnecessary work for yourselves.) The paths became compacted during winter so clearing them in spring takes effort. But after the paths have been cleared keeping them clean takes little effort and hardly any time. I allow weeds to again carpet my paths during autumn. I don't hoe them out then because these weeds won't form seeds until next spring; they also create useful biomass and prevent my boots from getting so muddy.

People these days lack knowledge about using hoes and about how to sharpen them. A dull hoe is worse than ineffective; it rapidly exhausts the hoer. Many discouraged hoers try to eliminate weeds by mulching paths (and beds), but weeds come up anyway unless the mulch is very thick. The soil under mulched paths still gets compacted by the gardener's feet so weeds that do manage to come up may not pull out easily. Unless raised beds have walls around them (a practice I do not recommend), some soil inevitably moves from bed down to path. Unfortunately, a mixture of fertile soil and mulch makes an excellent weed-growing medium.

Grass competition especially stunts vegetables. Most grasses aren't easily hoed out after they have grown for a few weeks. So after the spring clean up I rigorously eliminate grass when it is still small.

Some grass species spread by putting out underground runners (stolons); any piece of stolon left in the soil can start a new plant. Gardeners call these aggressive types witch grass, or twitch, crab, quack, couch, or cooch. Or use rude words to describe them. Some grasses leave behind tiny tubers that put up leaves. I prefer to admire all of them as an example of God's handiwork. The only practical way to eliminate these kinds of grass without poisoning them with something that can also poison you is to methodically dig up the infested area about 150 mm deep, patiently teasing out every fragment of underground runner. And then practice extreme vigilance for another year after that. Oxalis is one weed I can't defeat by hoeing or poisoning; every tiny bulblet forming below the plant must be patiently dug up. And they can be found as much as 100 mm below the surface.

To eliminate persistent weeds, every leaf that the root or even small piece of root puts up can be hoed off just below the soil line within a day or two of appearing; then the root's food reserve becomes exhausted. It will take more than a few weeks of repeated hoeing to completely kill them. I have eliminated horseradish, dock and comfrey this way. The key to success is applying a *sharp* hoe within a few days of seeing yet another emerging leaf.

Some weeds make and spread seeds within a few weeks of coming up. Included in this group are capeweed, groundsel, spitweed (looks like land cress). These pernicious species should not be permitted to survive long enough to make seeds inside the garden or even close to it.

When following my spacing recommendations for the first time the plants may seem rather far apart for their first month but hoeing easily keeps them weed-free. Only an occasional weed nestled hard against a vegetable seedling must be hand pulled. In their second month the vegetables form a leaf canopy that covers the whole area and prevents hoeing. The canopy's shade also suppresses weeds that manage to sprout under it. An occasional weed still emerges above the canopy and should be hand pulled when it is spotted. There won't be many like that and they'll pull out easily because all the hoeing that went on before the canopy formed; the leaf canopy also prevents rain or irrigation from compacting the soil.

After mid March I always feel lazy although I continue to hoe beds that are overwintering small plants. Otherwise I let the weeds alone. Autumn weeds grow slowly and won't make seed until spring; the crops for mid-winter harvest already are way ahead of them. It's also better for the soil to go through winter covered with green, even with weeds. Like an intentionally sown green manure, weeds reduce soil compaction from winter rains, make biomass, prevent erosion, and leave the soil looser next spring.

Thinning

I'd like to think the word "garden" derived from *guard*—fend off moisture stress, insects, wildlife, wind, protect from frost in spring. Protect from strong competition. But eliminating weeds may not reduce competition enough. The crop does far less well when it competes too much with itself. Crowded root vegetables grow more top and less bottom. Densely packed bush bean plants form smaller, often tougher and frequently misshaped pods that take more time to harvest, top and tail. Tomatoes, peppers, eggplant, zucchini, cucumber, and broccoli all produce well until the root zone allocated to them gets crowded; then fruit set (or broccoli side shoot production) greatly slows and quality drops.

If every seed sown would shoot and form a desirable plant then there would be no need to thin. But effectively using vegetable seeds requires that five seeds must be sown so that three seedlings emerge. If two of these three seedlings aren't removed, then they all struggle. I've met gardeners who resist thinning as though it were phytological murder. I entreat you, oh gentlest of persons, please reconsider the nature of plants. Thinning seedlings is not like drowning unwanted kittens. Vegetables *don't mind being thinned.* They know that thinning helps them. Left to their own devices, wild plants will strew—scatter is too refined a term for this—strew seeds far more densely than a gardener ever will. Wild plants thin themselves in far less merciful ways than you ever will.

Consider wild cabbage. After overwintering the plant forms sprays of small yellow flowers. Each one becomes a skinny pod containing half a dozen seeds that mature in summer. Some pods split open as the seeds ripen; escaped seeds sprout if there's an unusual summer rain. But these early starters soon die or get permanently stunted if the rest of the summer proves rainless. Some seeds remain securely within their pod where they are protected from the first showers of late summer. These seeds sprout after the seed pod gets thoroughly soaked, by which time the soil has become properly moist. Often all the seeds within a single pod sprout at once and come up in a cluster. Imagine the intense struggle as many clusters of seedlings fight it out to only a few plants.

I see great wisdom behind this struggle. Brassica seedlings are weak and small. By coming up in tight bunches they combine forces so that a cluster may push aside an obstacle and reach the light where a single seedling would fail. Then the cluster proceeds to compete for water, nutrients and light. The seedling that is best adapted to the current circumstance dominates the space. The others die. Do they die in slow agony or die peacefully, having fulfilled their function in the Great Scheme of Things?

A wild cabbage plant may disperse 1,000 seeds so that one of them survives to make the next 1,000 seeds. Perhaps all 1,000 embryos in those 1,000 seeds are at peace with the process; perhaps all are entirely unaware; perhaps all of them are immortal parts of the cabbage spirit. You choose.

I hope that's sufficient argument to convince even the gentlest of readers that thinning aligns with God's plan. Thinning is merciful.

I'll give you a few guidelines: When growing small plants in rows from seeds thin the row for the first time soon after emergence; your intention is to eliminate seedling clusters so that no plants quite touch each other. In their second week most kinds of vegetables begin to grow rapidly. During the first two weeks some weak or damaged seedlings disappear by themselves. Time to thin again so that none are touching each other. Continue to remove the less desirable plants until the intended interplant spacing has been arrived at. When sowing cabbage family plants on positions like 600 mm x 600 mm, sow five or six seeds on each spot; three or four seedlings will come up. Thin these gradually to prevent severe competition. End up with one plant per position by the time it has four fully developed leaves. I call this approach *progressive thinning.*

The vegetable by vegetable growing instructions in Chapter 9 mention if the species makes seeds by exchanging pollen between plants or if it mostly or exclusively pollinates itself. Vegetables that are pollinated by wind or insects should be thinned differently than self-pollinating species. From a self-pollinating species expect that almost all the seedlings will grow at the same speed and will closely resemble each other. Reducing competition is the main reason to choose one seedling over another when thinning.

However, when you sow a bee- or wind-pollinated species the seedlings will have differences. If it is a well-bred high quality open pollinated variety there only be an occasional off-type plant but there will be variations in how vigorously the seedlings grow. Between 10 and 20 percent of them may be slow-growing inbreds (see Chapter 5) that almost eliminate themselves. The majority of plants will be in the middle-range of vigour. A few seedlings may be much more vigorous than the others; these tall poppies should be thinned out when spotted. I know doing that runs against the apparent logic of choosing the strongest plants but these super growers are less likely to prove true to type. Unusually vigorous individuals probably result from an unintended cross with a different variety or else got crossed with a wild plant in the same family or else are mutants. Pull them out! Grow your crop from average seedlings; these have the highest probability of being true-to-type.

Seedlings from F_1 hybrid varieties should be uniform in all respects. F_1 hybrids grow more vigorously than OP varieties, and that includes seed germination; when using hybrid varieties you can sow fewer seeds.

Seedlings become what I call *well established* once they are large enough to not disappear as a slug's breakfast or to wither and fall dead from damping off disease. Vegetable seedlings certainly are well established by the time they have grown three (pairs of) regular leaves. Well established seedlings may safely be thinned to their final spacing.

Light

The word "cultivation" is taken by most to mean hoeing, ploughing or otherwise stirring the soil. Considered more broadly, the term means improving growing conditions from the plant's viewpoint. Growers cultivate plants by increasing soil moisture, we increase and balance soil nutrients, limit competition, increase the quantity of oxygen and organic matter in the soil. We can raise temperature with cloches and greenhouses. But we can't afford to increase the amount of light although light intensity has much to do with plant growth.

I apologize for belabouring the obvious but sometimes great wisdom can be discovered by reconsidering what everyone already knows. Around mid August some strength returns to Tassie's sun; vegetables that overwintered start growing again. So I fertilize them. The first spring bulbs shoot up at this time, indicating that the soil has warmed enough to sow strongly frost-tolerant crops like peas and broad beans. In a few more weeks the soil will be warm enough that I sow lettuce, mustard greens and spinach.

By mid-September direct sunlight feels quite warm on my face. Biennial weeds—dandelion, chicory, wild radish—are growing fast now so I sow biennial root vegetables—beets, carrots and parsley. Overwintered cabbage family plants start flowering; I take this as a sign to sow broccoli, cabbage, kohlrabi and radish. The sun continues to strengthen; frost danger well and truly ends. Now I eagerly sow fruit-bearers like French bean, pumpkin, zucchini and set out tomatoes. It isn't just frost risk—fruit making crops need intense light.

I start most autumn and winter crops in January so that they enjoy three good growing months before light energy declines too much. With the exception of brussels sprout, if autumn/winter crops are started in mid-December they will mature too soon; they will grow beyond being good eating in autumn. Some winter vegetables may be started mid-February. By May they'll be full size, or nearly full size.

By mid-March light energy has lessened so much that tomatoes don't taste nearly as good as they did a few weeks earlier, peppers get smaller and less sweet (or less hot). Cucumber succumbs to powdery mildew. Zucchini and pumpkin get that disease before the end of March even if there is no rain or heavy dew. The causes of powdery mildew *seem* to be colder nights, heavy morning dews, daytime humidity and exhaustion after such heavy bearing. Actually, lack of light energy is the major factor that lowers overall resistance.

Some leaf vegetables grow (slowly) during sunny winter days. There is not enough light energy in winter to accumulate surplus sugar so carrots and swedes do not enlarge much; winter glasshouse tomatoes do not taste good unless they are, at great expense, kept warm *and* provided with intense artificial light every day the sun is not shining. During a more cloudy than usual winter outdoor crops may cannibalise their own leaves. Weakened by light starvation plants often get diseased in winter. The detailed planting schedule/calendar at the beginning of Chapter 9, page 120 allows for all this.

Tools

This section addresses lack of experience with gardening tools.

The hoe

There are many hoe designs. For removing small weeds from beds and paths I prefer the stirrup hoe which has a sharp thin blade that slides just below the surface on both the push and pull stroke. This design is unknown to many gardeners. The common garden hoe also slices off weeds but only when pulling; the strokes must be short, semi-chopping motions because this tool tends to mound up soil in front of the blade. The common hoe is the best design for cleaning compacted paths by scraping the weeds tops off their roots as you pull the blade towards you while simultaneously pressing its sharp edge down firmly.

Chopping big weeds with a dull hoe is beyond tiring. Cutting off young weeds with a sharp hoe takes no more effort than using a vacuum cleaner. In order to cut weeds a sharp blade must glide just below the surface without pulling itself in deeper or lifting itself out. For that to happen the blade must lie flat on the soil's surface when you are standing erect and comfortably holding the handle close to your body (see drawing on the next page). But one factory-made hoe must fit all bodies. So the blade of the common hoe is attached to the handle by a swansneck, which is a rod of mild

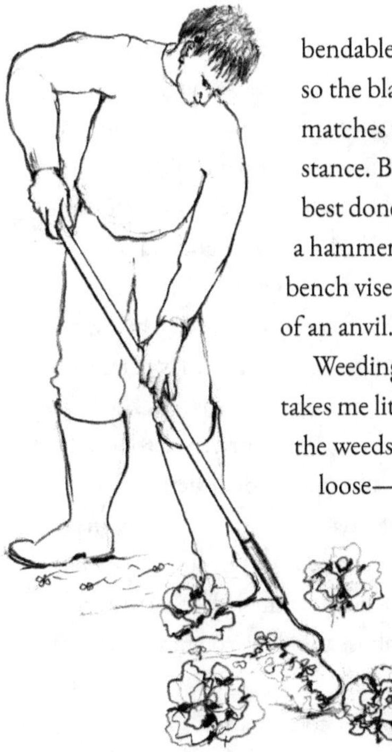

bendable steel that can be adjusted so the blade's angle of attack matches the user's comfortable stance. Bending the swansneck is best done by tapping it firmly with a hammer when it is held in a stout bench vise or held against the corner of an anvil.

Weeding with a sharp blade takes me little time or effort when the weeds are small and the soil is loose—which is the case *because* I thoroughly weed the garden once a week. But if two weeks should pass between weedings it'll take four times longer and be much more effort.

The common garden hoe will be entirely dull when you buy it; usually there isn't even the suggestion of a bevel ground into the edge. Any gardener who doesn't sharpen a new hoe soon discourages themselves and then adopts far less desirable and expensive alternatives when the only thing they needed was a metal file.

The first time a new tool is sharpened there's usually a lot of metal to grind off. For doing this use a large, new (still sharp) metal file with a stout handle. Lock the handle in a bench vise and patiently a grind down the *outside face* until a 15° bevel is formed, resembling a wood chisel. If you don't have a vise and can't imitate the stance of the ex-martial artist shown, ask someone else to stand on the handle while you file. When the entire bevel is perfect then remove the very thin metal burr that filing only on one side inevitably forms by giving the opposite face a few light strokes with the file pressed almost perfectly flat against the blade. *Do not grind a bevel into that side.* With the burr removed, a 15° edge should almost slice your finger if you press hard.

Filing an effective bevel the first time makes a person sweat. You must *concentrate* on holding the file at exactly the same angle through each and every stroke or else the edge will never get sharp. Don't forget that metal files get dull with use. Files get entirely dull overnight if you let them rust. The only other garden chore that is as exhausting as weeding with a dull hoe would be making the initial bevel with a dull file. And don't do what may seem to be the easier, quicker way—making the bevel less acute so that there's less metal to grind off. Do that and you'll make weeding into much more work than any effort you saved when filing.

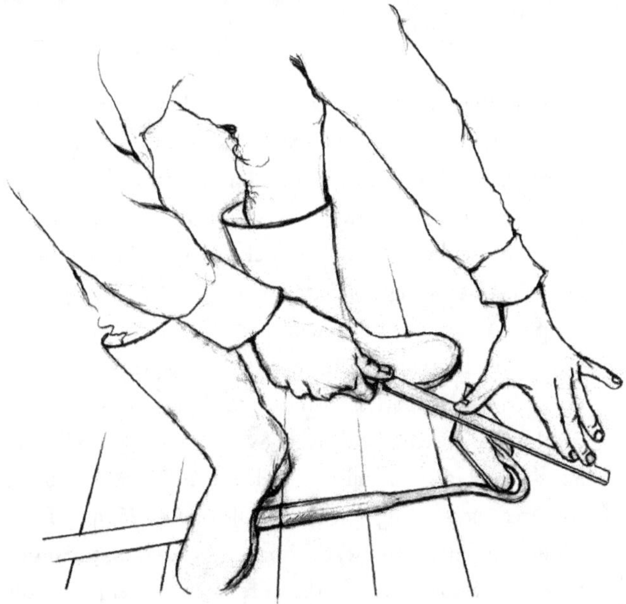

A cheap hoe usually costs you far more energy than any money it saved. Inexpensive hoe blades are made of soft (mild) steel because it is quick to shape, easy to weld and far less costly compared to tool steel. If filing the initial bevel goes rapidly then you've got mild steel that won't get very sharp no matter how skilfully you wield the file. I once used a cheap hoe like that; it had to be resharpened after weeding only one 30 metre long row and path. Tool-grade steel takes more time and effort to sharpen the first time but will only need resharpening once each spring if your soil is free of stones.

I think any gardener who uses a hoe should own at least two kinds:

The common garden hoe (illustrated on this page) works by pulling the blade towards you. Compared to pushing, pulling is much more controllable and far less tiring. It is "common" because the design is so useful and if made properly, is very strong. It slices, scrapes and chops, makes furrows and can push soil back into furrows after seeds have been sown. It should be almost unbreakable unless it is a very low priced imported imitation.

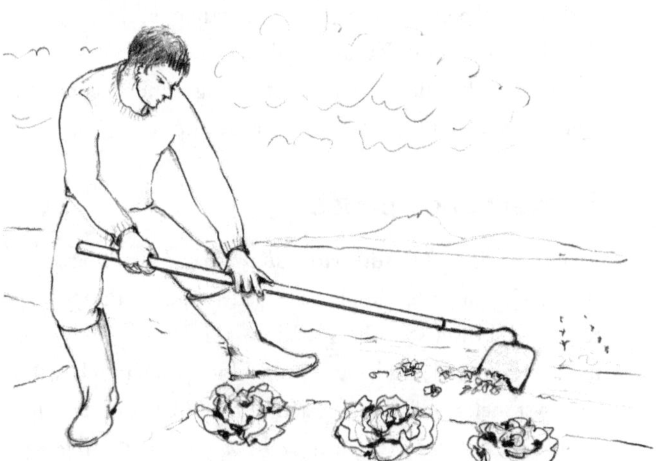

Scraping weeds on compact soil by pushing down (front hand) and pulling (mostly rear hand)

After the paths have been cleaned and spring crops are up and growing I prefer to weed beds and paths with a stirrup hoe although I could do all that with a common hoe. When I was a young man this design was sold as a Hula Hoe because the "U" wobbles back and forth just enough to keep the blade's angle of attack ideal for either the push or the pull stroke. The bottom of the "U" is the cutting edge. Beware of cheap imitations that do not wiggle. They are not even worth 90% less than the real deal. The best stirrup hoe I know of is imported from Switzerland and is sold by Southern Harvest and also by Delquip in Deoraine. There are three widths, I suggest the middle one—125 mm. The wider one is tiring to use; the smaller one uses up too much time. In my hoe collection there are several other push-pull hoes with propeller-shaped blades that work nearly as well as a stirrup design.

Hoes that only cut on the push-away stroke, sometimes called the Dutch hoe, are exhausting and hard to control; I don't recommend them.

The garden knife

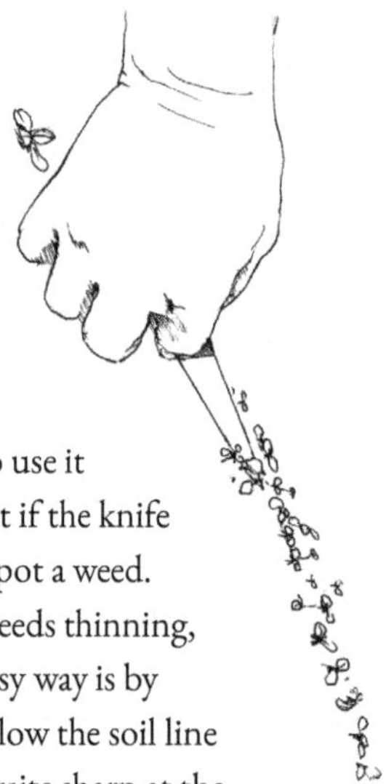

Kitchen peeling knives make valuable garden tools. Mine has a red plastic handle that helps me spot it when I forget where I'd last put it. Of course I use this knife for harvesting but the most valuable application is for thinning young seedlings. I can also use it to detach leaves from growing point if the knife happens to be in my hand when I spot a weed.

When a recently-emerged row needs thinning, the slow way is with fingers. The easy way is by cutting surplus seedlings off just below the soil line with a small, pointed knife that is quite sharp at the tip—like a mini-hoe. Running a sharp knife through soil rapidly dulls it, which is why a sharpening stone is kept by the wooden gate post that the knife is stuck into.

Shovels and spades

Digging is my pleasure with a *sharp* spade or combination shovel. Digging tools should have blades made of thin tempered springy steel that gets almost knife sharp and holds its edge. But spade blades are always blunt when purchased. To dig stoneless soil file a very acute chisel-like bevel (around 10°) *on the surface facing away from you when you're digging* (see illustration on this page). For a stony garden I'd make the bevel about 15°.

Shovels and spades are not the same thing. Shovels have broad blades that can lift a lot of loose sand, gravel or compost—like big spoons. Most shovelling effort is done with arms and core muscles. Spades have flat or slightly curved narrow blades attached to the handle at an angle best for bring pushed into firm soil with leg strength and body weight. A spade can slice into (moist) sod and turn over a chunk of it but a spade can't efficiently fill a wheelbarrow or spread what is in that wheelbarrow. Because I'm constantly switching from one task to another and because my beds have not been compacted by my own feet, my preferred tool is the combination shovel, which is an intermediate design that digs and also moves loose material. Sometimes this design is called "farmer's friend." One caution: At big box shops I have seen low-priced farmer's "friends?" with blades that are too wide to push in easily and whose too thick too heavy blade is attached to the too-heavy handle.

When digging with a spade or combination shovel its blade is push-kicked into the soil with leg muscles combined with total body weight. The larger the person is and the more expert they are at doing a front kick then the wider the blade they can wield, and all things being equal, the faster the digging goes. I weigh 80 kg; I can push-kick a combination shovel blade 250 mm deep into my soft soil. If I only weighed 55 kg I'd do better with a the narrower curved blade of a "plumbers friend." Plumbers use these to uncover leaks or tidy up ditches before laying pipe in them. Repeatedly pushing with the sole of your shoe or boot is more comfortable when the blade's upper edge is rolled over.

If I were teaching a child to garden I'd make a strong 100 mm wide spade on a short handle by patiently grinding down a full sized tool. I would not discourage a child by giving them a worthless toy.

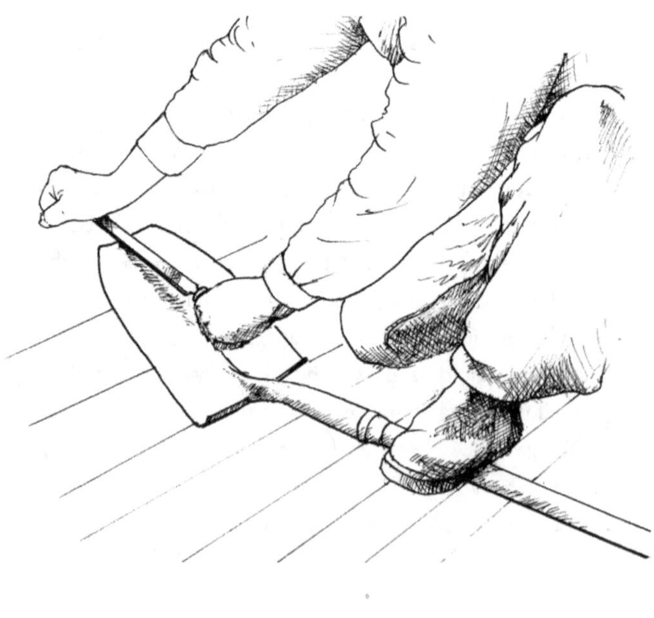

Shovels and spades come with either short or long handles. Short handled tools soon make my back tired. A short handled combination shovel carried in a car boot might be useful when camping or in a roadside emergency but for serious digging give me a long-handled tool. For moving loose materials buy the lighter weight shovel that's honestly strong. When it comes to digging, a bit more metal helps withstand the stress. However, extra weight tires me sooner. That's why I prefer composite handles over wooden ones.

Spading forks can be pushed in to their full depth with less force than a spade requires. Forks work most efficiently when soft soil flows between the tines—usually this means naturally loose sandy ground or garden soil that already contains an excessive amount of compost. The fork does poorly when used to break up big chunks—a combination shovel does that task better. When buying a digging fork make sure your foot can get good purchase. Beware of buying a cheap fork, be it new or used. The tines must be very strong or else they'll bend—and that means you want a forged fork of the highest quality. Even a properly strong fork may bend a tine when only one of them pulls against a much harder spot than the other tines are dealing with. A bent tine can straightened by inserting it part way into a 400 mm length of galvanized water pipe and pulling it back into line but once a tine has been bent it will be easier to bend the next time. That's why I'm always doubtful when inspecting a used garden fork being sold at a market stall.

Rotary cultivators

You can rent a powerful rotary cultivator for one day in order to convert grass into a new garden. Gardeners operating on less than 100 square metres do not benefit much from owning a rotary cultivator. Before I reached the age of 70 I grew 40- ten square metre beds without using a powered machine because only one or two of the beds were dug in any given day.

A self-propelled rear-tine rotary cultivator (usually around seven horsepower) can pulverize the top 150 mm of a 10 square metre bed in under five minutes. A front-end five horsepower machine can work the same area in about 20 minutes and may well dig it 50 millimetres deeper. To put that in perspective, at age 82, using a sharp combination shovel and two hours of my limited energy I can dig in fertilizer an honest 250 mm deep as I loosen a 10 square metre bed, then spread a 100 litre wheelbarrow load of compost over the top and rake out a seedbed. When I was under 70 I could do the job in one hour.

I owned a seven horsepower Honda rear-end tiller when I grew a variety trial grounds in Oregon. Every time I considered getting another one in Australia (until the year I approached age 70) I would recall how much time it took to guide the machine out to the garden and then back into the garage. The time and effort it took to clear vegetation tangled around the digging tines. There was the effort to turn it around at the end of the row or bed, the smell of engine exhaust and my hands tingling for several minutes after finishing. Then I'd recall the quiet pleasure of digging by hand and meditatively raking out a seedbed . . . and I'd conclude I didn't need a tiller. And I'd remind myself that if more gardeners knew how to sharpen their tools there'd be a lot fewer powered cultivators sold. Then ageing made it necessary to either buy a rotary cultivator or else reduce the size of my garden. This time I purchased a front-ender, a less costly design better suited to an oldie's home garden.

I am confident that Honda still makes the strongest and most dependable garden tillers under 8 horsepower. A Honda may cost you double the price of seemingly equivalent consumer grade home garden gear but Honda tillers are designed to withstand the thousands of running hours required by *market gardeners* and small-scale farmers. The self-propelled Honda I owned in Oregon worked a ¾ acre trials ground for the last three years I owned Territorial Seed Company. After I sold the business that tiller worked my one-third acre vegie garden for six more years. For about three of those years it also broke a lot of thick paddock sod when I was learning how to create total food self sufficiency by growing broad beans, chickpeas, wheat, millet and quinoa, each one in its own 200 square metre plot. During those years I changed the engine oil every 25 running hours and always changed it at the beginning of spring. I cleaned the air filter at each oil change. I also installed a new spark plug every spring, needed or not. Once I had to replace a clutch cable. And about year six I had to replace all the digging tines because the original set had been sanded away. Had I taken this machine to Tasmania 25 years ago I am sure that tiller would still be starting on the first pull and I'd be ready to replace the tines yet again.

Front-end tillers can make tighter turns and dig deeper than self-propelled rear-end models. They also take more skill and strength to operate. Most of them dig 600 mm wide. With my 5 HP Honda it is possible to remove the outer tines, reducing the digging face to 300 mm. Set up that way it penetrates a few honest centimetres deeper and gets there faster but is harder to steer. Front enders cost less than half the price of a rear-ender. So they're preferable, especially so when the gardener digs no more than 20 square metres at one go.

Front enders have down points. The bed has to be fairly free of vegetation or else their slow-moving tines get tangled up and stop digging. On the other hand, the slow moving tines are easier on worms. An inexperienced uninstructed operator soon tires after trying to control a front-ender by force. However, with a few hours of practice they'll drive one with little effort. The trick is to set the drag bar deep enough that it can almost completely prevent the rotating tines from pulling the machine forward faster than it can dig. It should not be slowed by a soon to be exhausted person pulling the machine backwards. The speed of forward motion can be changed by gently lifting up or gently pressing down on the handles to raise/lower the drag bar. Forward direction can be made to curve by tilting the handles, much like a motorbike takes a curve. Done with poise, controlling one does not take much effort.

Rear-end self propelled designs are best for working more than 20 square metres at one go. They demand less skill to operate—point them in the right direction and the machine does the work. They even roll themselves out of the shed and out to the garden. I should mention here that rear-enders spin their tines more rapidly; for this reason they get criticized for killing earthworms but in my experience, they never seem to eliminate the earthworms.

If I reach age 90 and am still able to garden I may replace my front-ender with an electric-start rear ender and change my gardening style to single long rows as recommended by Dick Raymond the American garden writer. Back in the 1970s Raymond made planting beds the width of the tiller's tines (600 mm) and paths between beds the same width, using the tiller to weed paths and for chopping in old vegetation and green manure crops back into the beds—no heap composting necessary. All an old codger has to do is to hold one handlebar and walk slowly behind it. His books (used) can still be found on the internet and are worth a read.

Rakes

Rotary cultivators usually make a fine seedbed that at most needs only smoothing with a rake before sowing or setting out seedlings. A recently spaded bed can be raked to form the level fine textured surface inch that seeds germinate well in. Most kinds of soil are left with small lumps in the fine stuff after digging or rotary cultivating. Raking can comb lumps out of the surface inch as it blends in compost at the same time. This is accomplished by slowly moving the rake back and forth such that the teeth tease lumps up to the surface and pull them over the edge of the bed. This action requires total concentration on controlling how deeply the teeth penetrate. The teeth must glide through loose soil without pulling up a mound ahead of the teeth. Done right, making seedbeds goes quickly. I point out here that raking out seedbeds only works well if the bed is raised enough that lumps can be deposited on the path below. It usually takes me five minutes to groom the surface inch of a 10 square metre raised bed into a level, fine-textured medium resembling potting mix.

The rake should come with a handle around 300 mm longer than a common hoe handle. Increased handle length counterbalances the working end so that you can more easily control how deep the teeth penetrate. If you try to control the depth the teeth go in by strength of wrist then you'll soon tire. Instead, one hand, the "front" hand, *loosely* grasps the handle close to the tool's natural balance point. This front hand supports most of the weight and also acts like a pivot or fulcrum and sometimes like a guide that the handle slides through. This hand controls how deeply the teeth penetrate. The rear hand holds the handle *firmly*; this arm does most of the pushing and pulling. Both arms move in harmony as you groom the bed's surface. Used this way, stress on the wrists is minor and endurable for long periods. You'll soon discover why you should slightly bend your knees into what martial artists call a horse stance when raking out a seedbed. Raking excellently requires putting so much attention on the soil flowing between the rake's teeth that I usually do not think when doing it.

There are two rake designs, the bow rake and the "T" rake. The comb of a "T" rake is welded at its centre to a stout metal strip (similar to a hoe's swansneck but it is straight, not bent) that usually anchors in a reinforced slot cut into the end of a long wooden handle. Because so much stress is placed on the middle of the "T" the comb is usually made of thick steel which means the working end of the tool weighs more. Because of the heavy comb I can't reach out as far with a "T" rake. Because of its simpler construction, the "T" rake usually costs less than a bow rake.

The bow rake's comb is attached to the handle by a pair of thin curved springy rods welded to its outer upper corners. This tool is lighter in your hands than a "T" design. I prefer a bow rake. But bow rakes are not easy to find these days.

Most rakes have a comb 14 to 16 inches wide. There are unusually wide rakes that might seem to work faster but actually are front heavy and prove exhausting if you use them to make seedbeds. Similarly, someone with arms and wrists that aren't strong might look for a rake with a narrower comb.

Chapter 2

Soil

. . . only after the supply of organic matter has been adequately provided for, will the full benefit of artificials [chemical fertilizers] be realised. There appears to be a great field for future experiment in the judicious use of artificials to land already in a fair state of fertility.

Sir Albert Howard, ***The Waste Products of Agriculture,**** 1933.

There are a few districts on our planet where nutrient-dense vegetables can be grown without fertilizer, compost or animal manure. A few thousand acres in Fiji along the Sigatoka River's floodplain is one of them. The Sigatoka's watershed mostly consists of superminerlized ultrabasic volcanic rock, a rare kind. Every few years a cyclonic flood deposits a layer of ultrabasic sand and silt over the valley floor. During the season of high heat and humidity all the fields are taken over by weeds and grasses that grow chest high. When the cooler dry season arrives this natural green manure is plowed under. The warm soil rapidly decomposes that organic matter and the intense biological activity breaks down ultrabasic silt so rapidly that huge quantities of plant nutrients are released. Vegetables have been produced this way in the Sigatoka Valley for about 100 years. Before the Aswan Dam was built the enormously productive Nile Valley was remineralized by an annual flood. Some excellent soils get regularly replenished by highly mineralized volcanic ash, although not all volcanic ash is nutrient-rich.

In climates where there is enough rainfall to support a forest—like most of Tasmania—soils that form gradually out of the underlying rocks are not nearly as fertile as the Sigatoka Valley even if the parent rocks are well mineralized because rain over geologic time leaches out plant nutrients. Producing nutrient dense vegetables in Tasmania requires 1) upping soil organic matter without trying to supply most plant nutrients from decomposing organic matter and 2) generously replenishing and balancing plant nutrients. These nutrients include copper, zinc, manganese, boron, molybdenum, sulfur, nitrogen, phosphorus, calcium, magnesium, potassium and sodium. Adding miniscule quantities of cobalt, selenium, iodine, nickel, chromium, etc may also be needed. Every one of these elements is vitally important. If any of them are more than slightly short or more than slightly excessive then both nutrient density and plant health decline. The health of livestock grazing on plant nutrient deficient soil and the health of humans substantially eating from that soil also declines. Human lifespan declines too.

Mineral fertility

The intensely farmed red soils of northern Tasmania developed out of a type of basalt that could supply adequate calcium, copper, boron, potassium and phosphorus (and too much magnesium) except that these soils have been strongly depleted (leached) by rain. Industrial farming—which essentially is soil mining—has further lowered fertility. Not very many home gardeners live on this valuable agricultural soil. Most Tasmanians live on soils formed from rocks that provide fewer plant nutrient elements than the aforementioned basalt and also provide too much magnesium. Large areas of Tasmania's soil developed out of sandstones that are extremely short of all nutrients except iron.

In order to produce highly nutritious vegetables and fruits Tasmanian gardeners must remineralize with a plan, with understanding of what is missing and what it takes to replace these elements.

Remineralizing with organic matter

Livestock produce manure whose plant nutrient content resembles the soil it derived from. Manure from Tasmanian grazing-animals lacks phosphorus, calcium, boron, copper; and molybdenum, and contains considerably less potassium than manures from elsewhere usually provide. Compost made from Tasmanian grass eater manures does not balance Tasmanian soils.

Compost made of forestry wastes does not make Tasmanian soils produce nutrient-dense foods. Tasmanian native forests still stand only where the soil is too infertile (and sometimes too rocky) to farm. Tree plantations are established only after a farmed field has become so depleted that it can no longer be used profitably. Like the soils it derives from, compost made from forestry waste is inevitably low in most plant nutrients and high in a few—this compost is out of balance.

Soil that is built up with compost and lime can produce large-sized good looking vegetables—all that organic matter does bring some plant nutrients with it. Compost does make the soil more friable and there may be a great many earthworms—but the vegetables do not provide anything close to maximum nutrition. Nor will they taste as good as vegetables and fruit can taste. Tasmanian vegetables fertilized only with compost can be slightly more nutritious than what the industrial food system offers at the supermarket.

Remineralizing effectively

I said in the Introduction that I divided gardeners into two groups—serious and casual. Casual gardening doesn't improve the family's health very much even if the small percentage of their year-round food that is produced in their own back yard is highly nutrient dense. But there can be a noticeable health gain when a family provides more than 25% of their year round dietary from their own remineralized soil. For the serious food gardener I have written a book about soil fertility management called *The Intelligent Gardener.* It explains how to interpret a soil test and from that information bring a specific soil into the kind of balance the produces highly nutrient dense food. It is not possible to compress that book into one chapter of this book. Nor is soil analysis a necessary skill for beginners or casual gardeners.

An uncomplicated way for Tasmanians to significantly increase the nutrient density of garden vegetables is to use one of my two complete organic fertilizer recipes (COF). Both versions of COF are simple enough to make for yourself and are straightforward to use. COF is ideal for novices. COF strongly inclines the soil towards a balanced abundant mineral content—but being a one-size sort-of-fits-most method it won't exactly balance anyone's soil.

My first COF recipe appeared in 1984; it was primitive but it grew bountiful crops in the heavily leached soils of western Oregon and Washington, USA. The recipe has been steadily improved since then. COF works! It's convenient. And economical.

The COF recipes in this book are designed for the average Tasmanian soil. They include a *light dose* of agricultural lime—around one half ton per acre when a full dose of COF is spread. Repeated light liming gradually and gently saturates the soil with calcium. Gypsum in COF insures that the plants will find enough available calcium. Gypsum also allows plants to manufacture more sulfur-containing amino acids that make the plant far more disease resistant and provides the consumer with better quality proteins. I include enough zinc, boron and copper in COF to prevent gross deficiencies, similar to the Minimum Daily Requirement approach when taking vitamin supplements. COF supplies what it takes to make food producing plants far healthier and the vegetables they provide far more nutrient-dense.

Complete organic fertilizer and some compost—but not too much compost—is all a new garden needs for the first five years. After that many applications, doing a soil test and adjusting the COF recipe to match the test result would prevent building up nutrient excesses.

The basic theory behind COF was developed by an agricultural scientist and farm advisor named Victor Tiedjens. If you want a full explanation, best to get it direct and unfiltered, see Tiedjens' *More Food From Soil Science** and *Olena Farm.**

Lime and pH

Tasmanian soils are acidic because they have been leached by rain. Soil acidity is measured as pH. A pH of 7.0 is neutral. Over 7 is alkaline; you won't find alkaline soil on Tasmania unless you put in way to much aglime. Below 7.0 is acidic. Most of the ungardened Tasmanian soils I have tested have a pH of 5.25 to 5.5. Acidity below 5.0 can be harmful because the availability of toxic elements like aluminium and sometimes manganese increases so much that food crop species are poisoned. The very best results for most vegetables happen when soil pH is only slightly acid, around pH 6.4. The way to get a Tasmanian soil to pH 6.4 is by getting a proper soil test, and then guided by that test mixing *the right amount* of agricultural lime into the topsoil. But it isn't quite that simple.

There are two types of lime: ordinary agricultural lime and dolomite. We have plenty of both kinds in Tasmania.

A great many garden writers and popular TV presenters have wrongly asserted that dolomite lime is the best kind to use because it provides magnesium, which is a essential plant nutrient, as well as providing calcium. Dolomite also raises soil pH about 20 percent more than the same amount of agricultural lime does. Seems like such a good deal!

Please take my warning to heart: dolomite lime worsens Tasmanian soils that contain very much clay. Excess magnesium makes clay particles strongly attract each other; then the whole soil body shrinks, becomes tight, airless, inhospitable to root development, prone to form clods and stick to boots—the opposite of what it takes to grow great vegetables. When a Tasmanian gardener uses dolomite lime on soil containing more than ten percent clay (that naturally contains too much magnesium) then they soon feel compelled to remedy its tight airless nature by bringing in large amounts of compost. This action unbalances the soil's mineralization pattern even more than it was at the start. You could say that putting too much magnesium into clay addicts the garden to compost, the making or buying of which makes a great deal of unnecessary cost and work—and lowers nutrient-density.

The parent rocks that formed Tasmania's volcanic soils provide plenty of magnesium. Rather than add magnesium, the agriculturalist's problem is how to eliminate some from the subsoil so that it'll loosen up, hold more air and allow better root development. The main Tasmanian exceptions requiring magnesium are coastal sands, light loamy soils around Mole Creek that form out of very pure limestone that lacks magnesium and soils formed out of sandstone.

LIMING

Unless your soil has been adequately limed in recent years it is safe to assume your soil needs lime. This is also true of soil from limestone around Mole Creek.

The quantity of lime needed and the correct kind of lime to use depends upon the amount of clay in the topsoil and sometimes on the nature of the subsoil.

A loam soil by definition contains at least 10 percent clay but no more than 40 percent. When starting a garden on loam it's smart to spread and dig in 25 kg of *aglime* per 100 square metres (1 generous ton/acre). And from that point on use COF. Or do not spread lime but double the amount of aglime in COF for the first year.

If it is clay or clayey topsoil first spread and dig in two tons of *aglime* per acre (50 kg/100 square metres) and also double the quantities of aglime and gypsum in COF for the first two years.

On any sand or loam topsoil with clay below (duplex) do not use dolomite lime.

Does your garden seem to need endless quantities of compost to keep the soil friable? Am I describing your treadmill? The way off it is simple for most—abandon dolomite lime in favour of ordinary aglime. A sticky soil can become naturally crumbly after adding enough aglime lime and gypsum. But it can take a few years for calcium to replace enough magnesium to loosen topsoil; much longer than that to loosen a sticky clay subsoil such that vegetable crops can put roots into it. And even longer than that if very much dolomite has already been spread. If you're wondering how calcium can replace magnesium please read *The Intelligent Gardener.*

Supplying essential plant nutrients

Most farm advisors focus on five chemical elements—calcium, magnesium, nitrate, phosphate and potassium—because if these five are sufficiently provided and the other nutrients aren't catastrophically short, then the crop will be profitable. This is the degree of soil fertility most farmers try to achieve. However, if at least twelve plant nutrients are made abundant—not just barely enough to prevent obvious deficiency symptoms—and in the right balance—then the yield might not be all that much higher but the nutritional quality and flavour definitely will be far better and there'll be far fewer insect or disease problems. Five nutrients must accessible to plants in quantities ranging from hundreds to thousands of kilograms in a hectare of topsoil. These are nitrogen (N), phosphorus (P), potassium (K), calcium (Ca) and magnesium (Mg). Other elements, sometimes named "trace elements," should be present in quantities ranging from seventy five kilograms per hectare down to four kilograms per hectare. These include sulfur (S), sodium (Na), iron (Fe), manganese (Mn), zinc (Zn), copper (Cu) and boron (B). Micronutrients must be present in quantities less than two kilograms per hectare. These include molybdenum, selenium, iodine, chromium, nickel and cobalt.

In the 1970s when I was learning to garden, the organic movement strongly asserted that *all* synthetic soluble fertilizers damage soil and harm the soil ecology. Organic certification authorities are smarter these days. The truth of the matter is that most soluble plant nutrients (be they synthetic or naturally occurring) strongly encourage soil life when they are in concentrations the biology is comfortable with. Some chemical fertilizers do harm soil organisms or otherwise degrade the soil. These include di-ammonium phosphate (not mono-ammonium phosphate), gaseous ammonia and muriate of potash (KCl). Urea may be damaging, but about that complexity I am uncertain.

Vegetable gardeners can afford the higher cost of using organic materials to supply slow-release nitrogen. Rock powders and mined salts can effectively supply phosphorus, calcium, magnesium, potassium, boron and sulfur. Effective sources of iron, manganese, zinc and copper are salts made with sulfuric acid; another manufactured salt, potassium sulphate, is the equal of the mined version, but less costly. That's why synthetic sulphate salts are now okay for certified organics.

Balanced soil

Balanced soil provides nutrients in proportionate amounts—such as: for every unit of available phosphorus there is 1/10th as much zinc; for every unit of calcium there is a proportionate (and much smaller) quantity of magnesium. Some soil analysts think these proportionate relationships should extend to other plant nutrients. For instance, boron should be proportionate to calcium, copper proportionate to zinc, iron in balance with manganese.

The idea that soil nutrient balance leads to food nutrient density was first proposed in the 1950s by William Albrecht, a health-minded agronomist. Albrecht asserted that we should fertilize soils in humid temperate climates so they offer up in plant-available form: 68 percent calcium, 12 percent magnesium, 3-5 percent potassium and 1-2 percent sodium. When the soil achieves this balance *and there also is an abundance of the other essential nutrients*, food crops develop the most proteins, vitamins, phytoprotective substances and provide the minerals essential for human and animal health. Crops growing on soils like this yield a lot, they strongly resist disease and insects.

To learn more about this I suggest starting with William Albrecht's *Soil Fertility and Animal Health.**

Harvesting vegetables with less than ideal nutrient density is the usual Tasmanian home garden result. The only effective way I know to remedy this is to bring the soil into balance with fertilizers.

The word fertilizer is correctly defined as *a concentrated source of plant nutrients.* Some organic folks growl at the word because they believe adding more organic matter is the only right way. To this sort of person the word "fertilizer" connotes chemical, synthetic, artificial, harmful. Actually, synthetic fertilizers are not the only kind. Finely ground limestone is a powerful calcium fertilizer. Oilseed meals—the residue remaining after extracting seed oils—are potent, slow release nitrogen fertilizers. Tasmania produces non-GM canolaseedmeal. Blood-and-bone (meatmeal) is a very potent nitrogen source. It comes from local abattoirs. Soft rock phosphate and reactive rock phosphate and guano are crushed rocks that release phosphorus for many months. Gypsum, a slightly-soluble crushed rock, provides a steady supply of sulfur and calcium. For micronutrients we have Tasmanian-produced kelpmeal.

Working out which plant nutrients a particular soil needs is a complex subject that casual gardeners need not bother with because most soils in those parts of Tasmania where people grow gardens are chemically similar. Because of this similarity I could concoct a pair of fertilizer recipes that conveniently bring most Tasmanian soils into better balance.

New gardeners have so much to learn I urge them to use COF for the first few years and then investigate soil testing and soil analysis if their garden supplies a major part of their family's food.

Complete Organic Fertilizer (COF)

The ideal fertilizer for garden vegetables and small fruit would be an odourless coarse dry powder that provides a long lasting steady release of balanced plant nutrients that bring forth a large yield of nutrient-dense food. It should not harm leaves if some got sprinkled on them and should not damage plants or soil microlife if spread several times heavier than the recommended rate. It should not interest pets or wildlife. It should not be so concentrated that it is hard to spread uniformly. It should not have an unpleasant odour. A single application before sowing should steadily feed most crops from start to finish. It should be compounded from substances acceptable for certified organic production. All this describes COF.

COF provides Tasmanian gardens with nitrogen (N) and phosphorus (P) in abundance; it provides about half the total amount of potassium (K from the Latin *kalium)* a crop needs, only half, because the gardener brings in potassium with compost. COF also supplies enough calcium to slightly more than replace what winter rains leach out. It contains enough gypsum to feed plenty of soluble calcium and sulfur the current crop; enough zinc, copper, boron and molybdenum to prevent a damaging deficiency should the soil be majorly short; and delivers a scant whiff of iodine, cobalt, selenium, etc.

COF can be easily compounded at home. You measure every ingredient by volume and then blend them thoroughly. Boron, molybdenum and sulphate salts of zinc, copper and potassium are apportioned with kitchen measuring spoons and scoops. The other dry powders are measured by the litre or half litre, the same way liquids are measured.

Enough fertilizer to cover 10 square metres does not fill a ten litre plastic bucket to the top. Precise measurement is not essential; anything that comes out to be within ten percent of the recipe's suggested proportions will work excellently. Complete mixing is crucial; don't rush this step. If most of the copper or boron should land on one small spot it might harm whatever tries to grow there. I find the best way to compound fertilizers is to measure each ingredient into one bucket and then when the wind is not blowing hard, pour these materials from one bucket into another, back and forth, eight times or more.

About COF ingredients

Spreading oilseed meal plus aglime at 850 gm per $10m^2$ and some decent compost usually grows a great-*looking* garden. Adding some bloodandbone causes nitrogen to be released more rapidly in chilly soil, accelerating spring growth. Adding phosphate fertilizer, gypsum and kelpmeal builds resilience and greatly increases nutrient density, something you'll experience as better flavour. Because gardeners bring in compost that provides some potassium, the amount of potassium I put in Tasmanian COF is just barely enough. The quantities of copper, zinc and boron are small enough to not create an excess yet the amounts are large enough that the flavour of your vegies may improve and there'll also be fewer insect and disease problems. Your particular soil probably could use more of some of the plant nutrients than COF provides and may not need any of some others in it but this can only be discovered from a lab soil test. Without that test it would be foolish to add more than what is in COF because excesses of some of these elements have long-lasting negative effects.

Oilseedmeal is the residue left after extracting vegetable oil from seeds. Most kinds provide 5 to 6 percent nitrogen, 2 percent phosphorus and 1 percent potassium. Seedmeal stores for years if kept dry and protected from mice and rats. Seedmeal is rough textured, irregular—grippy you might say. It helps finely ground fertilizers to blend in uniformly.

These days, mainland-sourced soy, cotton, and canola meals almost inevitably come from genetically modified (GM) crops. I do not eat GM foods as they are now. I might if genetic modification meant greater nutrient density across the board and the result had been rigorously checked for safety with multigenerational animal feeding studies that should show excellent reproduction and increased life span. Which is not the case these days. Some people object so strongly to GM foods they resist using the waste products of GM crops as fertilizer. But as fertilizer I have noticed no difference using either Tasmanian GM-free canolaseedmeal or GM oilseed meal from the mainland. I accept that GM oilseed meal will contain detectable traces of glyphosate whilst non-GM oilseed meals carry traces of different herbicides that probably cost farmers more than glyphosate and may be even more toxic than glyphosate.

TP Jones (now Nutrien), a farm supply business in Youngtown (Launceston), usually had the best retail price for

Complete Organic Fertilizer Recipe

To make the right amount of COF for 10 square metres of most vegetable crops, measure out and then uniformly blend these ingredients. Before sowing, uniformly spread the full amount: A few pages further I provide an alternate recipe for sand soils without a clay subsoil.

NITROGEN

4 litres of canolaseedmeal (2,400 gm)

or else

3 litres canolaseedmeal (1,800 gm) ***and***
1 litre blood-and-bone (700 gm). This variant works better in the chilly soils of spring and for side dressing.

CALCIUM

½ litre agricultural lime ***(not dolomite)***,
best ground finely, #65 ***or*** #100 (850 gm)

and

½ litre agricultural gypsum (600 gm)

PHOSPHORUS

1 scant litre of colloidal (soft) rock phosphate (1,000 gm)

or else

the same amount of reactive rock phosphate (RRP)
or high phosphate guano

POTASSIUM

½ cup potassium sulphate (150 gm)

TRACE ELEMENTS AND MICRONUTRIENTS

Garden centre
10 to 11% purity boron fertilizer (20 gm)

or else

Organibor (15 gm)

and

2 teaspoons zinc sulphate (10 gm)
2 teaspoons copper sulphate (15 gm)
½ litre kelpmeal (400 gm)
⅛ tsp sodium molybdate (0.5 gm)

Tassie-grown canolameal. Now I think all the Nutrien shops can sell it. The price of canolameal by the 25 kilogram bag is about the same as the price of Dynamic Lifter, Rapid Raiser or other pelletized composted chook poo by the 25 kg bag. If you consider that Tasmanian canolameal is about 5.5 percent nitrogen whilst pelletized chook poo averages around 3.5 percent nitrogen, then evaluated only by nitrogen content, canolaseedmeal costs less.

In the unlikely event you're offered a choice of seedmeals and their protein content is stated, use whichever contains the most protein for the least money (protein releases nitrogen as it decomposes in soil). Any oilseed meal providing over 25 percent protein will act like fertilizer if you spread enough of it. Canolameal, at 35 to 40 percent protein, works really well. The quick rule is every 6.2 percent of protein releases one percent nitrogen.

Tasmanian canolameal is produced by the Macquarie Oilseed Company near Cressy; it comes in 25 kg woven poly feed bags with Macquarie's name printed on them. Macquarie will sell direct to individuals (or groups) that buy at least one ton and may sell a bulk cubic metre at a significantly lower price per kilogram. A few garden centres and farm suppliers offer it; I'm sure more of them would if enough readers of this book request it.

Bloodandbone comes from local abattoirs. The bags I buy at my local farm supply shop say 10 percent nitrogen and 4 percent phosphorus—twice the amount there is in canolameal. Bloodandbone releases nitrogen much faster than oilseedmeal does so I include some when preparing cold soil in spring and also to get a quicker response from side dressing. However, bloodandbone releases too rapidly to serve as the main source of nitrogen.

Lime. COF includes two calcium fertilizers: agricultural lime (aglime) which is finely ground limestone rock—calcium carbonate; and gypsum—calcium sulphate—which can either be a finely-ground naturally occurring rock or an industrial by-product that comes with the risk of heavy metal contamination.

Agricultural lime is insoluble. Aglime needs from a few weeks to ten years to break down in soil depending on the fineness of the grind. Coarser stuff feels gritty like beach sand. Coarse grinds cost less and are best for paddocks because larger quantities of slower releasing material can be spread less often, more economically. For COF you want quicker release; use a finer grind like #65 or best, use #100. The fineness of aglime is expressed by the sieve it will pass through. Number 10 (#10) will pass through a mesh of 10 fine wires per inch; #65 passes a screen with 65 fine wires per inch. There are also very expensive microfine aglimes; these will pass a #300 screen. A small quantity of microfine lime rapidly pushes up soil pH but only for a short time. Please do not use #300 for COF.

Limestone rocks always contain useless impurities and often contain some magnesium; every quarry is different. When farmers buy aglime they'll ask for a lab analysis showing overall purity and the percentage of magnesium carbonate. I've already mentioned that are strong reasons to not add magnesium to some Tasmanian soils. I prefer aglime quarried at Mole Creek by Silbelco. It is sold with the makers name printed on 25 kg sacks. Mole Creek lime is 93 percent calcium carbonate and less than one percent magnesium carbonate. Do not use quicklime, burnt lime or hydrated lime.

Lime that contains more than two percent magnesium carbonate (and less than 13 percent) should be called "dolomitic lime." Pure dolomite is 24 percent calcium and 13 percent magnesium. Dolomite lime in Waratah poly bags is always found at garden centres.

Agricultural gypsum is finely ground soft rock made of calcium sulfate. Gypsum can also be a manufacturing residue. The natural sort meets organic certification requirements. Waratah distributes gypsum that is mined in South Australia. The byproduct sort can bring toxic heavy metals with it; I would not use this kind for fertilizer even if it was much less costly.

The modest amount of aglime in COF gradually balances the topsoil. You won't significantly over lime by repeatedly spreading COF because most nutrients become more available to plants as the soil becomes increasingly saturated with calcium, so after using COF for a few years you'll get the same result from less of it. Don't forget—abundant calcium is not forever. When winter rain passes through soil it leaches calcium. When I lived in western Oregon I learned that the average soil there is leached of about 300 kg/ha of calcium every winter; most of Tasmania gets slightly less winter rainfall than Oregon does; our soils lose slightly less calcium. Unless you know for sure that your garden has recently been limed heavily I suggest that you include the small quantities of lime and gypsum I prescribe when making COF.

Phosphate rock or guano. Tasmanian gardeners have access to three natural phosphorus fertilizers: guano (fossilized sea bird poop), soft (sometimes termed "colloidal") rock phosphate (SRP) and reactive rock phosphate (RRP). Soft rock phosphate is broadly useful and economical. I've purchased SRP by the ton shipped direct to me by Nutri-Tech Solutions in Queensland. Around Hobart, buy from ActiveVista in Longley (www.Activevista.com.au). East coasters contact Frank Giles in St. Marys, 0419-372-192. Frank is a soil consultant and Nutri-Tech representative. Nutrien in Youngtown stocked SRP when they were called T.P. Jones. I don't know what Nutrien is offering. Soft rock phosphate releases phosphorus enormously more rapidly than the hard form.

Hard rock phosphate (HRP) is the crude feedstock used to make chemical phosphate fertilizers. HRP contains more elemental phosphorus per dollar than SRP does but even when HRP is ground to talcum-powder fineness it still is extremely insoluble and thus of little value as garden fertilizer. The only way I know to get a phosphorus response from HRP is to include it while building the compost heap because heat and intense biological activity make some of the phosphorus become available.

Phosphorus from guano costs more than it costs from SRP but guano provides ocean-sourced micronutrients. Farm supply shops sometimes sell guano by the 25 kg bag.

Reactive Rock Phosphate provides about the same amount of phosphorus as SRP. RRP is sold by the 25 kg sack by Kelpomix in Devonport and sold in larger quantities by AgriFert in Somerset. I use RRP. To learn more about this unique material visit www.bioag.com.au and read their info sheet about RRP.

Potassium. There isn't nearly enough potassium in oilseed meals. Kelpmeal provides some too but kelp costs far too much to be used to supply that element. Potassium is inevitably added from landscape yard compost. Because most Tasmanian soils are more than a little short of potassium, gardeners should supplement organic matter inputs with potassium sulphate.

Kelpmeal seems expensive and seems to do little you can directly observe. So people may be tempted to leave it out of COF. However, kelp used generously and repeatedly provides useful amounts of all the micronutrients that both plants and humans need, like iodine, chromium, nickel and cobalt. Natural hormones and growth regulating substances in kelp boost plant fortitude. Kelpomix, Activevista and many farm suppliers distribute Tasmanian kelpmeal.

Trace elements. After analyzing a few hundred Tassie soil tests I now assume Tasmanian soil will test deficient in copper unless it previously grew an orchard. Almost all Tassie soils are quite short boron. Your soil's need for zinc is less certain. The quantity of zinc in COF won't harm a soil that already is adequately endowed but may make a huge difference where it is deficient. One precaution about zinc sulphate. This salt picks up moisture from the atmosphere and becomes damp. Its better to store this material in something airtight. Mixing damp zinc sulphate into COF is okay; there isn't enough moisture in the little bit needed to cause problems.

You'll find trace element fertilizers in 500 gm packages at large garden centres. When remineralizing a quarter-acre or larger it makes economic sense to discover by soil test what and how much is actually needed and invest in 25 kg bags from a farm supply shop or a ServAg outlet.

Boron. Borax comes from a mined salt deposit. It is soluble in water and contains between 10 and 11 percent boron. There's a story about borax that is worth an extra paragraph. For many years I used laundry borax to make up COF. Then an Aussie doctor discovered a link between boron deficiency and arthritis. He started prescribing a few milligrams of boron per day to arthritics, and these patients soon felt better. And that's only one of the many reasons you want plenty of boron in your food.

I was expensively going through three or more half-kilo packets of garden centre borax every year so I frugally bought a 25 kg lifetime-supply of Solubor, which is 22% boron so when using Solubor to make up COF I put in half the weight I would with borax. However, Solubor is not kosher for certified organics because it isn't a natural substance. Recently I discovered a natural *slow-release* boron fertilizer called Organibor. Boron is highly leachable so it is far better to have it released over months. Organibor must be purchased through a farm supply shop as a special order item in 25 kg sacks.

Using COF

Initial soil preparation: For the first crop of the season uniformly spread a full batch of COF over 10 square metres of raised bed or else over a strip 600 mm-wide and 16 metres long if you garden using long rows with paths between them. One batch of COF spread on 10 square metres abundantly feeds *low demand crops* such as carrot, beetroot, parsnip, parsley, bean, pea, lettuce, endive and escarole and starts off crops that will need more nutrients applied after they have grown for a few weeks.

Side dressing means spreading fertilizer on the soil's surface above the plant's root zone. The growing instructions in Chapter 9 state if the vegetable is a low, medium, or high demand crop. Medium-demand and high-demand crops start out better when they're fertilized like a low demand crop but are side dressed after they're up and growing.

One full dose of COF pushes plant growth for two months and then the effect diminishes. Side-dressing a half-dose of COF produces a growth response that lasts one month and then diminishes because the actively feeding part of the root system will have extended beyond the side dressed soil whilst the larger plant can make use of far more nutrients than you spread a month previously. When a high demand crop should be growing fast I side-dress more COF every few weeks. Side-dressing is best applied in a ring just beyond the plant's drip line, covering the ground that the roots will expand into during the next few weeks. The first side-dressing should be few tablespoons of COF in a small ring close to each seedling or as a narrow band close to the row. The plants will be much bigger when they get side dressed a second time so you'll spread a larger amount over a larger area. There is no absolute requirement to hoe-in or rake-in side-dressed COF. If you can work it in shallowly it'll start releasing nutrients a few days sooner.

The growth rate of heat loving crops inevitably slows around mid February; slower growing plants do not need as many nutrients. So side dress frost-sensitive crops for the last time around the middle of January. That way the effect of this side-dressing tapers off as growth must slow down. Autumn and winter crops slow their growth early in April;

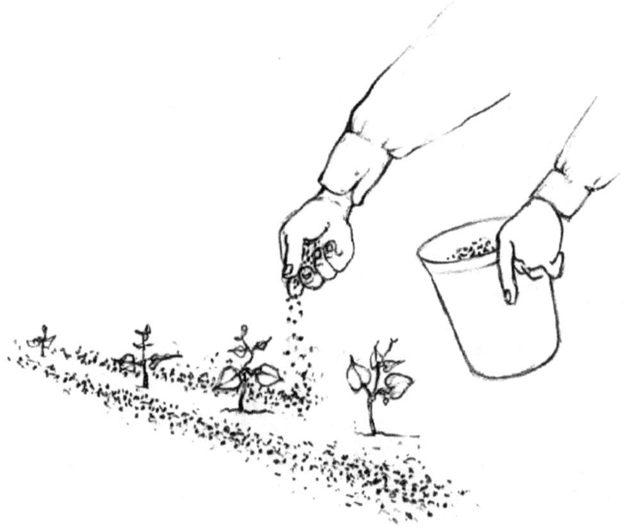

these should be side-dressed for the last time early in March. Overwintered crops begin growing fast when the first spring bulbs emerge; they'll benefit enormously from being side-dressed at this time.

Subsequent crops: Many of the beds in a Tasmanian vegie garden could (and should) produce more than one crop per year. Every new crop should start with a full dose of COF unless the first crop was something quick and very low-demand, such as rocket or radish.

Transplanting. Prepare the bed for a low-demand crop. At each position that a large plant is to grow, scoop out a hole about 75 mm deep and 200 mm in diameter. Put a handful of additional COF in the bottom of the hole. Using your fingertips or a trowel, mix in the COF. Then refill the hole and put the seedling in this extra fertile spot.

Hills. Sometimes I make extra fertile low mounds for sowing sprawling vegetables like zucchini, pumpkin, melon or cucumber and also for transplanting tomato seedlings. I suggest also making hills for the larger cabbage family vegetables when it is a new garden whose soil hasn't yet come into balance. First, spread and work in the usual quantity of COF over the entire area the crop will eventually fill with roots. Then make an extra-fertile spot for each plant. Using shovel or spade, remove two large scoops of soil from a spot and set them next to the shallow hole you just made. In the bottom of the hole put a generous handful of COF and a shovelful of your best compost. Mix them in with the spade. Then push the soil you removed back over the spot; this forms an approximately 450 mm diameter low mound (hill) with extra high fertility starting 75 to 100 mm below the surface.

To make seeds germinate well in that hill, first slightly compress the soil in the hill's centre; this helps keep the spot moist while the seeds germinate. (see Chapter 6). I do this by making a fist and gently pressing it into the mound's centre. I don't press hard and I stop pushing as soon as I feel resistance; the goal is firm soil not hard soil. Then place seeds on the bottom of this depression and cover them to the appropriate depth with loose soil.

Sometimes unsettled spring weather keeps me out of the garden. I get behind. Instead of digging and fertilizing entire beds before making hills, I just dig and fertilize the hills and immediately sow seeds or transplant into them. Weeks later when I am ahead (and not a behind) I spread COF and dig or hoe it in between the hills.

Sandstone (and other sand) soils

Tasmania has areas where the soil formed out of sandstone. Near the Bass Strait are many acres covered with deep wind deposited sand. There are many homesteads on sandstone hills emerging out of the agricultural red soils around Deloraine. I've lab tested sand soils around St. Helens and visited gardens on deep coarse sands along the East Coast that developed from granite. I have tested sand soils near Hobart. All these soils severely lack plant nutrients. They also hold little moisture and because they do not contain clay they have little ability to hold on to plant nutrients that gardeners put in. Sometimes they have a reddish-brown subsoil that seems like clay to someone that doesn't know soil very well but actually the material is sand that has been cemented into hard stuff by iron leached from above and deposited below. And sometimes near Bass Straight and on King Island, leached iron and sulfur combined to form an impervious black subsoil layer under sand soil called "coffee rock," which is composed of iron pyrites and is extremely acidic. It makes for very poor drainage. This layer shouldn't be disturbed because when it gets broken up it'll release sulphuric acid that kills all plants exposed to it.

Sands grow much better vegetables when they are fed more organic matter than a heavier soil needs. Growing excellent vegies on sand soils can be a lot like practising hydroponics with dry powders—to get a nutrient-dense result you must repeatedly feed all the plant nutrients in small doses. My regular COF recipe works well in sand but the alternate recipe on this page does better. Spread and work in the entire amount on 10 square metres before planting. With all crops, including low-demand crops, be prepared to side-dress COF every few weeks and/or side-dress every time plant growth slows.

COF for Sand

4 litres oilseedmeal (2,400 gm)
¼ litre *dolomite* lime (350 gm)
¼ litre agricultural lime (350gm)
¼ litre agricultural gypsum (350gm)
½ litre soft rock phosphate *or* guano (500 gm)
½ cup potassium sulphate (150 gm)
½ litre kelpmeal (400 gm)
2 tablespoons ferrous (iron) sulphate (30 gm)
1½ tablespoons ma*n*ganese sulphate (30 gm)
(not mag*nesium* sulphate)
3 teaspoons zinc sulphate (15 gm)
2 teaspoons copper sulphate (15 gm)
1 tablespoon borax *or* Organibor (20 gm)
⅛ tsp sodium molybdate (0.5 gm)
Mix these ingredients so they're uniformly blended.
Spread on 10 square metres.

Liquid fertilizer

Gardeners make liquid fertilizer by soaking animal manure, compost and/or leaves in water. We dilute worm bed drippings. We dilute fish and kelp extracts. Any of these are poured over plants (drench), sprayed on leaves (foliar feed) or put directly into the root zone (fertigation). This boosts growth for a week or two.

I've experienced that fish and kelp extracts are not as effective as full-spectrum soluble chemicals because they have insignificant levels of trace elements and because it is impossible to soak much phosphorus out of an organic material. If you should encounter a liquid "organic" concentrate providing more than one percent phosphate, be aware! Most of that P came from phosphoric acid. In my opinion, diluted phosphoric acid is excellent fertilizer. Until recently, organic certification authorities ideologically banned phosphoric acid because it isn't a naturally occurring substance. They now reckon phosphoric acid can be kosher when it is "used to prevent fermentation." Amazingly, the amount that stops spoilage just happens to be the exact amount needed for better fertilization.

In my opinion, the best concentrates at the garden centre in the year 2025 are Miracle Gro and Maxicrop Seaweed Plant Food Concentrate. Neither of them provides the ideal NPK ratio for most vegetables, which is 1-2-2 (5-10-10 or 10-20-20). Both do supply useful amounts of trace elements. Either of these products strongly pushes plants forward.

Liquid kelp

Kelp has long been used as food, for fertilizer and in more recent times for the extraction of alginates—which are valuable chemicals with a wide range of industrial uses. Kelp also contains natural growth regulators and hormones that help crops resist stress and diseases. Kelp extracts that retain the alginates and the hormones (not all do) make seedlings develop stronger roots. Kelp also provides the full range of micronutrients because it grows in sea water. If you make COF but can't afford kelpmeal, try foliar feeding liquid kelp every few weeks.

Some kelp extracts are made with residue from alginate extraction. Unfortunately, the valuable hormones and growth regulators went with the alginates; by-product liquid kelp still has value, it contains the minerals, but liquid kelp works much better when it hasn't been denatured. Don't expect recyclers of alginate-extraction waste to tell you that's what they are doing. Tasmania has been blessed yet again: we have several makers of high quality kelp extract including Sea Sol in Launceston, Marrawah Gold and The Marrawah Kelp Company.

Foliar feeding

Leaves can intake plant nutrients that are dissolved in water. Foliar feeding works best when leaf breathing pores (stomata) are open, which happens when moisture stress is low, such as early morning and on overcast humid days. Fertilizer solution is sprayed on leaves until drops start falling from leaf tips; then the spray moves on. The very small quantity of fertilizer that gets sprayed on leaves provokes as much growth as though much more of it had it been put into the soil. However, the effect only lasts one week. Assimilation of foliars can be increased by adding a water softener that allows the droplets to spread out over leaves in a thin film rather than beading up and rolling off. Ordinary dishwashing liquid does this. The amount to put in the spray tank varies by brand but it will be only a few drops per litre. If frothy bubbles form whilst filling the spray tank then too much detergent was used.

Plants that already are making rapid growth can be made to grow even faster by foliar feeding them every seven days. When heat lovers start ripening fruit their growth rate slows so from this point foliar feed every two weeks. Slow-growing autumn/winter crops could use a foliar feed every two- to three weeks until mid-May, but there is little point in foliar feeding after that because growth pretty much stops no matter what is done short of putting plants under plastic.

Until the 2015-16 growing season I had rarely bothered with foliar feeding. I thought that balancing soil nutrients was enough. But then I experimented with foliar feeding two related substances: liquid fertilizer concentrates and aerated compost tea—ACT. Both of them produced a noticeable increase in growth rate and both improved flavour.

I now believe that no matter how fertile or how balanced the soil is, no matter how vibrant the soil ecology, it is not possible for a plant to draw all the nutrients it *could* use from the soil. Plants enjoying balanced soil that is in good tilth will resist most diseases and insects, they will be nutritious and delicious. Foliar feeding an already healthy plant like that creates obvious improvements by the following day—growth noticeably speeds up; the head of broccoli forming soon after a foliar feed tastes sweeter.

Used as foliars, the aforementioned Miracle Gro and Maxicrop work better than fish and/or kelp, but I much prefer using a product made by Nutri-Tech Solutions (Qld) called "10-10-10." (The same stuff is variously named as though it is especially for "vegetables," "berries," "vines" or half a dozen other crops. All of them provide the same fertilizer at the same price but are labelled with different directions for use.) Nutri-Tech's concentrate is far less costly per diluted litre of spray than what you'll find at the garden centre. T.P. Jones sold 20 litre containers but now that they have been gobbled up by Nutrien I can't say if they will continue to do so. Frank Gilson is the Nutri-Tech rep in St. Marys. (0419-372-192).Activevista sells Nutri-Tech products. Nutri-Tech sells a 5 litre container online.

Contact: www.nutri-tech.com.au

Nutri-Tech recommends diluting 10-10-10 to foliar feed vegetables at 10 ml/litre. I think this is too concentrated for a mixture of species because spinach, beetroot and silverbeet (and maybe others) get slightly bruised by 10-10-10 at this concentration. So I dilute it to 7 ml/litre. *Do not spray the undersides of the leaves.* I suggest regulating foliar feeding according to this principle: if the season allows the plants to make rapid vegetative growth then spray every time the total plant mass doubles (every seven days during summer). If the crop is forming or ripening fruit, spray every two weeks. Fruit trees—spray every two weeks from petal drop until about a month before harvest.

Aerated Compost Tea

Completely finished humified compost shelters a complex microecology consisting of beneficial microbes, fungi, protozoa, etc. Plants grow much better when their root zone is densely populated by an ecology similar to this. An unnecessarily laborious and counter-productive way to build a high population of beneficial soil microorganisms is by spreading and working in very large quantities of high quality compost—I mean amounts like 20 dry-weight tons per acre per year. I have known gardeners who make and spread more than that amount. Every year. Their plants grow large and look good.

So why do I disdain this approach? Making that much great compost means doing a lot of (unnecessary, as I'll soon explain) work. What you buy at the landscape yard is not great compost. It also does not bring with it a full microecology. Chapter 3, "Composting" has a lot to say about this. I say using this much compost is impractical because your garden and its surrounds and your lawns and ornamental gardens combined can not generate all the raw materials needed to make that much, which means spending considerable money to import compost feedstocks. I think importing is risky because some broadleaf plant herbicides that are used on paddocks have made gardens incapable of growing any vegetable except corn, and alliums for several years until the herbicide residues break down. This happens when using manure from animals that were grazing paddocks sprayed to eliminate invasive weeds. I've also heard of gardens ruined for years to come by mulching with contaminated grain straw.

Building soil fertility with organic matter would not be dangerous or costly for a family farm's food garden because a few percent of their own farm's total biomass production could be made into compost without damaging the farm itself. Even it costs nothing but labour I think the practice is counter-productive. Because bringing that much organic matter into a garden almost certainly will create soil imbalances that lower the nutrient density of the family's vegetables, thus undermining the intention behind making so much compost.

Aerated compost tea is another way to positively shift the garden's soil ecology. Making ACT doesn't require nearly as much work as making compost and it won't chemically imbalance the soil.

I apologize in advance for the brevity and incomplete nature of my discussion of aerated compost tea. I have only limited experience and do not want to write a book report. But I feel compelled to encourage the use of ACT because it did improve my own garden's performance.

Aerated compost tea is not soaked compost tea. As I mention in "Chapter 3, Composting," gardeners have long made effective liquid fertilizers by soaking animal manure/compost/green leafy materials in water and then pouring the resulting extract (after being diluted) over plants and into soil. Aerated compost tea is something else. It is the result of a microbial brewing procedure that rapidly increase a complex ecology of beneficial microbes by jillions of times their starting number, all in 24 hours. The device that does this is termed a "bioreactor." An effective home garden sized bioreactor can be made from a 20 litre white plastic bucket and a few bits of gear from a pet shop.

Benefits of ACT

When aerated compost tea is sprayed at low rates, like 100 litres per acre, it inoculates the soil with the same beneficial ecology found in high quality compost. ACT affordably helps paddocks, orchards and cultivated farm crops grow better. In the garden ACT may gradually change the soil as though a lot of compost had been worked in. When ACT is sprayed on plants it heavily inoculates their leaves and stems with beneficial microbes and chelated nutrients that have become part of microbes. This improves growth rate and overall plant health because plants must use part of their energy budget to resist diseases. ACT puts high concentrations of beneficials on their leaves that outcompete and eliminate harmful organisms and this lessen the plant's burden for awhile.

Finally, ACT that is cultured in a solution of balanced plant nutrients will create a markedly greater growth response than had that same nutrients been sprayed as a foliar feed without first brewing microbes in it. Nutri-Tech similarly converts the chemical nutrients in their 10-10-10 into complex organic molecules by using humates and fulvic acids.

How to make and use ACT

All you need is a small quantity of excellent compost to use as a starter, two- 15 to 20 litre plastic buckets and some hobby fish tank accessories. One bucket serves as the bioreactor, the second bucket upside down next to it makes a secure platform that allows the airpump to be supported as close as possible to the brewer. Also needed are four air stones and some air hose. To maintain the brewing medium at or slightly over 20°C use a thermostatically controlled fishtank immersion heater that is a size or two larger than what would keep tropical fish comfortable in a 20 litre fishtank in the house.

This is the procedure in short: Microbe food is dissolved in water, a starter culture is added, an air pump vigorously and constantly oxygenates the warm brewing medium and soon there are jillions of microbes.

Starter culture

It is essential to start the brew with high quality compost that recently finished, that has remained moist since finishing and has not been packaged in an airtight plastic bag (which soon kills most of the microbes). I opine that the best starter is humified compost such as I make mostly from vegetable crop waste. If the starter compost dried out and/or sat around for many months after finishing then the surviving ecology will be less complex and the resulting ACT less effective. I have made excellent ACT from the cow-horn compost that is used by my Biodynamic friends to stir into BD-500. I have suggested to them that ACT can be thought of as BD-500 taken to the next level. They didn't appreciate my assertion. An attractive-looking airtight plastic bag of industrial compost conveniently purchased from the garden centre won't have many living microbes left in it and is unlikely to brew an effective batch of ACT.

The crumbly worm castings from the bottom of a worm bin makes excellent ACT starter. I think every gardening household should use worm composting to dispose of kitchen waste.

Market gardeners who regularly brew ACT purchase starter cultures in dry powder form, much like bakers buy yeast. These provide diverse ecologies of beneficial microbes. Nutri-Tech sells these. Sometimes an ACT brew is inoculated with specific microbes that suppress specific diseases.

The amount of compost starter needed to inoculate a brew is 2.5% of the volume of water (for up to around a 1,000 litre brewer). Thus, to brew 20 litres of ACT x 2.5% = roughly 2 cups of compost starter. Fifteen litres of ACT is not quite enough to treat a one-eighth acre food garden.

Water

The brew must start in water that is free of chlorine because chlorinated water kills a great many microbes. One type of chlorine used to sanitize mains water can be eliminated by running air bubblers for two hours before introducing the inoculant and the nutrients. I can't say anything for very certain about what's in *your* municipal water other than it almost certainly has fluoride in it—so you shouldn't be drinking it or even washing your body in it.

Fill the bioreactor bucket no more than three-quarters full because foam sometimes develops on top. So a 20 litre plastic bucket can brew 15 litres of ACT.

Special brews

ACT can be used to control diseases. Interventions with specific microbes at key points in the crop's growth cycle often are as effective as fungicides but without suppressing the entire microecology the way chemical fungicides do. And ACT costs next to nothing compared to chemicals. Advanced brewers may incorporate specific trace elements into a microbial brew because providing those nutrients at that moment makes a huge difference.

Nutrient solutions

Internet publications and videos suggest using many different materials and recipes when brewing ACT. Some of these recipes provide enough nutrients to breed up a very high concentration of microbes, but only if there is enough oxygen to sustain them. The higher that the concentration of microbes goes, the higher their demand for oxygen becomes. Market gardeners and orchardists who brew ACT invest in quite noisy (not suitable to suburbia) high capacity air blowers that can fully oxygenate a rich brewing media in 1,000 litre shuttle tanks.

A suburban home gardener attempting to make more litres of ACT at one go than an aquarium shop airpump can thoroughly oxygenate is inviting failure. Making the brewing medium too nutrient-rich also leads to failure when there is insufficient oxygenation. The home gardener's fundamental requirement is to multiply a diverse ecology of beneficial aerobic microorganisms until the brew arrives at an effective concentration. If the ACT a home gardener produces is only half as potent as what might be possible to achieve— what of it! It'll still produce a remarkable result.

Tim Wilson (whose useful website will soon be referenced) and Tad Hussey (who runs KIS Organics near Seattle), are crop advisors in the Cascadia Bioregion. They assert that the only material needed to brew home garden ACT is molasses. I urge you to follow their lead, at least until you have experienced several successes with it.

Please brew microbes in molasses dissolved into the brew water at 0.5% (5 ml/litre). Add nothing else!

I am fully aware that my recommendation disagrees with Dr. Elaine Ingham. You will find many Elaine Ingham videos on youtube. I think these should be seen by all who are interested in ACT. Although I see value from looking at this material I should tell you that I do not agree with Ingham that ACT makes fertilizing the soil unnecessary. Maybe this may be true in the Someday Isles. It is for sure not true regarding Tasmanian soils. What is obviously true is that Ingham's simplified assertions attract a large followership. Also indisputably true is that Ingham has products to sell to you and gets paid handsomely for presenting.

Incidentally, I define the word *charlatan* as someone—qualified or not—who oversimplifies a subject so it appeals to the scantly educated and seeks to personally profit from so doing. I am not accusing anyone of being a charlatan because that could be construed as defamation. I am merely informing you that I define the word differently than the dictionary does.

Ingham brews beneficial microbes in a solution made from organic fertilizer concentrates that all by themselves could function as a potent foliar spray or soil drench. Microbes convert those plant nutrients into amino-acid chelates that plants use more effectively than simple chemicals. Because there is so much microbe food available during an Elaine Ingham style brew, a very high level of oxygenation must be maintained or else the brew goes anaerobic. If that should happen, even briefly anaerobic, not only does the process fail, but what results might damage plants and gardens. To keep control of this risky business a microscope is needed and checks must be made every few hours during the brew cycle.

The method this book proposes will not make as potent a brew as Dr. Ingham tantalizes us with, but the approach is nearly foolproof. And potent enough for the home gardener.

Air supply

Tim Wilson advises using an air pump that supplies 1.4 litres to 2 litres of air bubbles per minute for each litre of brew when it is at a temperature high enough to make the microbes reproduce rapidly. A four-outlet home aquarium air pump (all four outlets combined) usually puts out 10 litres per minute, which is enough flow to fully oxygenate maybe six litres of a nutrient-rich growing medium (similar to Ingham's recommendation). Ten litres per minute does adequately oxygenate 15 litres of molasses-only brewing solution when *the temperature stays below 22°C.*

It is essential to have an air stone on every one of those four outlets. It is essential to keep the air lines as short as possible because the supply tubes from an aquarium shop pump to the airstones are very small diameter and strongly reduce air flow. That's why I position the air pump as close to the brewing solution as possible.

To brew larger quantities of ACT at one go requires a much larger air pump, and these are not found in pet supply shops. They are noisy (maybe noisy beyond the tolerance of neighbours) and they won't be cheap.

You may wish to learn more, and in that case I suggest starting with Tim Wilson's web page (http://www.microbeorganics.com/).

Temperature and oxygen demand

Most of the microbes involved in an ACT brew are bacteria and fungi. Fungi rapidly form thready hyphae which thicken the brew like starch thickens soup. Bacteria can divide every 20 minutes. These organisms increase to very large numbers within 24 hours; then we then declare the brew "finished" and spray it on the soil and plants.

The amount of time required for each microbial doubling and the quantity of oxygen consumed by the brew are determined by temperature. Oxygen demand by microbes approximately doubles for every 10°C temperature increase whilst at the same time the capacity of water to dissolve oxygen decreases with increased temperature. Allowing for the limited airflow provided by a four-outlet fishtank airpump, I think a bucket brewer should be run in a temperature range of 18°C to 22°C for 24 hours after it is inoculated with compost. A few degrees warmer would be okay in the beginning of the brew but not okay towards the end when there will be so many microbes that increasing the temperature will increase demand for oxygen above the level the equipment can sustain it. A 50 watt fish tank heater should be able to maintain 15 litres of brewing solution at 20°C in an unheated out building in summer. If the ambient temperature drops below 10°C then the brew bucket can be wrapped with an old blanket or thick towel. Or a higher wattage fishtank heater can be used. If the brew should fall below 20°C the only "harm" is that the concentration of microbes will be lower—but the brew will still be effective.

The microbes in a finished brew are consuming oxygen at a high rate so the brew must be sprayed or drenched soon after turning off the air bubbler. Less than 20 minutes would be okay; immediately is best. As soon as I turn off the airpump I pour the contents of my brewer through a fine mesh tea strainer into a 14 litre backpack sprayer with a filtered nozzle that won't block up and immediately distribute the entire brew.

A brew should not be allowed to go on past the point all the food has been consumed because from this point the microbes must eat each other and consequently, the ecology gets ever more simplified. Without a microscope it is not possible to observe the peaks and valleys of the microbial ecology so it is simplest (and safest) to keep the brewing temperature moderate and distribute the entire lot after brewing for 24 hours.

A good brew finishes with a pleasant earthy aroma. If it smells sour or unpleasant at the end, don't use it; it might damage plants. There should be no need to invest in a microscope as long as the brewing medium is only molasses at 5 ml/litre, the brew is bubbled strongly, the temperature is held between 18°C and 22°C and the brew time is no more than 24 hours.

Mesh bag or free suspension

When starting the brew it is okay to toss compost inoculant into the water and let it float. I vigorously stir the inoculant with a stick for a minute when first putting it into the brewer. I think this helps knock microorganisms off the compost and into the nutrient solution. I believe the brew forms a higher density of microorganisms sooner by dumping starter culture materials into warm nutrient solution that is already being aerated. Bits of compost floating in the solution can't be sprayed or even poured through the small holes of a watering can. To filter the small quantity I am describing the best option is to pour the finished brew through a large tea strainer with a very fine mesh before putting it into the spray tank and also using a large-bore spray nozzle. Removing particles from ACT by the 1,000 litres isn't so easy. People who brew on that scale put the starter inoculant into a fine mesh bag, that dangles in the brewing vat like a big teabag. In that case the bag itself must have a very strong air bubbler inside of it, one strong enough to constantly shake up the material or else the microbes (especially fungi) may not be knocked loose to enter the brewing solution and/or the mass of compost in the bag will settle into an airless mass at the bottom of the bag.

Cleaning the brewer

Brewed microbes deposit a thick slime on all surfaces in the brewer. This slime is easy to scrub off when it is still moist but very difficult to remove after it dries. This slime could inoculate the next brew with undesirable microbes. So the brewing gear must be scrubbed clean immediately after the brew has been sprayed.

Take care to brush the airstones severely.

Large volume brewers do not use airstones. They manufacture a bubbler out of poly pipe with hundreds of tiny holes drilled or punched into it. On Tim Wilson's website you'll find plans to build small airlift brewers that aerate like a coffee percolator.

Frequency and method of use;

You can use ACT (made only with molasses) as often as you wish. I would find it interesting to construct a 1,000 litre shuttle tank brewer, make a new batch almost every day and make ACT the main source of irrigation for an entire garden. What a lush garden that would be!

In my opinion the most efficient way to use ACT is to spray it on leaves as though the plants were being foliar fed (spray until moisture starts to drip off leaf tips); I would not to spray ACT on bare soil as some do. I suggest spraying the entire vegie garden this way once each month. My eighth-acre of vegie beds plus a few fruit trees needed about 14 litres for one treatment.

The best time of day/weather to spray ACT is just before dark, or on overcast drizzly days. Moisture that is already on the leaves at the time of spraying gives the microbes time to find a niche and get established. Microbes that get washed off the leaves inoculate soil.

Some growers add foliar fertilizers and/or molasses and/or humic acid to finished ACT just before applying it. By doing before/after microscopic analyses Tim Wilson discovered that adding fish hydrolysate at 5 ml/litre killed or put to sleep almost half of the microorganisms he had just brewed. Now he always does foliar feeding separately from spraying ACT. And this is what I also recommend.

Molybdenum

Molybdenum is an essential plant nutrient that gets little attention or recognition. I once opined that molybdenum is almost always available in sufficient amounts in all soils; that Mo is rarely a concern—much like silicon is also incorrectly said to be of no concern. In 2016 I was surprised to discover that smart Tasmanian cauliflower and broccoli growers apply sodium molybdate every few years to prevent strapleaf—a condition formally-educated agronomists term whiptail. Molybdenum deficient brassica leaves become extremely narrow, which means the plant can't manufacture as much sugar so it grows slowly, ends up being much smaller—and narrowed leaves fail to wrap the cauliflower's curds, causing them to become yellowed and harsh tasting. Broccoli shows lack of Mo by making smaller narrower leaves and much smaller flowers. So in the spring of 2017 after checking that a moderate excess could do no harm, I applied a moderate amount of molybdenum to all my beds.

I did this without a soil test. Few soil labs will test for molybdenum in any case and frankly, there is no need to test because at the scale I operate it is cheaper to obtain one kilogram of sodium molybdate and apply enough to make the difference. I reckoned if one feed of Mo made no perceptible difference then it was not needed; so do not repeat. Other than a minor waste of money, no harm will be done because, as I just said, molybdenum at any reasonable level is not toxic to plants.

Garden centres do not sell sodium molybdate. Tassie farm suppliers sell one kilogram for over $100. Buy it online and you might save $20. I urge garden clubs and community garden committees to invest in a kilo and share it out. I urge garden centre owners to buy 1 kg and resell it by the 25 grams. I urge serious gardeners to invest in their own one kilogram lifetime supply.

The correct dose

The tiny amount of sodium molybdate in COF is enough. If you do not use COF I suggest intentionally remineralizing only that element. Here is how to:

Sodium molybdate is a dense substance; a little bit weighs more than you might think. Measure it carefully; distribute it uniformly. One level kitchen measure quarter teaspoon of sodium molybdate weighs about 2 grams. That much makes a generous feed for 10 square metres that should be repeated every three years. Dissolve 2 grams of sodium molybdate into 1 litre of warm water in a pump sprayer and *apply it to 10 square metres of soil*. Go over the entire 10 square metres least two times with that litre—thereby making sure it is uniformly distributed. If the area is growing a food crop when it is being sprayed, then mix the same amount of sodium molybdate into twice as much water and use a coarse spray—so that much of the water immediately drips from the leaves to the soil. Then immediately put another litre or two of plain water into the pump sprayer and go over the bed again, or else use a hose and nozzle to wash as much molybdenum off the leaves as possible. Washing it off the leaves is not done to prevent the plants from assimilating it. That much molybdenum would do no harm to the crop or to the eater of the crop. This method makes sure the material actually gets into the soil so crops following on for the next few years find it in their rootzone.

The iron-rich soils of Tasmania provide little available Mo because molybdenum combines with iron and becomes completely insoluble and thereby unavailable to plants in much the same manner that phosphate disappears from the soil test when it becomes iron phosphate. Molybdenum does not cling to clay; it readily gets removed by leaching. You can see why most Tasmanian soils can be significantly short Mo. Even if you're not using my COF recipe I urge you to find out if a dose of Mo will make a difference.

Soon after remineralizing my garden with molybdenum the following vegetable species showed noticeable improvement—broccoli, cauliflower, cabbage, brussels sprout, swede, lettuce, onion, beetroot, pea, spinach, tomato, all legumes. All the aforementioned brassicas formed larger, broader leaves that photosynthesized more sugar so the harvest was larger. Our broccoli now tastes even sweeter than before. Normally when I direct seed onion early in spring, frosts and who knows what else causes many seedlings to disappear in their first month. After Mo almost none of them died and I had to do a lot more thinning. So now I sow fewer seeds. Lettuce didn't grow noticeably better, but now our lettuce is sweeter. So are beetroot, carrot and peas.

How often should molybdenum be applied? Erica Reinheimer, who helped me write *The Intelligent Gardener,* is both a soil analyst in the United States and a serious vegetable gardener. In her country testing for Mo is readily available and inexpensive. As a test, once each year for five consecutive years Erica added half as much sodium molybdate as I just suggested. After five years her garden's test level for molybdenum has not significantly increased.

Biochar and wood ash

Ancient abandoned gardens in the totally leached Amazon rainforest are still fertile after 500 years of neglect because the soil there contains a lot of charcoal, lately termed biochar. Finding fertile soil in a tropical rainforest has raised great interest in biochar.

Charcoal holds on to plant nutrients much like clay and humus do so biochar greatly reduces leaching and stabilizes nutrient delivery by acting like bits of nutrient-saturated sponge that plants can draw from. Biochar remains in the soil for more than 1,000 years; we don't really know how long. Humus lasts 100 years at most. Non-humified compost, which is what can be purchased from landscape yards, decomposes completely within three years.

Frank Strie is Tasmania's biochar activist. He encourages commercial biochar manufacturing from farm- and timber processing waste with the side-benefit of co-generated electricity. I speculate that sandy farm soils amended with biochar would grow better crops than had the same feedstocks been returned to the soil as compost.

You could reduce airflow into your woodheater at bedtime so that the fire goes out sooner. Each morning remove charcoal but not the ash. Putting freshly made charcoal into soil and then immediately trying to grow something there creates a shockingly bad result because raw biochar so powerfully intakes plant nutrients from the soil that crops can't grow. But when biochar has been saturated with plant nutrients before going into soil it then serves as a self-recharging nutrient source. One way to precharge new charcoal is to first soak it in water for a day (to keep the dust down) and then grind it to the size of rice grains with an electric kitchen garbage grinder attached under an old sink. A small amount of water must be run through the grinder with the charcoal. Then mix it into a compost heap when the heap is being formed. During the composting process biochar saturates itself with plant nutrients. I reckon that including up to 5 percent raw biochar by starting volume will not slow the composting process. I am a believer in the "a difference that makes no difference is no difference" principle, so I put woodstove charcoal into my compost heaps without grinding it first. Some of it crumbles by itself, especially when I dig and rake seedbeds. Resistant larger bits get raked out of seedbeds onto the paths where my feet break them up. Eventually it all crumbles.

I once experimentally precharged finely crushed charcoal by soaking exactly half a bucket of it in NTS 10-10-10 solution that was three times the recommended strength (30 ml/lt). The soak went on for weeks because the biochar kept expanding. Eventually it filled 2/3 of the bucket and stabilized. The soaked biochar was then drained, briefly rinsed, dried in the sun and became five percent of a container growing medium. I got a remarkable result!

Biochar is a new topic. I don't yet know if hardwood versus softwood charcoal matters very much. Or if char made from crop waste (like rice hulls or almond hulls) is better than charcoal made from wood; some say it is. I don't yet know the ideal temperature to target while making the charcoal nor the best possible way to precharge biochar. I don't yet know if any amount of biochar could be too much. My guess at this point: Tasmanian soils comprised of more than

20 percent clay will not hugely benefit from biochar after it has released the nutrients it was precharged with. However the performance of sandy soil should steadily improve as its biochar content increases. I speculate that sand soils could benefit from having one-quarter by volume biochar in the top 30 cm. This much char would stabilize crop nutrition as though there were an similar proportion of clay in the sand. Unlike clay, biochar would not act to reduce soil air or turn the sand into something resembling concrete when it dried out. I hope biochar soon becomes inexpensive enough that gardeners can buy it from landscape yards by the metre.

Since we're talking charcoal, what about that wood ash I mentioned a few paragraphs back. Many garden books recommend using wood ash as fertilizer because it is mostly oxides of calcium, potassium and magnesium, which makes them extremely alkaline. But Tasmanians should avoid bringing more magnesium into garden soils containing very much clay and it's a reasonable speculation that since our soils are naturally magnesium-rich, so are our wood ashes. If there is much clay in your garden I advise spreading ashes *very thinly* under native ornamentals or else send them to the tip. But if you garden on sand I suggest putting ashes into the compost heap.

Compost as fertilizer

Before COF I depended on an American compost product similar to Dynamic Lifter or Rapid Raiser. The results I got from that fertilizer certainly impressed visitors to my trials ground. Chicken manure and sawdust composted together can make a nitrogen-rich fertilizer with a useful amount of phosphorus in it. Chook poo compost is potent because poultry mainly eat seeds, not leaves. So chicken manure compost contains a nutrient profile similar to the 5.5 percent nitrogen oilseedmeal I base COF upon, but chook provides only 3.5 percent nitrogen because the chickens have already had first go at extracting nutrition from it.

But here's the important however: as the nitrogen concentration of an organic material increases the growth response it produces when decomposing in soil increases even faster. You'll become a much better gardener if you'll take a moment to contemplate this principle. Eight to twelve litres of Dynamic Lifter holding 3.5% nitrogen mixed into 10 square metres of topsoil creates a growth response similar to what is produced from four litres of canolaseedmeal holding 5.5% nitrogen. Seedmeal works out to be much less costly. And seedmeal doesn't have a strong odour. I may be old but I'm still flexible—both mentally and physically. If a 25 kilogram bag of chook poo pellets sold for half the price of canolaseedmeal I would be using chook in addition to canola.

As the nitrogen concentration in organic fertilizers decreases, the growth response they produce diminishes even faster. Materials containing less than two percent nitrogen do not create a noticeable growth response unless they go into very warm soil. Materials containing one percent nitrogen actually slow growth when mixed into soil. Properly made garden waste compost usually provides around two percent nitrogen. This prompts better growth during the two warmest months of Tasmanian summer—if at least 100 litres of it are hoed into 10 square metres. And what about the rest of the year?

Spring crops grow slowly in Tasmanian gardens that are fed nothing but average compost. This persists until the soil approaches its annual peak temperature, which happens around Christmas. That's when the corn patch turns dark green and gets to growing fast. Other heat loving crops also start growing fast at that time. If heat loving species could have made more progress before Christmas they'd yield sooner and produce more. That's one reason to use both—COF to supply plant nutrients—especially nitrogen—and compost to feed the soil ecology.

Composts made of mostly municipal green wastes, paper and sawdust usually provide around one percent nitrogen. Composts like this increase soil organic matter and bring in some plant nutrients, usually way out of balance, but they do not make crops grow fast; in fact, when compost like this is mixed into soil it can temporarily act like anti-fertilizer. If I wanted my garden to grow strongly with much of this stuff in the soil then I'd also have to put half-again more seedmeal than the usual into each batch of COF.

Soil organic matter

COF can not maintain soil health by itself. Preparing seed beds, hoeing weeds, digging—all these actions increase the rate at which soil organic matter decomposes. Using nitrogen fertilizer triggers a large increase in the microbial population which eats soil organic matter. Digging and hoeing temporarily increase soil air which allows microbes to reproduce faster and eat more. So vegetable gardeners must take steps to maintain organic matter or else the soil ecology declines, plant health declines, the friability and moisture holding capacity most soil types decline.

Carbon in soil organic matter fuels much of the soil's ecosystem just like human bodies can be fuelled by carbo(n) hydrate foods. Soil that contains little or no clay will almost completely consume landscape yard or garden centre compost within a few years. In soils containing more clay a small fraction of that carbon transforms into humus, which is a relatively stable substance that provides great benefits for many years before it fully decomposes. Either way, short-lasting or rather more permanent, the presence of decomposing organic matter makes an enormous difference in how soil behaves and how it grows crops. But the presence of humus makes the greatest difference.

Humus has been studied for well over a century but we still do not know its chemical formula (or should I better say formulae). We cannot synthesize it. All humus is dark-coloured (brown or black), spongy (holds a lot of moisture) and has powerful, positive effects when mixed into soil.

When raw organic matter is added to soil most of it is initially digested by small soil dwelling animals such as earwigs, slaters, millipedes, worms, slugs and snails. Their excretions and their dead bodies are in turn eaten by microbes and fungi. Each eater derives its energy (burns carbon) from the organic matter it consumes, uses nutrients from the organic matter to build its own protoplasm and excretes wastes that are in turn eaten by a complex ecology of even smaller life forms. After everything has finished dining and dying, most of the carbon has been converted to carbon dioxide gas and the mineral nutrients in that organic matter have been liberated; any remaining indigestible residue is humus.

N. S. Krasil'nikov was a brilliant Soviet-era soil microbiologist and author of the classic book *Soil Microorganisms and Higher Plants**. He asserted that soil fertility is "determined by biological factors, mainly by microorganisms . . . . Were this microlife eliminated the soil would become an object of geology (not biology)." He measured soil quality by the number of microorganisms per gram of soil; there is always a close match between this number and productivity.

Of the many useful effects accomplished by the soil ecology, these are of the most benefit to food growers—improved soil structure; suppression of soil-dwelling plant diseases; the bacterial creation of what Krasil'nikov named phytamins; some microbes manufacture nitrates from atmospheric nitrogen; other microbes liberate insoluble phosphates; microbes and fungi release plant nutrients from rock particles; soil fungi penetrate or closely associate with the roots of certain plant species and transport nutrients directly into the plant.

It would require another book much longer than this one to fully explain all these matters.

Phytamins—plant vitamins

Hydroponic lettuce from the supermarket tastes incomplete to me because it lacks tiny quantities of essential somethings that Krasil'nikov named phytamins—plant vitamins. Plants need phytamins to be fully healthy as much as animals and humans need vitamins. That's why the smartest hydroponic growers supply phytamins by adding brewed organic concoctions to their nutrient tank.

Plants can't make their own phytamins any more than humans can make their own vitamin C. Plants entice soil dwelling microbes to supply them. The plant's root tips and root hairs exude watery substances that establish a chemical environment immediately around the root that strongly favours specific (beneficial) bacteria and fungi as well as feeding them sugar that the plant considers is excess to its requirements. Root exudates can also suppress disease organisms. It's a fair exchange; the cultivated microbes create phytamins and humus and release nutrients out of the soil in plant-available forms. If the amount of soil organic matter declines so does the microbial population and so does plant health. To learn more, do a web search for "regenerative agriculture."

Tilth

Soil is a complex mixture. The largest proportion of many soils consists of tiny rock fragments that have not yet been dissolved by weak soil acids and by microbes. Clay forms in the soil from chemicals released by dissolving rock particles. Soil contains fast decomposing organic matter and long-lasting humus; it houses microorganisms and a complex ecology of tiny living things; it holds water and air and plant roots. All these components work together to form what is termed "structure"—the gaps and spaces that provide air to roots, that allow moisture to penetrate rapidly and drain out freely. The coarser and more stable the soil structure becomes then the more oxygen there will be in the root zone and the better plants grow. Immediately after digging or hoeing it, a structureless soil provides roots with more air so the plants grow faster for a short while. But that kind of soil soon resettles, there's less oxygen and growth slows.

Microorganisms and worms create soil structure by producing slimy, gluey substances that strongly cement soil particles into irregularly-shaped crumbs that can be as large as rice grains. Soil crumbs do not pack tightly; crumbs make spaces for air and water. Earthworms leave a crumb trail behind themselves the crumbs are made by combining soil with decomposed organic matter as both of them pass through the worm's digestive system. Without a crumb structure the finer bits of silt and clay would sift into gaps between the larger sand particles and then there would be far less air in the soil. A crumbly soil is said to have good tilth. It can be worked easily and can be massaged into a finely-textured loose seedbed that doesn't quickly get tight, nor will a crumbly soil readily form a hard surface crust that prevents the emergence of seedlings.

Good tilth allows rain and irrigation to flow into soil more rapidly. When you see long-lasting puddles on farm fields after a heavy rain likely you are looking at structureless humus-depleted soil. Good tilth also prevents surface crust from forming after rain or irrigation. Crusting does more than stop fragile vegetable seeds from sprouting. Crust seals the surface, reducing the amount of oxygen in soil. That's one reason I advise gardeners to rake compost into the surface rather than dig it in; a crust can not form when the top inch contains that much organic matter. There's another benefit from improved tilth: well oxygenated micro-organisms thrive. So in an airy soil more nutrients are released from decomposing organic matter. More soil air means more phytamins get manufactured. Well oxygenated root systems expand faster. *Plants grow no better above ground than their roots manage.* I often reflect upon how oxygen in soil may be one of the most important plant nutrients.

So, how much organic matter does garden soil actually need?

Decomposing organic matter releases plant nutrients. The rate of decomposition depends upon temperature. *In warm soil* compost can nourish vegetables as well as or better than concentrated fertilizer— if the compost contains all needed plant nutrients in reasonable balance. Compost also feeds soil microorganisms whose activities are essential to plant- and soil health. The founders of the organic farming and gardening movement convinced us that soil couldn't possibly be given too much compost. Their early books and subsequent publications of the organic movement's followership suggest that gardeners should make and spread as much compost as possible. A corollary of this belief is that soil fertility should be gauged by worm count because worms multiply rapidly when they are fed plenty of partly-decomposed organic matter.

Rather than sheepishly accept what gardening authorities tell us, please consider it afresh. Is there a point of diminishing returns, where putting in more and more results in less and less benefit? And perhaps more important: could we put in too much?

About the possibility that any amount of soil organic matter could be excessive, I have already explained that the plant nutrients in compost and in animal manure are out of balance. Adding large quantities puts the soil similarly out of balance; this lessens plant health and lowers nutrient density. In the next chapter I will explain how some kinds of industrial composts worsen soil that contains more than a little clay. Still, vegie gardeners must bring in organic matter because food gardening accelerates the loss of soil organic matter. Interesting problem!

Here's a worry-ending rule: "Tasmanian gardens on heavy soil (more than 20 percent clay) need seven to eight percent organic matter as it is measured by a routine laboratory soil test. Gardens on sand and other light soils containing little or no clay need five to six percent. So when starting a brand new garden spread a layer of industrial compost 25 mm thick, mix that into the top 150 mm of soil. To maintain sufficient soil organic matter after that large initial dose, provide an annual addition of industrial compost 10 mm thick." You might like to know that 10 litres uniformly spread over one square meter makes a layer 10 mm thick.

But following Steve's Rule is not nearly as useful as understanding what's behind Steve's Numbers.

The amount of soil organic matter that should be in vegie garden soils varies according to climate. Hans Jenny explained this in *Factors in Soil Formation,** published in 1942. Jenny said, "Within regions of similar moisture conditions, for each drop of 10°C in annual average soil temperature the average organic matter content increases two or three times." I will unpack that.

Humid climates grow more biomass than semi-arid or arid climates do. All vegetation eventually decomposes back into the soil. The rate of organic matter decomposition in soil doubles with every 10°C increase in temperature. Cool moist climates produce nearly as much biomass per year as warm moist ones do, but rot it slower. Consequently a mild humid climate like Tasmania develops higher levels of soil organic matter than mainland soils east of the Great Dividing Range. As one goes further north on the wet side of the Range there is ever less soil organic matter naturally present. Where there is enough rainfall to dry farm west of the Great Dividing Range unirrigated soils have even less organic matter.

Hans Jenny was American. He points out that soil moisture levels are similar along the entire Mississippi River, however the average soil temperature decreases as you go further from the Equator. Jenny said he found two percent organic matter in sultry Arkansas, three percent in Missouri and over four percent in Wisconsin. Productive Tasmanian paddocks on heavy soil naturally develop five to six percent organic matter; Tasmanian paddocks on sand or other light soil have four to five percent.

There are other factors involved. Highly mineralized soils grow more biomass so they develop more soil organic matter compared to nearby soils with less mineralization. The soil's air supply strongly influences how rapidly organic matter rots away so sandy soils that naturally hold more air than heavier soils inevitably contain less organic matter. But the most powerful influences are moisture and temperature.

Without human intervention the amount of soil organic matter at any place stabilizes at its own ecological climax. A close approximation of climax-level soil organic matter is found in paddocks that aren't over-grazed and where any hay made from that land is fed back to livestock on the same land. One morning I was leaning on my hoe staring intently at nothing, and . . . . this insight appeared! *A thriving vegetable garden needs roughly the amount of soil organic matter you'd find in a highly productive paddock nearby or maybe just a little more than that.* Aligning this insight with Hans Jenny's data, a vegie garden needs two to three percent soil organic matter in a hot humid climate like northern coastal New South Wales. In a very hot desert I'd have to import enormous quantities of compost foolishly trying to lift soil organic matter above one percent.

The most important thing about the amount of soil organic matter in any soil is *how much of it decomposes every year.* For only by decomposing does organic matter release plant nutrients; only by being consumed does it support the microecology that so markedly contributes to plant nutrition; while consuming organic matter the soil ecology aggressively breaks down rock particles and releases the plant nutrients they contain. And builds soil structure.

Gardens on heavy Tasmanian soil must hold around seven percent organic matter in order to decompose enough of it each year to support excellent plant and soil health. Because a Tasmanian sand holds more air it will decompose enough SOM if it is at five percent. These levels are adequate for all Tasmanian soils except for heavy clays, which are a special case to be discussed later and at some length.

I like to think in numbers. To simplify the arithmetic, let's incorrectly assume that Tasmanian gardens should hold ten percent organic matter when seven percent actually is a gracious plenty. And let's overestimate again: suppose a Tasmanian vegie garden decomposes ten percent of that ten percent soil organic matter each year. So what does that mean in practical terms?

First imagine the *furrowslice*—the layer of topsoil 150 mm thick that a conventional plough turns over. The furrowslice is where almost all the soil's organic matter naturally resides. Varying somewhat by the type of soil and also on how much air it holds, an average furrowslice hectare weighs about two million kilograms (2,000 tons). Ten percent organic matter in 2,000 tons of soil amounts to 200 tons of once-living, partly decomposed material. This amount changes a hectare of dead dust into a potentially productive soil that only needs to have its mineral nutrients balanced.

Suppose as a consequence of one year's vegetable growing that an over-estimated ten percent of the garden's soil organic matter decomposes into plant nutrients and carbon dioxide gas; so the annual loss amounts to 20 tons—20,000 kilograms per hectare. One hectare equals 10,000 square metres. There being 1,000 x 10 square metre areas in one hectare, that loss amounts to 20 dry weight kilograms of organic matter lost from each 10 square metres of garden bed.

When I uniformly spread 50 wet kilograms of high quality compost (roughly 30 kg dry weight) over a 10 square metre bed the ground is barely covered. But for the purpose of *maintaining* soil organic matter in an ongoing vegetable garden that seemingly insignificant amount spread once a year will more than do. If I were starting a new garden and I wanted to quickly convert that soil into a thriving vegetable garden with abundant soil organic matter then I would cover the soil 25 mm to 50 mm thick with the best compost I could buy and mix it into the furrowslice. Only once.

Steve's Principle

When starting a new garden where lawn or pasture now grows, spread a 25 mm layer of municipal/industrial compost or partly-decomposed stable manure or feedlot manure that does not contain raw sawdust or distinguishable woodchips. ***Or else*** spread a 50 mm layer of compost-like industrial waste like poppy mark or mushroom compost. Dig that into the top 150 mm. Clay soils could use 75 mm of this the first time.

•

To maintain soil organic matter in an established productive Tasmanian garden, once a year spread a layer of humified (for a discussion of what "humified" means see Chapter 3) compost 5 mm thick or else spread industrial compost 10 mm thick. You'll get the most benefit when compost top-ups are not dug in, but raked into the surface inch where decomposition is the most rapid.

Green manuring/cover cropping

Fertile soil that is thickly canopied by actively growing vegetation is rapidly producing new organic matter. So green manure crops should be overwintered on as much of the garden as is conveniently possible. A green manure also dries out the topsoil sooner in spring and this topsoil gets thickly filled with quick-to-rot roots that make the soil crumble into a beaut seedbed. My favourite green manure is cereal rye, aka corn rye. The root system of cereal rye is so dense and decomposes so quickly that after mowing and removing the straw the entire furrowslice (and deeper) becomes a fine seedbed almost by itself. Cereal rye quickly dries out heavy soils. This is especially useful because heavy soils tend to form clods if worked when too wet, but as I just said, rye's root system is so fine and so dense that the soil forms a seed bed almost by itself. A green crop also prevents winter rains from compacting the beds. In spring and summer, fast growing green manures like buckwheat or rocket can be squeezed into short-term vacancies. (See Chapter 9/Legumes/Green Manures for full information.)

Dolomite lime worsens some soils

The organic farming and gardening followership worships compost and recommends spreading even more of it to solve most problems. Unfortunately for us Tasmanians the organic movement's founders did not know that too much magnesium makes clay tighten up, get sticky, relatively airless, prone to form clods and stick to your boots.

J.I. Rodale was the most influential American in the early days of the organic movement. Rodale was the wealthy owner of an electrical parts manufacturer. He transformed himself into a full-of-himself garden guru when he began publishing *Organic Farming and Gardening Magazine* in 1942; Rodale Press issued many books thereafter. Rodale, always the businessman, considered dolomite to be an extraordinary good value because it supplies both magnesium *and* calcium *and* raises soil pH 20 percent more than the same quantity of ordinary aglime—all those extras for the same price. So Rodale Press publications praised dolomite and the people who established the organic gardening tradition on Tasmania were educated directly or indirectly by Rodale. I think that's why aglime is not as easy to find in our garden centres as dolomite is, even though dolomite worsens many Tasmanian soils.

Digging in a large dose of compost immediately loosens a sticky loam or clay soil. By "large" I don't mean enough compost to slightly more than maintain the site's natural ecological peak soil organic matter level, but considerably more. However, repairing sticky soil by blending in large amounts of *industrial/municipal* compost usually means getting on an unnecessarily steep treadmill that resembles drug addiction because more than half the industrial compost available in Tasmanian *actually contains way too much magnesium.* My next chapter has much more to say about why this happens.

Magnesium added to a sand- or sandy loam topsoil quickly leaches into the subsoil. If the subsoil is clay or clayey then putting more magnesium into it makes it become even more airless—if that be possible. Aglime added to a topsoil with some clay in it gradually loosens the topsoil because calcium released from the lime slowly replaces excess magnesium, which then leaches into the subsoil. If you regularly repeat adding as much aglime as the soil can accept without going out of balance, some of that calcium may leach into the subsoil where it very slowly makes magnesium leach even deeper down. This extends the depth plant roots can penetrate. Moving magnesium deeper is a slow process; it can take decades when our only tool is aglime. When a clayey subsoil holds excess magnesium (and the greatest part of Tasmanian subsoils are like that) it'll be airless, dense, near-impossible to stick a spade into, inhospitable to root activity. In other words, high subsoil magnesium blocks crops from making roots there. If dolomite lime is added to the topsoil then the subsoil never improves; it may worsen.

Most vegetable species can make roots over one metre deep when the subsoil provides oxygen. If you wish to confirm that vegetables can do this please consult John Weaver's classic book *Root Development of Vegetable Crops.** Some drawings from Weaver's book are reproduced in Chapter 9 of this book. Bill Cotching was the DPIWE's main soil scientist for many years. His book *Soil Health For Farming In Tasmania* asserts that the maximum rooting depth of most crops in our state is about 600 mm (Bill's book a free download at www.billcotching.com).

A deeper root zone makes a huge difference in crop performance. The faster way to open a subsoil to root penetration is by adding both lime and many tons of gypsum per acre to the topsoil. But the cost of importing gypsum from South Australia is way beyond the farmer's budget. I suppose that is why farming in Tasmania is limited to the top 600 mm. However, gypsum is within a gardener's budget. No matter if the subsoil opens slowly after many many small doses of aglime and gypsum from COF or opens up as fast as possible by finding out by soil test how much lime could be fed to the topsoil without overloading it and approximately how much gypsum is needed, as roots penetrate deeper you'll notice the flavour of carrot, beetroot, parsnip, endive and escarole all improve; all these crops feed primarily in the subsoil.

One of the smartest things any gardener can do is to dig a deep hole and discover their subsoil. If it's sand then there's no harm in using dolomite, in fact, Tasmanian sands can be short magnesium. This is why the COF recipe for sand soils contains some dolomite. If it's Tasmanian clay subsoil I can safely assume it already contains plenty of magnesium. If it's tight, sticky airless clay I assume it holds way too much.

Do not use dolomite unless you're certain it is right for your soil; if your soil gets sticky, tight and dries into something hard, try once-off spreading three or four times the amount of gypsum I put into COF. And if that don't fix it study my book *The Intelligent Gardener.*

Mulching plus and minus

Gardeners, especially those on sandy soil, spread mulch to keep the surface moist in summer. Mulchers have been provided with many convincing reasons why they should make mulch permanent—and thick. Reasons such as not having to dig ever again. And no longer having to make compost. And henceforth be unconcerned about soil fertility because decomposing mulch does all that so have no worries!

Mulching does keep the surface damp which especially helps crops that feed close to the surface. Many Tasmanian topsoils are "hydrophobic," meaning they become reluctant to take up moisture after getting dry. Irrigation initially beads up on the dry surface of a hydrophobic soil and runs off, possibly eroding the bed. This especially dismays gardeners when they put down water rapidly with hose and nozzle. Mulch cures hydrophobia (but there is another way, see Chapter 5). When some clay soils dry down they become rock hard and shrink so much that deep cracks open. Mulching hides the cracks. Some weeds still emerge even through a thick mulch. But because of the mulch you can't use a hoe (fortunately most kinds of weeds emerging through mulch can more easily be pulled out). Soil that goes through winter covered with mulch will be much slower to warm up in spring; this greatly slows the growth of heat lovers until well into December.

Permanent mulching is an effective method to grow vegetables *in some climates.* In 1961 Ruth Stout introduced the entire English speaking world to permanent mulching with her best selling book *Gardening Without Work.* Ruth lived in Connecticut, USA, where summer months resemble eastern New South Wales; during summer mulch rots rapidly enough to act like fertilizer. Connecticut gets so cold during winter that invertebrate decomposers feeding on and sheltering in the mulch die off in the rock-hard frozen soil. This last thing is crucially important.

Followers of Ruth's no-digging method start a new garden by laying down thick flakes of straw or spoiled hay like overlapping shingles. These smother the existing vegetation. Any weed emerging through the mulch is telling us that the mulch is too thin at that spot so the gardener kills the weed by placing a straw flake on it. Under permanent mulch the surface inch becomes soft enough to dig with a teaspoon. To transplant seedlings, the mulch is pulled back exposing a bit of crumbly loose soil; as the seedling grows the mulch is pushed back around it. To plant seeds in rows, a narrow band of soil is exposed by raking back the mulch; a furrow is scratched in the soft, humusy earth. Mulch is pushed back against the seedlings after they've grown a few leaves. And that's it. No fertilizing, no manuring, no weeding, no making compost because all crop waste is spread over the mulch and becomes part of the mulch. And there's no watering either, at least not in Ruth's Connecticut garden where it normally rains enough in summer to support a mulched garden. If the soil starts out too infertile to grow much of anything then the gardener can one-time-only spread chicken manure or seedmeal under the initial layer of mulch. After that, rotting mulch maintains enough fertility to grow attractive looking food (but probably does not produce highly nutrient dense vegetables).

This method works throughout most of the northern United States and probably southern Canada as well. *It does not work in most of California nor in the Cascadia Bioregion.* I know this is so because I tried permanent mulching in Southern California (climate like Adelaide) and tried it again in western Oregon (climate like Tasmania). Both times I experienced the same catastrophe. Without a severe winter that freezes the soil rock hard for months, permanent mulch provokes a steady and unstoppable increase of slugs, snails, sow bugs (aka pill bugs, wood lice, slaters) and earwigs (pinchbugs). These primary decomposers are present in all gardens; at the population density normally found they rarely cause noticeable damage. But if you spread mulch where winter is mild, where the ground doesn't freeze, then these creatures encounter an unlimited food supply and excellent shelter. By the second summer of permanent mulching sowbug, earwig and gastropod populations reach plague levels. They then start eating everything tender, including lettuce seedlings, ripening tomatoes, etc. Another problem arises from how seedy most Tasmanian grass hay is. I think it is so seedy here because our rainy springs delay cutting hay until after seeds have formed. Other climates allow pasture grass to be cut and dried before it starts forming seeds. When Tasmanian grass hay becomes mulch a thick carpet of grass emerges.

It is easy and quick to cure the mess. Simply rake up all the mulch and make a compost heap with it located at least ten metres away from the garden. In a few days there'll be far fewer slugs and snails in the garden; slaters and earwigs will mainly be found in and immediately around the compost heap, which, in my opinion, is where they are useful. If you feel you must mulch, then spread *grain straw* in December *after* the topsoil has warmed up enough to allow heat lovers to make rapid growth. And make sure the straw does not contain seeds from the cereal crop that produced it. One indication that the soil has warmed up enough to be mulched is that pumpkin and cucumber vines will have started running. And when you do mulch, don't try to stop weeds with it, only spread enough to keep the surface damp—then you can slide a hoe under it. And when you are doing the autumn clean up, *rake up what's left of the mulch and put it into the compost heap that you should be building in this season.*

Eliminating sod

Converting grass into a vegie garden can be hard work. Permanent mulchers use an easy fix—kill the grass with a thick layer of mulch. That way doesn't always work. Grass finds it way up through mulch if the material used isn't dense enough. Some put a sheet of black plastic over the grass until everything dies. That does work. I've seen grass killed with overlapping layers of cardboard that stay in place once they've been sprayed with water.

I no longer eliminate sod with glyphosate, often called Roundup. I once thought glyphosate was safe enough for starting a new garden or to terminate a many-years-long rotation into grass and return the plot to vegies again. Like every sinner I had my justifications—I was spraying it but once in a blue moon; the garden still grew excellently after I did. And at the time there was falsified evidence asserting glyphosate's harmlessness. Actually, both glyphosate itself and its breakdown residues are toxic. They also lower the nutritional quality of food crops by preventing the uptake of trace elements.

Fusilade is much safer than glyphosate although it only kills grass. It is especially useful if twitch grass is present because it wipes out the underground runners. I've never seen this herbicide sold at garden centres; it can be found at farm supply shops. Unfortunately the smallest amount you can buy is enough to spray a farm field.

Here's an old fashioned method needing only hand tools. Methodically cut chunks of sod about 50 mm thick and 100 mm to 150 mm deep using a sharp spade. Neatly place them upside down and tightly against each other for a month such that most of the grass dies from lack of light. Then reinvert these chunks while digging slightly deeper. After a few such turns there will be a deeply dug friable garden bed. In order to achieve a fine seedbed by tomato-planting-out time it's easiest to have begun digging the previous April.

The digging/inversion method gets much more laborious when there is twitch grass. Fragments of twitch continue to resprout for a long time. Their runners have to be patiently located and then teased out of loose soil. Every root piece not found has the potential to grow new leaves and spread rapidly. It may take several slow careful diggings before almost all the twitch runners have been removed. Fortunately, twitch does not go deeper than 150 mm. I would spray with Fusilade two weeks before the first digging.

Where there are no stoloniferous grasses I prefer to break sod with a rotary cultivator. It should be a rear-end self-propelled design, not front-end—sometimes I did this with a hired tractor because my gardens were large. Tilling readily kills most broadleaf weeds and most kinds of grass but will not eliminate stoloniferous grasses.

With a walk behind tiller it is best to till and then cross till. First, using a lawn mower cut the vegetation close to the earth and chop it into short lengths so it won't tangle in the rotating tines. Better, rake it up for making compost, then till. Set the tiller's drag bar so that the tines only penetrate three centimetres below the surface. Give the sod a once over. It may *seem* nothing much happened. Then immediately go over the same ground again but this time do it at right angles to the first tilling. Do not change the drag bar setting. This time the tiller goes down a few more centimetres. (Make the first time north/south; the second time east/west.) A third time done at right angles to the second pass may have the tines reaching as far down as they'll go. Much of the vegetation will die. Another tilling or digging by hand done a month later eliminates most of the rest of it.

Compaction

Your *topsoil* may be compacted. Livestock could have compressed it. Other causes of topsoil compaction include the heavy machinery that prepared your building block. Rotarycultivating or spading 150 mm deep *one time* repairs topsoil compaction. Food gardens are sometimes grown on land that had been repeatedly plowed. The weight of the plough's bottom compressed the soil just below it into something permanently hard—a "plowpan." I had one on my property at Elkton, Oregon. It was about three cm thick starting about 150 mm down.

The easiest way I know of to check for a plowpan is to bore a hole with a hand-powered fence post augur because its speed of penetration slows greatly when there is soil compaction. If, when you get down to about 150 mm the going becomes slow and then when you penetrate a few more centimetres the soil gets much softer, there is a plowpan.

Farmers shatter plowpans with a subsoiling "shoe" that rips through the soil about 30 cm below the surface, lifting the earth a few centimetres, fracturing the plowpan. The gardener accomplishes the same thing with a sharp spade that can be worked full-length into the soil, and then levered back. You might not be able to loosen slices more than 50 millimetres thick without breaking the spade's handle but the task is not extremely hard work when you take small bites. The whole job goes a lot easier if you rotarycultivate first.

This task has to be done only once. You should not invert the soil when breaking a plowpan, because most of the soil's organic matter will naturally be in the furrowslice and that's where you want to keep it.

Clay

Rocks become soil when running water, wind, freezing, thawing and naturally occurring weak acids cause them to fragment (weather) into little pieces. Soil particles are classified by their size.

Stones don't support food crops. A few stones don't matter. Having a great many stones interferes with digging and hoeing.

Sand particles are large enough to feel gritty when rubbed between the fingers. When viewed through a 10x magnifying glass they have sharp corners and flat surfaces because they recently (on a geologic time scale) broke off of a larger rock. Sand-sized particles are slowly dissolved by weak acids in the soil.

When sand particles have weathered down small enough we call them *silt.* Pure silt rubbed between the fingers feels smooth, like baby powder. Viewed through a microscope, silt particles are rounded and smooth, their sharp edges have been dissolved away. Eventually, silt particles entirely dissolve.

The elements dissolved out of sand and silt go through complex chemical recombinations in the soil and become *clay.* Clay is made of thin flat crystals that stack themselves in layers like pages in a book. Clay crystals are so small it takes the most powerful electron microscope to capture an image yet it is easy to intuit the nature of clay in soil because slate and shale are kinds of rock formed by subjecting clay to heat and pressure. These layered rocks fracture into thin sheets much like the clay crystals they started out as.

Clay crystals stack tightly like a deck of cards, so clay soils usually are dense and airless. Clay occupies gaps between silt and sand particles, filling up spaces that could hold air. Topsoils containing clay would be relatively airless except that microorganisms and worms combine clay and sand and silt and humus into irregularly shaped crumbs that don't pack tightly.

Clayey soils hold much more water than does a soil composed primarily of sand and/or silt. Sand and silt particles may be compared to books firmly closed with water adhering to their covers, spines and sides. Clay is like that book with all the pages slightly separated. If sand's ability to hold water were expressed numerically as one, silt would be around two, clay four to six and, pure humus six to eight. So clay soils sustain plants better between rains or irrigations but in spring they are slow to dry down and, because they hold so much water, they are slower to warm up, which makes spring crops grow slower and heat lovers mature later. In Chapter 9, page 145, I discuss in detail how the amount of water in soil influences its temperature in spring.

Some clay soils drain well and naturally develop an open structure; these can grow useful vegetables but only if they are managed skillfully. Clayey soil must be dug/rotarycultivated at the right moisture content. If clay is worked when it is too moist in spring it forms rock-hard clods that may not disintegrate until they have gone through another winter. Clods act like stones that do not allow root penetration or let seeds germinate. Conversely, clay becomes dust if it is rotary cultivated when it is dry. (No one *could* dig it with a spade when dry; maybe it's possible with a pickaxe.) That dust sags into a thick gooey soup the first time it gets wet and then becomes rock-hard and airless when it dries. After irrigation or rain the surface of a recently loosened up clayey soil often gets sealed over by a hard crust that prevents the emergence of sprouting seeds. A crust also lowers the amount of oxygen below.

Clayey soils can make excellent paddocks because sod keeps the surface open; the sod's root system creates permanent structure that increases soil air; and grasses don't mind having their roots waterlogged for a few days during periods of heavy rain. Free draining clays can grow excellent orchards.

My ideal vegetable soil would contain 20 to 25 percent clay and the rest would be approximately equal amounts of sand and silt—with eight percent organic matter in Tasmanian conditions. Soil like that would be digable when wet, would hardly form a clod no matter what you did, would hold quite a bit of moisture and wouldn't lose so many nutrients every winter because the fertility you put in would cling to the clay.

If you must grow vegies in clay, best apply some wisdom and be prepared to spend some money. The first step is to make sure it really is a clay soil.

Testing for clay content

A clay soil by definition contains more than 40 percent clay. It is possible to knowledgeably roll a handful of moist soil into a noodle and thereby assay what sort of particles it is composed of. Bill Cotching's online book *Soil Health For Farming In Tasmania* excellently describes how to. Gardeners, lacking experience, show me samples of their "clay subsoil" only to have me tell them it actually is sand cemented into hard reddish brown chunks by iron compounds that were leached from the sand topsoil. People living on the Chudleigh Valley floor think they have a clay soil. Actually, "Chudleigh Mud" is 50% fine sand and 50% silt—zero clay. The silt particles sift into gaps between sand grains, making it heavy, dense, airless—like clay. When Chudleigh Mud gets quite wet the water lubricates the silt particles in it, then the sand particles slide easily against each other and the material feels like oily clay if you kneed a lump in your hand. But the lump dries out quickly and easily is made to crumble to powder in the hand after it has dried.

There is a simple scientific test you can do with a glass jar that accurately reveals the percentage of sand to silt to clay in a soil sample. Please don't be off-putted by the formal name for this procedure—"soil fractional analysis." Dry 500 ml of soil (no pebbles, no roots, no obvious organic material) and crush it to powder. Don't dry it to zero moisture, just make it dry enough that you can break it up to particles no larger than sand grains. Then put the soil into a one-litre glass jar with a tight fitting lid. If you don't have a grease pencil or waterproof marking pen that will write on glass, then you can make marks on a vertical strip of adhesive tape affixed to the outside of the jar. Mostly fill the jar with water leaving 2 cm of air space at the top and then add *a few* drops of low-sudsing liquid dishwashing detergent to soften the water. *Do not use so much detergent that shaking makes suds.* If bubbles form you'll have to start over. Now tighten the lid well and begin shaking; shake hard, shake vigorously. And keep on a'shakin'. And then shake some more. You want to make sure every soil particle has been separated from every other soil particle, that every soil crumb has been disintegrated. (The detergent helps this happen; suds from too much detergent would stop this from happening.) Shake *very hard* for up to ten minutes; to break up the crumbs in a clayey soil can take a lot of force. Then put the jar in bright light where it won't have to be disturbed.

Exactly two minutes after you stopped shaking make a mark on the side of the jar at the point the soil has settled out so far. To see where this is you may need a powerful torch to peer into the murk. That mark shows the amount of sand particles. Being large, they settle out of suspension the most rapidly. Then wait exactly two hours and make another mark at the depth to which more soil has deposited. That mark shows the amount of fine silt particles resting atop the sand.

If the soil is all sand then the water will be almost completely clear in two minutes. If the soil is a mixture of sand and silt, or all silt, it'll all settle within two hours. But if there is much clay, depending on how fine the clay is, you may have to wait until the next day, sometimes wait two weeks to get the final result.

When the water has finally cleared, draw another line. That layer holds the clay. On the very top you might find a thin layer of jelly-like organic matter. Now measure the thickness of each layer. A bit of arithmetic will convert these thicknesses to percentages of sand, silt and clay. If the water won't ever seem to clear the soil is almost certainly all clay of the most minute type.

If the soil is more than 40% clay and drains well it'll be a difficult garden but doable. If the soil is all- or mostly all clay that drains well after days of heavy winter rains and you *must* grow vegetables in it—not grass or fruit trees or perennial ornamentals—then you have big obstacles to overcome and I recommend "the better way.". If it is a very fine clay that takes days to settle out of suspension you have my sympathies.

The poor solution

Encouraged by a great many trendy gardening books and magazines, you are going to turn your claypit into a Garden of Eatin' by incorporating heaps of organic matter, thereby converting it into synthetic loam—at least the top layer will seem loamy for awhile.

Start by spreading aglime. Acidic clay soils will ravenously grab most of the plant nutrients you put in and will not release much fertility until its hunger has been satisfied by feeding it large quantities of calcium, which is inexpensively obtained from agricultural lime. If the shake test shows that the soil is about one-half clay and the soil hasn't been limed in the last five years, then spread and dig in 50 kilograms of agricultural lime over each 100 square metres. If the soil contains two-thirds clay make that 75 kilograms per 100 square metres. If it is all clay, spread 100 kilograms. *Do not spread more lime than that unless you or a soil analyst knows from a complete soil test that even more calcium is needed!* Do that liming with ordinary agricultural lime. *Do not use dolomite lime unless you discover a significant magnesium deficiency by laboratory soil testing,* which would be highly unlikely in Tasmania.

When lack of calcium calls for much more aglime than there is in COF it must be thoroughly mixed into the furrowslice. The best time to accomplish that is autumn, giving the soil an entire winter to adjust. From this point onward the aglime and gypsum in COF will maintain and build upon the improvement and it won't matter if COF is dug in or not.

Tillage: Make sure a clay soil is close to the right moisture for tillage. Don't rush it but don't miss it either. The window of opportunity for working clay is brief. There's a quick "ready-to-till" test. Holding a small handful of loose soil, make a fist; squeeze the soil into a tight ball. If it won't hold a ball shape after releasing your hand then it is too dry to till. If it makes a ball but that ball won't crumble easily then it is too moist to till and will form clods if you till it anyway. If it makes a ball but that ball crumbles with moderate pressure from your thumb, then it is at the right moisture content to work.

Organic matter: When the moisture content is correct to till then spread aglime and a 25 mm thick layer of industrial compost. Till them in immediately because if it rains before you get around to it then the compost left on the surface acts like a mulch that prevents the soil from drying down again. Semi-decomposed horse/cow/sheep manure 25 mm thick (not chicken) or else mushroom compost spread 50 mm thick can also serve. Then dig it all in. I'd rent a large walk behind or tractor-pulled rotary cultivator. If this happens in autumn you can also establish a green manure.

In a clay garden's first year it'll probably help a lot to side-dress low-demand crops as though they were high-demand crops, partly because it takes a year or two before clay soaks up enough calcium from lime and other plant nutrients to release plant nutrients easily, and partly because all that organic matter you tilled in may trigger a gigantic microbial bloom that by itself ties up plant nutrients for a few months. That's another reason it is best to start a new clay garden the previous autumn.

Once you've established the garden there's still going to be more ongoing work than with a lighter soil. The organic matter you've put in will seem to disappear rapidly. Clay vegie gardens seem to need a great deal of compost, at least for the first few years.

Clay gardens are especially good candidates for slightly raised beds because tillage gets easier by not stepping on the growing areas. In fact, by using raised beds, by almost always overwintering green manures on any area not carrying a food crop, by alternating food crops with green manures and by mixing compost and COF into the surface with a hoe when preparing seedbeds, you may never need to deeply dig that stiff soil again. Handled this way, clay can grow most kinds of vegetables.

The better way

Rain water percolating through the topsoil in temperate climate regions transports newly formed clay particles downward, and deposits them in a distinctly different layer we call subsoil. The technical name for this is a "duplex" soil. Tasmanian red krasnozems uniquely do not do this; instead they gradually get more clayey as you dig deeper. Given geologic time eventually all the sand and silt in topsoil becomes clay or else erosion carries it away. Eventually there is only clay from the surface down to bedrock. If you encounter clay at the surface, why not consider it to be the subsoil that long ago lost its topsoil. So bring in enough topsoil to make a generous layer atop the clay. Generous—at least one spade's blade deep. Make it 400 millimetres deep if you've got deep pockets.

Buying topsoil is risky because what is called topsoil at landscape yards may actually be an artificial growing medium manufactured from coarse sand and compost. Before buying some I suggest doing a quick soil fractional analysis at the landscape yard. Arrive prepared with a tight-lidded jar holding a few drops of dishwashing detergent, add the "soil" they want to sell to you and water. After a 30 second shake and only a 30 second wait, if it is a synthetic growing medium you'll see coarse sand on the bottom and compost floating in the water. People often fill raised beds with this stuff. During the following two years most of the organic matter in it decomposes, the growing medium shrinks until mostly sand remains. If you think to blend this stuff into an existing clay soil, keep in mind that after the organic matter has decomposed, an equal mixture of clay and sand often forms something like concrete when it is dry.

I just stated that my ideal vegetable soil would be 20 percent clay. You already have the clay. If you were to cover that clay with a layer of genuine topsoil 300 mm deep and if that topsoil were less than 20% clay, then when digging deep you'll inevitably mix in a bit more clay, to your benefit. Worm activity also does that. It might take a few years but soon the imported sandy loam will contain enough clay that it won't dry out so rapidly.

Genuine loam topsoil costs less than compost—if you can find it for sale—and loam works out to be a far better value because ongoing you won't need nearly as much compost than had you tried to improve your clay pit with compost. The vegetables will be more nutritious from a loam topsoil and I guarantee they'll grow a lot bigger. And don't forget the definition of the word "loam" means at least ten percent clay.

What if the "loam" topsoil being offered is actually an impoverished hydrophobic sand topsoil. You have a way to check; do a soil fractional analysis before buying it.

The best way

A laboratory soil test reveals the amount of calcium and magnesium already present and how much more aglime that clay needs. The test also reveals what other nutrients are lacking and how much of them will be needed in order to remineralize and bring the top 150 mm of it into good balance. You spread and dig all that in 150 mm deep and most often the clay loosens up—flocculates is the technical term for this. Flocculated clay may grow decent vegetables but clay never grow stuff like loam. You'll always have to take some care not to dig it when it is too wet. It'll always be slower to warm up in spring; the vegetables will be smaller than they might have been on a loam soil.

Most gardeners never experience clay flocculation because they do not add enough of the right sort of lime to make it happen. Smart advice about liming says to never exceed four tons per acre (100 kilograms per 100 square metres) *in a single application* because when aglime is mixed into acidic soil it triggers a great deal of chemical activity that can hugely distort the soil ecology and temporarily reduces the availability of plant nutrients. That is why it is far better to work large doses of aglime into clay in autumn so the soil chemistry will stablilize by next spring. Some acidic clays have an *enormous* capacity to hold more calcium. I tested one on a property overlooking the Tamar; it had a lime requirement of 15 tons per hectare, and 15 tons provides only enough calcium for the top 150 mm of soil. If that gardener could have dug lime in deeper than 150 mm I'd have prescribed proportionately more.

Before importing loam and using "the better way" I suggest first reading my book *The Intelligent Gardener,* doing a proper lab test on the clay, spreading aglime according to the test result (and any other elements the test indicates as being needed) and rotarycultivating it in thoroughly. Then even if the clay doesn't behave quite like vegetable-growing topsoil a year later it still will serve as a much better subsoil when you put a foot of genuine loam on top of it.

Chapter 3

Compost

Increasing the amount of soil organic matter . . . is of great importance.
The addition of clay to sandy soil may be as important as the addition of organic matter itself.
A certain quantity of stable manure or compost or mass of plant residues can be converted into this type of complex [humus] *only when it is composted with a certain amount of clay before it is applied to the soil.*

Selman Waksman. ***Soil Microbiology.*** 1952.

In the early 1990s I wrote a practical potboiler called *Organic Gardener's Composting.* * After it went out of print I put the book online for free download. The State Library of Tasmania has many similar books; all of them convey about the same story, all provide diagrams for multi-bin systems and give step-by-step recipes for building layered heaps. They have tables listing the carbon-to-nitrogen ratio of compostable materials and the average nitrogen content of common manures. Expect a composting book to introduce you to enclosures, worms, tumblers, and the usual side-paths. If you've haven't yet read a basic compost making book be warned that I am not going to explain all that again in this chapter. Instead I'll assume you already are acquainted with the conventional wisdom so I'll only make overall comments and general suggestions.

Making Great Compost

Garden books usually give the impression that compost can be made in a variety of ways but the end result of all these approaches will be effective. In my experience this belief is incorrect. I will soon share some of my experience. Most such books suggest that compost brings with it all the plant nutrients a food garden needs. This could be true in a few rare districts; generally this belief is not correct. I explained why this is so in the previous chapter.

Garden composting manuals do not address the crucial question of how much soil organic matter is needed in each particular climatic area as I did in the previous chapter. Instead, gardeners are advised that more is always better. If the garden doesn't grow well enough—put more organic matter on it. Uncharitable soil analysts that balance soil nutrients call people who think this way "more-on-its." I call them "misinformed."

The worship of compost is at the core of the organic farming and gardening movement. First and foremost the organic movement is about health. The history goes back to the mid-1830s when a new method of transport called the railroad made fresh vegetables and fruits available in every English market town and affordable to all but the very poor. Naturally the British people become much healthier. But after World War I their collective health declined. Noticeably. Obviously. Degenerative diseases that once were very rare became commonplace. There were similar increases in livestock diseases and food crop diseases.

In the mid-1930s an earnest conversation started in England about reversing that health decline. It was clear to the perceptive that the cause was the use of chemical fertilizers that had become readily available and were inexpensive when World War I ended. Reducing the use of chemical fertilizers, returning to the use of animal manures as fertilizer, returning to green manuring and long rotations out of food crops and into grazing instead of using chemicals to grow cash crop after cash crop; using a new composting method developed in the late 1920s by Sir Albert Howard that made powerful compost from farmyard manure, living soil and crop wastes—all these remedies were proposed. I invite you to read the books, magazine articles and assorted documents from the key people creating that social movement in the Soil and Health Library.

I mentioned J. I. Rodale before. He was a businessman with a personal interest in healthy living. He knew nothing of farming and gardening before he got involved with this English social health movement. His awakening happened during the Blitz of 1940 when Rodale was in London to sell stuff to the British, just like a lot of other Americans were doing at the time. There he met Sir Albert Howard, the founder of the British organic farming and gardening movement. They became friends.

Howard inspired Rodale; he enthusiastically promoted the organic movement in the United States. Rodale purchased a hobby farm with very good soil located just outside Philadelphia, Pennsylvania. Now his daughter could keep a horse and he could become a gardener. Sir Albert taught Rodale that adding plenty of compost would loosen his garden soil and magnificently feed his vegetables. He soon experienced the truth of those assertions.

In 1942 the first issue of Rodale's *Organic Farming and Gardening Magazine* came out. You can read the first eight years of that magazine and a handful of Rodale's books on Soil and Health Library's website. I put them there so that you can assess Rodale's character for yourself. I see Rodale as a passionate forceful advocate of simple easy-to-grasp doctrines, just the sort of person to start a mass movement—which he did with great success.

I subscribed to his magazine in 1973. At that time it had a circulation of over one million. I soon became a worshipper at the shrine of organic. I had recently started a small graphic arts business that was growing rapidly; we had saved some money. Inspired by the idea of food gardening and the health it brought we made the down payment on an old cottage on a one acre block in the far fringe of LA. There I made huge compost heaps because Rodale's magazine of the 1970s repeatedly pointed out that my neighbourhood was full of organic treasures going to waste, we should convert these free materials into black gold that would grow nutritious food. Free and cheap rarely inspire me but healthy always does, so I bought a ute. This being prior to the era of wheelie bins, I started prowling the neighbourhood on trash pick-up day, bringing home bags of grass clippings and leaves from deciduous trees. I mixed trash-day collections with sawdusty horse manure from a local stable and my own garden wastes, weeds, grass clippings and the droppings from under a few meat rabbit cages and tried to keep everything moist. My heaps sort of decomposed. By the second turn the stuff had turned brownish and it grew vegetables acceptably well in southern California because the soil there is quite warm most of the year. I now know that my compost seemed to work because I also put enough nitrogen-rich cottonseedmeal into the beds to compensate for the undigested sawdust. Had I not done that my vegies would have been stunted.

I homesteaded in Oregon a few years later. I still believed that growing healthy vegetables required incorporating large amounts of compost. I took full advantage of a large stable nearby that gave away limitless compostable material free for the hauling. It was slightly damp Douglas Fir ("Oregon") sawdust with about 20 percent by volume horse poops; it smelled vaguely of ammonia because it had soaked up urine. I watered heavily as I heaped it up but the pile didn't get even slightly warm. After a few years the material had shrunk a bit and turned a brownish colour. The horse poops had vanished. It was loose and crumbly. So I declared it to be compost and stupidly dug it into my garden. It grew vegetables only because I tilled in lots of nitrogen-rich cottonseedmeal.

During those early Oregon years I also made compost from garden and kitchen wastes. That heap eventually did become very average compost but most of the original starting volume had vanished. My main mistake at that time was failing to put enough soil into the heap as it was being built. I had read that the bits of soil inevitably clinging to the roots of weeds provided all the microbial inoculation a heap needed and that the reason for including soil was to inoculate the heap. That idea made sense to me because at the time I made my own beer and had seen one tiny crumb of yeast become 20 wildly foaming litres of wort overnight. But this opinion is only partly correct as I will soon explain.

Ten years later we bought a house and 16 acres of Malabon Silty Clay Loam, a productive CLASS I alluvial soil. I did not make, buy or use compost when I was gardening on that property. I imported no manure. The method I used then involved the use of COF and a many years long rotation into grass that is discussed in Chapter 4, "Planning."

In short, I made poor compost, or none, from 1974 until 2007. Only in recent years have I made it excellently. Am I a slow learner? Well, maybe. In any case, it took me 33 years to grasp that *making highly effective compost requires including a significant quantity of garden soil when building the heap; to make the best compost that garden soil (or you) must provide some clay.* These days I could make excellent compost with almost any type of garden soil because I could buy a sack of bentonite clay from a farm supply shop to include in compost heaps if the soil had little or none. So can you.

Heap size

Compost forms when soil-dwelling microbes, fungi, microanimals and worms rapidly consume a heap of crude organic matter. Their activity can generate quite a bit of heat; self-generated heat causes them to work even more rapidly. There's a scientific principle about this: the speed of biological chemical reactions doubles and redoubles with each 10°C increase until temperature goes so high it harms the biology.

A large heap provides so much insulation that the core temperature may exceed what most microbes and fungi can tolerate. When excessive temperature ends decomposition it almost always has also dried out the heap. Biological activity does not resume at a high level until the material is moist again.

A small heap doesn't heat up enough or for long enough. A cold heap takes a long, long time to finish. It's basic arithmetic: heat radiates from surfaces whilst the surface area of a cube, rectangle or sphere increases less rapidly than its volume increases. Everyone intuitively understands that a heap of steaming hot mashed potatoes cools off faster when it is spread out on the plate. Same with composting. A heap with a starting volume under three cubic metres won't get hot enough, or if it does get properly warm then the amount of time it stays hot will be too brief.

The composting ecology breathes oxygen, burns carbon and you could say the heap itself exhales carbon dioxide. Insufficient air exchange would reduce the microbial population but serendipitously, internal heating makes the carbon dioxide rich air within the heap rise and exit the top, thereby pulling in fresh, oxygen-rich air. If the heap is too large there won't be enough air exchange in its core and then microorganisms that thrive without oxygen take over. Anaerobic compost is not desirable; I have a hard time even calling the gooey black stuff that comes of anaerobic conditions "compost."

The smallest effective home-garden heap is a circular mound about 1,800 mm across at the base and 1,500 mm high (when you first build it). You can extend that steep-sided hill into a long windrow. Make it narrower, and the heap may not heat up enough and definitely will cool off too soon; make it more than 2,100 wide at the base or over 1,800 mm high and the core may not breathe well enough.

So how large a food garden does it take to build a minimum sized heap from only garden waste? And how often will that much garden make enough crop waste to build another heap? I can best answer those questions by sharing my own experience. My previous house was on a quarter acre building block less than half covered by structures; almost all the rest was sunny and grew ornamentals, fruit trees and housed eight chooks. Our vegie garden completely occupied an adjoining quarter-acre block. Vegetable crop waste from the quarter acre food garden plus the non-woody trim, weeds and deadheading from the house block made two compost heaps each year. There was a substantial autumn garden-clean-up heap of about six cubic metres starting volume and a spring clean-up heap that was barely large enough to reach minimum starting size. During the last few years we've gardened at Chudleigh; here our 150 square metres of actual food growing beds plus litter from a chookhouse plus the trim from Annie's flower beds generated one heap once a year that is slightly more than minimum-size.

Already heating compost heaps that have new material piled on top as it becomes available do not make great compost. Far better that all crop waste is first dried as it is collected. A heap is assembled all at once when enough of this "hay" has accumulated.

If the property is too small to generate three cubic metres of dried crop- and ornamental wastes at least once each year, then why not consider composting as a convenient way to recycle, not as a way to manufacture the best possible soil amendment. There are compost tumblers that quickly convert small amounts of crop and kitchen waste into something similar to industrial compost. And you could use worm (vermi)composting which actually does result in pretty good stuff. You also could import grain straw or other materials to include when building your own compost heaps.

Bins/containers

Because I just mentioned compost tumblers, I expect some readers may be wondering: 'if I do not have enough material to make compost in a heap could I make a smaller quantity in a bin that retains heat?'

In my experience composting enclosures at their very best, all things considered, do not make a better product than heap composting does. Bins and composting containers do make a backyard look tidy but they also make turning heaps more difficult and, in my opinion, are an unnecessary expense unless you make them of recycle or make bins out of square straw bales that eventually become part of a compost heap.

Enclosures restrict air flow into the heap. In order to overcome this, gardeners put flexible slotted field drain pipes or plastic gutter down pipes with holes drilled into them under the heap before it is built. Or else build the heap on top of a slightly elevated screen or grid that lets air enter freely from the bottom. Or else turn the heap every few weeks. How-to-make-compost books are full of ideas like these.

But I don't see the sense in first creating the problem of insufficient air due to solid side walls and then cleverly solving it when the problem never had to exist in the first place.

You do not have to allocate a lot of space for heap composting. My previous composting yard measured 4 metres by 7 metres; that was enough space to process all the non-woody wastes generated by three-eights of an acre of food crops and ornamentals. There was room for two working heaps and twice a year there was one smaller heap of finished compost waiting to be used. There also was an ever expanding stack of dried garden wastes for building the next heap.

My working heaps are covered—top and sloping sides—with loose *grain* straw that is at least 300 mm thick or with tight flakes about 100 mm thick laid like patio pavers over the heap at the start. When composting in bins it's wise to thickly cover their tops with straw. Straw's properties are truly amazing! Straw insulates the heap and yet it allows plenty of air to flow through. A thick straw blanket retains internal moisture while also shedding rain, thus reducing leaching. Raking straw off the heap is a quick and easy task. I do this immediately before turning or using the heap. During the months that new straw insulates a heap it loses rigidity, stops being such a good insulator and is ready to become an ingredient in the next heap. I use about six bales of wheat straw to cover every heap.

I think a straw covered mound looks pretty.

Starting carbon to nitrogen ratio

Compostable organic matter is mostly made of plant fiber (structural material) and protein. Fibers are carbohydrates composed of carbon and water. Proteins are mostly carbon combined with nitrogen. The total amount of carbon in any kind of organic matter reckoned against the amount of nitrogen in it is called its carbon-to-nitrogen ratio or C:N. This ratio varies according to the material. The entire heap has an average C:N, which sums up the various materials in it. When I first read about how to make compost people were expected to remember the carbon-to-nitrogen ratios of many common compost feedstocks and therefrom, to guestimate the starting carbon-to-nitrogen ratio of the entire heap. In recent times garden writers distinguish high C:N materials from low C:N materials not by a numerical ratio but as being either "brown" or "green." Brown materials provide much carbon and little nitrogen. Green stuff has a good deal of nitrogen in it. This degraded understanding leads to errors, like this one: grass clippings at summer's end are green in colour but they are as low in nitrogen as cereal grain straw. They are "brown." On the other hand fresh green spring grass clippings that dry on the lawn for a day or two before being gathered up turn brown but this does not significantly reduce their high nitrogen content. They still are "green."

However we classify the raw materials, composting goes best when woody barky stuff is not part of the starting volume. Everything goes great when the heap is made from sun dried vegetable crop waste, grass clippings, leaves from non-native deciduous trees and *non-woody* waste from ornamentals. I urge you to include nothing that has developed bark! Leafy *young* green tips trimmed in spring from hedge plants may decompose readily as long as their stems have not yet formed bark. Reject sawdust, most kinds of tree bark, conifer needles, any sticks or twigs. Absolutely reject paper. In earlier times the glues in kraft paper cardboard were animal based and contributed enough nitrogen to allow it to decompose readily. Old organic gardening books recommend including cardboard. These days I suggest caution.

If you have woody material to dispose of and want to try composting it then I suggest grinding/chipping it first, put it in its own heap, include twice the usual quantity of soil (ten percent by starting volume) and double the usual amount of COF. Do not try this with chook poo pellets alone. Use the full COF recipe because woody wastes lack most plant nutrients but the microbes that consume the material must build their bodies of the same elements plants use to grow with. Expect a woody heap to take three or four turns (and remoistenings) and at least a year to finish (maybe two years) and do not plan to use that compost on vegetable crops. Use it to mulch plants with a low nitrogen requirement—ornamentals, fruit trees and bush fruit like currants or blueberries.

I emphasize: *making powerful compost requires having all the plant nutrients in the starting materials.* So I suggest fully remineralizing the lawn and its surrounds where there are no Australian natives. If you're a homesteader with deep pockets, then fully remineralize any land making organic matter (or manure) that you transfer to the food-garden by way of the compost heap. However, ornamentals and fruit trees that are provoked by as much nitrogen as a food garden gets respond by making rampant growth. Fruit trees will make less fruit and more wood. To remineralize orchards, small fruit, ornamentals and lawns I suggest using a variant of COF containing all the ingredients except that the quantity of seedmeal going into this special mix should be reduced by half. This special COF should be spread only once a year in early spring.

If you don't collect enough raw material from your own property to build at least one heap of sufficient starting volume then you can import material. Top of my list for this purpose is cereal grain straw. Barely on my list is straw from a grass seed crop. Absolutely do not use grass hay, especially if it is rain-spoiled hay that costs next to nothing. Grain straw decomposes nicely in a compost heap because it doesn't compact into a slimy airless mess. Grass hay and straw from grass seed crops compact severely. Put much of this in a heap and it'll become airless and require turning. Grass seed straw may or may not be entirely seedless (beware) but spoiled hay always brings heaps of viable seeds that you'll soon discover don't necessarily die from the heat of composting. Excellent compost can be made from a blend of four parts by volume cereal grain straw, one part fresh spring grass clippings, plus soil, COF and moisture. Lucerne chaff is equivalent to dried spring grass clippings or the best horse/cow/sheep manure. So is pea straw.

Corn and sunflower stalks, broccoli, kale and brussels sprout stalks should be cut into 300 mm pieces before drying them. Doing this makes turning the heap much easier.

Fallen leaves from deciduous (Northern Hemisphere) trees tend to pack tightly. When leaves form their own layer it blocks airflow in the heap so tree leaves should be dispersed throughout the heap. Running a lawnmower with a bagger over dry tree leaves greatly shrinks their volume and reduces their tendency to pack tight when wet. Eucalypt leaves and pine needles resist decomposition; these are best kept out of the heap.

Drying fresh plant waste by spreading it over already dried plant wastes causes different kinds of vegetation to end up in layers. So when you build a compost heap from one of these haystacks it is best to take material from an end or side, not from the top. Thus every part of the heap you're building gets roughly the same mix of vegetation. I learned this technique from Sir Albert Howard's finest book *The Waste Products of Agriculture.** Sir Albert took the art of composting to the highest level at Indore Research Station in India. I urge a thorough consideration of Howard's book to anyone that wants to make excellent compost.

Manure

Mixing animal manures into compost heaps lowers the overall starting carbon to nitrogen ratio. Fresh ruminant manures also contain digestive enzymes that accelerate heating up. Up to one-third of a heap's starting volume could be horse/cow/sheep/rabbit poo and another third might be the urine-soaked *straw* bedding it comes with. If the bedding was sawdust I'd probably reject the material unless it had been under chickens. However, composting nearly pure poo without bedding is not so straightforward because there is way too much nitrogen. Such a heap gets too hot. I soon have more to say about that.

Few gardeners these days know much about livestock, much less about their manures or about the fertilizing value of other crop wastes or industrially-manufactured composts. I hope the next batch of cautions and pointers assists you.

Horse manure

Before the automobile most horses were fed high protein hay and some wheat or oats so that they could work harder. Horse manure was strong stuff in those days; it was the most commonly used garden fertilizer. There were two types: "long" and "short."

Short manure is nearly pure poo. It was raked out of stalls without the bedding. It was swept up from city streets. In residential neighbourhoods any poo dropped by a passing horse was soon put into someone's rose bed. Expertly composted short manure sustained Nineteenth Century market gardens. Growers would deliver vegetables to the central produce market and return home with a wagonload of street sweepings.

When poo from well-nourished horses is composted with several times more soil than a vegetable crop waste heap needs, the result acts powerfully. It may still be possible to source potent short horse manure from a stud farm but the stuff produced by lifestyle horses grazing exhausted paddocks and sold by the roadside in recycled feed sacks is an empty imitation.

Long manure includes urine-soaked stall bedding. Urine contains about half the nutrients exiting the animal so soggy smelly bedding has great value. Long horse manure must first be heap composted or else sheet composted—which means spread over the field in autumn and immediately plowed or disced in so it will have decomposed by spring sowing time. Sheet composting was commonly done by farmers before the widespread use of chemical fertilizers but is no longer allowed in certified organics.

Tasmanian horses these days are bedded on sawdust. Raw sawdust takes a few years to decompose enough in soil to allow vegetables to grow well when not too much of it is mixed in. Otherwise, it takes even longer. I have already mentioned that the effect can be partly reversed by using large amounts of nitrogen fertilizer, seedmeal or pelletized composted chook poo.

In Tasmania's cool soils, expertly composted strawy horse manure by itself can supply enough nitrogen to grow low-demand crops such as turnip, swede, kale, broad bean, carrot and beetroot to an acceptable standard. If sawdust predominates, even if well composted, the result will not be this good.

Cow manure

Fresh cow manure is not quite as high in nitrogen as horse manure. If it has been well composted then the material grows low-demand crops fairly well. If much undecomposed sawdust or straw is present then the end product may act like the reverse of fertilizer.

Sheep manure

Sheep manure sold in sacks is short manure from shearing sheds. Usually sheep are shorn early in spring before the grass becomes nitrogen-rich so shearing shed manure may not be hugely potent. I would mix bagged sheep poo into a compost heap whilst it is being built. It is "green," but not powerfully so.

Rabbit manure

Bedding under rabbit cages adsorbs urine. I once fed meat rabbits on pelletized feed. I abandoned pellets because (too much) salt is added in order to create the illusion of weight gain from retained fluids. I prefer meat that doesn't release a lot of water when it is cooked. I soon learned to feed my bunnies on lucerne hay and vegetable trim instead of pellets. I spread wheat straw below their cages. When the odour got too strong the bedding was composted. According to Albert Howard I should not have used straw for this purpose. I could have removed a few inches of urine-soaked soil from beneath the bedding and used that for the soil component when building a compost heap. And then put new soil under the cages to soak up more urine.

Feedlot manure

Steer manure sold by the cubic metre at the landscape yard is already composted. The bedding was wood chips and bark. The stuff has already broken down enough to not shock the soil when mixed in but it has little potency. It maintains soil organic matter but when I depended upon feedlot manure it did not noticeably make my vegetables grow. COF did that. I worry that there may be persistent herbicide residues remaining in feedlot manure.

Poultry manure, pelletized

Pelletized chook poo makes potent fertilizer because chickens are mainly fed high-protein seed based foods. A seed must store enough plant nutrients to completely feed an embryo until it develops into a self-sufficient plant. And chooks make no urine so no value is lost that way. Chook poo is rich stuff.

Dynamic Lifter or Rapid Raiser contain sawdust bedding as well as poo but the high nitrogen content overcomes sawdust's growth-retarding effect. Because it is seed based, chicken manure contains much more phosphorus than grass-eater manure usually does. Chicken manure compost doesn't supply much in the way of trace elements but my soil testing shows it does have a lot of zinc. It does not eliminate the need for remineralizing with aglime. It provides some potassium, but not nearly enough. All factors considered I view pelletized chicken manure as slow-release nitrogen fertilizer with a phosphate bonus. Because the nutrient release goes on for 18 months I must spread more than twice as much weight of Lifter compared to oilseed meal in order to provoke a similar growth response. When I see a soil test showing excess phosphorus accompanied by excess zinc I query the gardener about chook poo. Every one of them has admitted to depending upon chook poo for many years. Excess phosphorus lessens nutrient density and interferes with zinc uptake. Maybe in this situation excess zinc is a plus, not a minus. Maybe. I advise moderation with Lifter or Rapid Raiser I think 10 litres per 10 square metres provides enough available nitrogen for the current crop and almost enough for another low demand crop following it.

Industrial composts

Tasmania has at least four municipal waste disposal businesses whose dubious composts are sold by the cubic metre at landscape supply yards and in 20 kg sacks at garden centres. "Gardener's Friend" in poly bags is this sort. Sea Greens from HALS, Brighton, is a better product when it is purchased by the cubic metre (more about that soon) but not that much better when it is in sacks. I have strong reservations about buying any maker's compost in sealed airtight plastic bags because without air exchange most of the microbes in that compost will be dead.

The product from McRobies Gully Waste Management Centre, Hobart is better than the other industrial composts because as best I can discover this maker does not include biosolids (more about that soon). Poppy pod waste (called poppy mulch or poppy marc) and pyrethrum waste are plant-nutrient-rich compost-like materials. They are spread by the truck load for farmers but they don't usually find their way into landscape supply yards—and probably shouldn't because if poppy and pyrethrum wastes are not spread promptly after being generated they soon settle into a hard mass that doesn't spread easily.

Mushie

Ordinary supermarket mushrooms are grown in grain straw and animal manure, usually chicken. The growing medium may contain oilseedmeal, grape crushings, gypsum, chemical fertilizers and lime. Producers may use chemicals to eliminate wild fungi and insects, so some organic gardeners reject mushroom compost.

Mushroom compost falls short of balancing soil by itself but it does encourage the soil biology extraordinarily well. I depended on mushie for many years because we could purchase it direct, 100 or more bags at a time, delivered to us for the same price garden centres paid. The bags were the same ones the mushrooms had been grown in so they were not sealed airtight; delicious fresh mushrooms emerged from some of these bags for weeks after we bought them. I dug in one bag per square metre plus the usual dose of COF ahead of each crop. With that combination the vegies grew more robustly than had they been given COF and industrial compost. I speculate this strong performance was due to mass inoculation of mushroom mycelia which temporarily suppressed ever-present soil diseases that plants constantly resist. This resembles how mixing antibiotics into livestock feed increases growth rate and weight gain by reducing the load on the animals' immune system.

Mushie has downsides. Left in its plastic bag for too many weeks it compacts and no longer spreads easily. So we tried to use all bags within a month of receipt. Occasionally a mushroom production house gets contaminated. When this happens the currently producing bags *and* the entire house itself are sterilized by heating them to the boiling point of water. Cooked mushie is no longer fluffy and won't spread easily. And it no longer has active mycelia so there's much less bang for the buck. Buying sterilized mushie can be avoided at the garden centre because the bag will be tightly sealed with duct tape.

In recent years mushroom compost at the wholesale price became unavailable to me although garden centres still sell it at retail. At the retail price I think mushie is too expensive.

At the landscape yard

If you put municipal compost into soil that contains more than a little clay it is crucial to not use too much of it, maybe it is best to not use it at all in that circumstance. For background on that please see the previous chapter for more about how clay soil is worsened by holding too much magnesium.

Waste disposal businesses earn most of their profit by charging to take away the materials they process into compost. They'll accept anything that'll legally disappear into a compost heap. Their waste stream includes chipped tree trimmings, green waste, paper of all sorts, restaurant and supermarket waste, cannery and fisheries wastes. All good so far! One feedstock they use has—for the purpose of preventing public revulsion—been given a carefully sculpted clean green innocent sounding name—*biosolids.* Google defines biosolids as wastes from sewerage treatment and water purification. The Pure Living Soil folks who make municipal/industrial compost in the Midlands evade the word biosolids by calling it "organic sludges." What is this stuff? Municipal reticulated water is processed to remove all suspended solids. Sewerage water also must be cleansed of suspended particles before it is discharged—this creates another biosolid. Both forms of biosolid contain a great deal of magnesium because MgO inexpensively makes particulates settle out fast.

Dulverton Industries near Devonport, Pure Living Soil and the Hobart municipality all include biosolids. The lab analysis provided by Pure Living Soil says their compost contains about 1% magnesium. Dulverton's lab analysis used to say 1% Mg but now they assert that their product has only about 0.4% magnesium. This down-revision of Mg content may be due to my communications with their management about the harmful effects of magnesium on heavy soils. I do not believe that all the batches of compost from this particular municipal composter have much less magnesium in them now than they previously had.

Glebe Gardens, Launceston, operates a retail garden centre on the North Esk floodplain where they also make compost from shredded (woody) green waste. Because Glebe can't make nearly enough compost to satisfy local demand it blends their own output with compost from Dulverton Industries. I have not seen an analysis of what Glebe sells. I expect it varies according to how much from Dulverton they blend in.

I advise not putting magnesium-rich compost into a Tasmanian soil containing more than 10 percent clay. However, on sand or sandy soils that *do not have a clay subsoil,* increasing magnesium does no harm. In fact, it might improve the soil by making the little bit of clay in it become more sticky, hold a bit more moisture, hold on the carrots better so that they don't get ripped out of the ground by a strong wind.

Industrial compost is not made for the benefit of food growers. It only has to be useful enough that people will pay for it and take it away. This is what Longley Organics' website has to say about it:

> In Hobart, Tasmania as in most modern cities there are numerous competitive recycling and upcycling commercial waste value adders (compost suppliers).
>
> Amongst the local compost oligarchy we find different sources of inputs and compositions, the things they seem to have in common are: regular independent testing, competitive prices and services and erratic results!
>
> Often the composts are still very hot, so little or no humic actions there. The demand must outrun the supply of these places, I"m amazed they can't stockpile more.
>
> As we have a soil testing service and our microfarm I am constantly being told of poor experiences with all of these composts, occasionally good by the same gardener, and amongst the Hobart growers we start to get a picture of the inconsistency.
>
> My best suggestion to growers is to stockpile the compost yourself for as long as possible.

The bottom line I draw from Longley Organics' elegant demonstration of damning with faint praise is that industrial compost is typically sold before it has finished heating. If you must use it let it rest in a moist heap for at least a few months.

Horticultural Supplies in Brighton produces Sea Greens compost. It is especially made for horticultural purposes. Their Biological Farmers Association (BFA)-certifiable feedstocks are pine bark, hardwood sawdust, cow manure, Marinova Organic seaweed extract wastes and coir (which I assume is recycled from hydroponic growers). These ingredients were carefully chosen by a qualified agronomist so as to produce an effective soil amendment. Compared to municipal compost this product has a better chemical balance for food growing, it also provides micronutrients from seaweed. Sea Greens compost does not contain far too much magnesium. I know many who have used it successfully. However, I must warn you that I also know bitterly disappointed people who generously added unfinished Sea Greens into their garden soil, which then greatly slowed growth for several months until the soil digested it.

Horticultural Supplies says to spread Sea Greens 30 mm to 60 mm thick and blend that in to a depth of 15 to 20 centimetres. On brand new gardens I suggest spreading it 25 mm thick the first time, digging that in to a shovel's blade deep and after that, *only once a year*, spread it 10 mm thick and hoe/rake it in. Sea Greens lab analysis says it is 0.23% magnesium. Dulverton's lab analysis says 0.38% Mg, which is half again more—and I doubt those numbers apply to all the batches Dulverton turns out. The compost from Soil First analyses close to 1%. I do not have current data about Hobart's municipal compost. If someone spreads 1% magnesium compost only 6 mm thick *one time,* that single application provides the maximum annual dose of magnesium a clayey Tasmanian soil could possibly accept without getting overdosed. Repeatedly spread compost like that on a heavy loam or clay soil and the garden (and gardener) becomes addicted to using ever-more compost. Here's how the addiction develops: the tighter the magnesium makes the clay in that soil become, the thicker and more often the gardener spreads compost to loosen it up. Which it does. Temporarily. However, after the compost decomposes the soil becomes even tighter than it was before. So the gardener uses even more next time. Repeat year on year. Like I said, addiction.

Humus formation requires clay

In order to maximize humus formation during composting about two percent of the heap's starting volume must be clay. Without clay the heap only produces partly-decomposed organic matter, not humus. And without clay *and* soil in the starting volume you also end up with a much less compost. Industrial composters can not include living soil and do not add clay when building a heap. Consequently, industrial compost continues shrinking rapidly after it cools down. This is equally true of Sea Greens compost. When you mix unhumified compost into soil it continues to rot, acting like low-grade fertilizer that provokes better plant growth for about two years, after which almost all of the organic matter will have disappeared. If the soil contains more than a few percent clay a small part of that organic matter may become stable humus as it decomposes in the soil.

Humus has the capacity to hold on to plant nutrients and then release nutrients to plants on demand—exactly like clay does. Humus enormously improves the performance of sandy gardens. Without humus (or biochar, which acts much the same way), plant nutrients soon wash out of sand.

Mixing sandy garden soil into a compost heap does not provide enough clay to encourage humus formation. Where a sandy topsoil sits atop a clay subsoil, one way to put clay into a compost heap would be to dig a small pit and mine some clay. Convert a quarter-bucket of clay subsoil into a nearly full bucket of clay soup with an electric-drill-driven paint mixer and some water. Dip a small broom or stiff long-bristled brush into the slurry and whisk sprays of clay over each layer of your heap as it is being built. How much clay do you need? About two percent by starting volume. Sand soil gardeners could include 12 to 16 litres of clay in each cubic metre of starting volume. Sodium bentonite, used to seal dams, is a useful form of dry powdered clay sold in sacks at some farm supply shops. Bentonite swells by more than 10 times when hydrated. Bentonite powder could be very thinly sprinkled over each layer as the heap is being built. Include one to two litres per cubic metre.

Sir Albert Howard made excellent compost with clay soil at the Indore Research Station in India. He had pits dug that were 3 metres wide x 15 metres long x 1 metre deep. These were partly filled with water and then urine-soaked clay soil taken from beneath his work oxen's loafing pen was stirred into the water until the pit was filled with nitrogen-rich clay soup. His one-shilling-per-day labourers then mixed in dry crop waste, letting the vegetation soak until it was both rehydrated and coated with clay. This material was then combined with fresh manure.

Soil in the heap

Proteins decomposing in a compost heap release their nitrogen component in the form of ammonia gas. If this ammonia is immediately captured by specialist soil-dwelling microbes that convert ammonia into nitrogen fertilizer then it remains in the heap. Otherwise it offgasses. A heap that even faintly smells like a horse stall that should have been cleaned out a few days ago is losing nitrogen. So that heap must burn off even more carbon before it stabilizes—in consequence it shrinks more.

Books about composting all agree that properly finished compost cools and stabilizes at 10- to 12 parts of carbon for every part of nitrogen. Compostable "green" materials contain 20 to 30 parts of carbon to each part of nitrogen. Brown materials range from 30:1 to 200:1. Fresh animal manures contain a lot of nitrogen; their ratio is less than 10:1. The heap should start out with an average carbon-to-nitrogen ratio between 25:1 and 35:1, best when closer to 25:1. To end up with compost that makes vegetables jump up and grow, the heap must burn off carbon until the ratio stabilizes at 12:1.

To keep the arithmetic simple suppose that the starting materials in a heap have an average C:N of 24:1. By the time the heap reaches 12:1 *at least half* of its starting carbon must have become carbon dioxide gas. Hopefully no nitrogen offgasses. However, if the heap releases ammonia gas then the 12:1 ratio is not achieved until even more carbon is burned off. There might be very little left by the time the heap stabilizes.

Blending in garden soil so it becomes about five percent of starting volume provides plenty of habitat for ammonia-capturing bacteria. Including that much soil also mass inoculates the heap with other essential bacteria. So I thinly scatter garden soil no more than a few millimetres thick over each layer as the heap is being constructed. My heavy loam soil contains more than enough clay.

Building a heap with more than five percent soil in it slows the fermentation much like the moderating rods in a nuclear reactor. That can be a good thing. A heap that starts out with too much nitrogen gets too hot. This often happens if a great deal of animal manure is in the starting volume or moreso, when someone tries to compost short horse manure by itself. In that case try starting with ten percent soil by volume, keep an eye on the core temperature to make sure the heap isn't overheating and/or drying out, and be prepared to turn and remoisten it every few weeks. If that heap doesn't burn itself out then it'll finish quickly. If it gets too hot then add even more soil next time.

Vermicomposting

One of the worst plagues a food garden could suffer would be a flock of English sparrows (aka in the USA as "flying rats") hanging around, making holes in silverbeet leaves, scratching up seedbeds to eat germinating seeds. People who carelessly feed backyard chickens attract sparrows. Cereal-based kitchen wastes interest sparrows. Cooked foods of all sorts appeal to rats and mice. Scattering these items atop the growing stack of drying ornamental- and food garden waste may not be such a good idea.

One way to keep vermin out of kitchen wastes is to put them straight into a covered worm bin. Large plastic composting enclosures sold at garden centres can be used as vermicomposters with a capacity around one cubic metre. I would not use them as enclosures for heaps that heat up. Even if one of these is filled up all at once they are not large enough to heat up for long enough. Worm bins steadily receive new material on top as worms eat the older stuff. When one of these bins is open to biologically active soil at the bottom it is rarely necessary to import redworms; a few of the right sort (not the common earthworm) will discover this rich food source and start multiplying prolifically. To get the compost ecology going sooner you can inoculate the first buckets of kitchen scraps—beg a hundred red wigglers from a vermicomposting neighbour. After redworms get established, wastes and grass clippings quickly disappear when tossed on top.

Large plastic bins make much better vermicompost by drilling about 50 ten-mm-diameter holes scattered on the sides. Holes facilitate air exchange; that helps the worms thrive.

People with small gardens that do not generate enough compostable waste to make at least one large-enough heap each year could put all their garden and kitchen wastes into large worm bins.

That free-to-download compost making book of mine has much to say about vermicomposting.

Final thoughts and suggestions

Nearly all gardeners make ineffective plant-nutrient-deficient compost. The typical heap starts out with too much woody material and not enough soil. This heap may heat up for a week or three, the material eventually resembles what gardeners have been told compost is supposed to look like, but the C:N hasn't yet dropped to 12:1. It'll be closer to 20:1. When this half-done compost is mixed into cool Tasmanian soil it does not rapidly release plant nutrients. I apologize for sounding negative; Mainland-based TV garden presenters usually are filming where the soil get much warmer than here.

Composting is a fermentation process. Foods and drinks are also made by fermentation. When I was a young man with a strong liver I brewed beer. My first batch was undrinkable. By the time I had made the sixth batch my homebrew was nearly as good as most craft beers—with higher octane than most of them.

Years later I started baking the daily bread using absolutely fresh flour that I milled on the day. My first attempt turned rock hard as soon as it cooled. Fortunately, almost anything made of fresh wholemeal flour is delicious when still hot from of the oven if you melt some butter into it. My sixth batch didn't turn hard when it cooled and it tasted okay but it was objectionably crumbly, more like cake than like bread. So was the tenth loaf.

That prompted me to learn few things about bread wheat—about its variable protein content, that virtually all wheat protein is gluten, that gluten makes the bread flexible instead of crumbly, allows big pore spaces to develop (light texture). I discovered unabashed irresponsible wheat ignorance at my local health food shop. All they knew was that their wholesale distributors provided two kinds of wheat for grinding into flour—organic and conventional; it was not their responsibility to know more. I contacted their wholesaler; they also had no idea of the protein content of either sort and also had no interest in sourcing wheat berries with enough protein in them to make decent bread, which is, at minimum, 14 percent protein. So I started buying wheat from a specialty home baking shop that sourced direct from a farmer growing on highly mineralized soil in a semi-arid climate. The shop owner proudly declared her hard red wheat to be 18 percent protein and the hard white variety she sold was 19 percent. These are extraordinarily high numbers. After making a few wonderfully light loaves with incredible crusts I had the basics pretty well worked out and could depend on an excellent result every time. Incidentally, after a century of soil depletion only the very best Tasmanian Midlands wheat achieves 14 percent protein. Most Tassie wheat these days has less protein than that and is feed to chooks.

Getting back to my point: because I made bread every few days, learning how to do it well only took me a few months. Making excellent homebrew took longer to learn because each batch fermented for a few weeks before it was ready to be bottled and in order to smooth out the beer needed to rest in the bottle for at least three months. Consequently, my beer making improved steadily over a few years (and by then my liver no longer coped so I quit drinking beer). Beer and bread are relatively easy ferments to learn. With proper ingredients the outcome becomes predictable. Switch to different wheat or use a different yeast and the dough may slightly alter its nature, but only a little.

Compost is also a ferment. However, it may take a gardener ten years to make and use ten heaps. The ingredients almost certainly will be different every time. Ordinary beer ferments quickly at room temperature; lager ferments slowly under cool conditions. If the baker is smart their yeast-dough rises in a warming oven. However, compost heaps that are made in autumn ferment during a cold rainy winter while heaps made in spring ferment through a warm dry summer. There are colder-than-average winters and hotter-than usual summers. How this constantly changing stream interacts with the ever changing feedstocks going into a compost heap is not predictable without a lot of prior experience and close observation. But I have accumulated some of both of those; here is a brief summary, much of it already stated in this chapter:

Size: The heap must be large enough to hold heat but the core must breathe. So a minimum heap should be a steep-sided flat-topped mound at least 1,800 mm across at the base but not wider than 2,100 mm. It should be at least 1,500 mm high at the start but no higher than 1,800 mm. It may be extended into a windrow. If you lack materials to make at least one minimum sized heap once a year I suggest you make vermicompost.

Air supply: The bottom layer of the heap should ideally be a 30 cm layer of corn stalks, sunflower stalks, brussels sprout and kale stalks, woody old broccoli plants or the like, cut into 30 cm lengths that are crisscrossed so they won't pack tight. This allows more fresh air into the bottom of the heap, which allows more warm air to rise out the top. If the bottom layer compacts too much then you'll have to turn the heap before it is finished. Turning is far more work than building it correctly in the first place.

Moisture: When building the heap, wet down each layer thoroughly before starting the next layer. I do this with hose and nozzle set to spray fine droplets. Best to have a helper spray water constantly as you build the heap. If you: 1) get the entire heap thoroughly moist at the start, and 2) incorporate enough soil, and 3) thickly insulate the heap with loose straw, then you may never have to turn and remoisten the heap.

Extra nitrogen: To make potent compost the heap must start with an average carbon to nitrogen ratio between 24:1 and 30:1. If it starts at 36:1 then the process takes longer and the end product will not provoke as much of a growth response. People with livestock, even just a few backyard chickens, should include manure in order to lower the starting C:N. Rather than go to the bother of finding and hauling animal manure to mix into a new compost heap, I suggest those without livestock sprinkle each layer with seedmeal or, much better, with about the same amount of COF you'd spread to prepare a bed for a new crop. On each layer! Men can conveniently fill empty milk bottles with their own urine in the garage or tool shed. I suggest pouring more than a few litres of aged (stinky) urine over each layer as you build the heap. The escaping odour only persists for a day.

Materials: Please believe me! To end up with effective compost do not put woody material or paper into the heap. Nitrogen-rich vegetation like lucerne or pea straw might be up to one-quarter of the starting volume in place of that much animal manure. However, these materials tend to compact and become airless. Don't use too much and disperse it through the entire starting mass. Most of the heap's starting volume should originate from your garden and surrounds. If you import materials then the best one is grain straw. Its carbon to nitrogen ratio is similar to a broad mixture of garden trim and waste. Do not use grass hay because wet hay compacts, becomes airless. And no matter what other composting books say, believe me: the seeds in grass hay do not all die from the heat generated. The worst material is woody—sawdust, planer shavings, bark chips—unless it has been well scratched by chickens for months and has become saturated with chook poo. Do not include twigs and sticks that have developed bark.

Insulation is essential. Cover the heap with a blanket of loose grain straw 30 cm to 45 cm thick. Immediately mist water over loose straw so it will not blow away.

Location influences core temperature and moisture loss. In summer it's best to compost in the shade but under a tree is not a good spot because tree roots will steal nutrients and suck moisture from the heap. But spreading a sheet of black plastic under the heap to keep out tree roots also prevents worms from entering and leaving and it is the worms that convert organic matter into humus. The winter wind lowers core temperature. Compensate for that with a 30+ cm layer of loose straw. The most convenient and least costly way to keep strong summer sun from baking a working heap dry or to stop winter wind from robbing core heat is to cover the heap with a thick blanket of loose straw.

Turning: I can't predict how often someone else should turn a heap. My location, my materials, my methods sometimes requires one turn after six months with a thorough watering while being turned, and a final turn-out after another six months that loosens the material and prepares it for spreading. I have been surprised by a few heaps that started in spring and were finished when I began the first turn in autumn. Most of mine need an entire year and one turn. If a heap dries out then it needs turning and remoistening. If the heap smells of ammonia it certainly needs turning, watering and could have its temperature lowered by having more soil mixed in as it is turned. If the heap cools prematurely then turning and remoistening it may cause it to heat up again for a short while. But high core heat is not necessary; as long as the core is moist, is getting sufficient air and was warm during the first month there is no absolute need to turn unless there's need for it to finish quickly.

Temperature (and duration): A heap whose core temperature never exceeded 55°C and that stayed warm for a more than one month may finish in less than one year; a cold heap takes longer. Either way makes effective compost. However, when core temperature exceeds 68°C the organisms of decomposition die. Fermentation doesn't resume after the core cools back down because high heat like that also dried out the core. Many garden writers imitate industrial composters, who, to make a profit, must make compost as fast as possible. So they bring core temperature as high as possible without killing off the biology and then using heavy machinery turn and remoisten the heap every few days. Industrial composters are not able to include living soil in their heaps so they ignore nitrogen loss. I think they release so much CO_2 that they could more usefully convert the material to biochar and co-generate electricity at the same time—which is often done in Europe.

I target core temperature at 50°C and opine the maximum core temperature should never be above 55°C, which happens to be the maximum temperature for bacterial ammonia fixation. A medium-heat heap takes longer to finish. But you'll end up with a larger volume of finished compost. And that compost will be more effective. A quick-easy way to check the heap's core temperature is to push a garden stake well into the heap when it is first built and leave it there. Gauge the core temperature by pulling the stick out of the heap and holding the heated end of the stick tightly in your hand; the stick should feel uncomfortably warm but not painfully hot. Then reinsert the stick.

If a heap fails to heat up enough then tear it apart and rebuild it while adding more green stuff, more manure, more seedmeal or COF. Make sure all the material is properly damp. Perhaps make the heap larger. Use an insulating straw blanket. If a heap gets too hot then the starting C:N was too low. Tear it apart, add more soil and remoisten; next time include less seedmeal or less manure or more brown materials.

Gardens without compost

I once owned 16 acres of deep black alluvial silty-clay loam, a highly productive Class I soil that already had withstood a full century of extractive farming. For at least ten years before I bought the land it had produced enough hay to profitably harvest and sell. Before that it grew plowed crops. Despite the fact that selling hay off the farm is the fastest known way to exhaust soil minerals, the grass on this field was still dense, abundant. The property was located 80 kilometres from any convenient source of organic matter. So I rotary cultivated some sod, spread COF and started gardening. I had an excellent albeit weedy result. It was excellent only because I knew how to wield a sharp hoe. The weeds were far fewer the second year but the garden's performance declined slightly; it seemed a good idea to shift to a new spot. And that is how I experienced the easiest way of all to grow highly nutrient-dense food. Do not make compost; do not import it. Just till in well-developed sod and add COF.

If you live on a few acres or more why not put most of an half acre into a wildlife fenced paddock-like reserve that accumulates organic matter. A Tasmanian vegetable garden that provides a generous half the entire year-round food supply for a family of four or five can be around 500 square metres. But instead of having just one such garden, aspire to having enough good land for four such gardens—maybe even eight of them. One garden currently grows vegetables, another grows fruit trees, berries, asparagus and other perennials that remain in the same place for many years; the rest of the space grows deeply rooting grass, clover and broad leaf herbs. For this method to work best no biomass should be removed from the reserve areas and everything possible should be done to avoid soil compaction, which means livestock larger than *a very few* chickens should graze different land. Instead of being grazed the grass area it is mowed like a hayfield but unlike a hayfield, everything lies where it falls. In order to produce the most biomass never mow closer than 100 mm above ground so that regrowth starts sooner. And it is slightly better to use a (heavy duty) lawn mower that chops up what gets mowed into small bits so it doesn't block the light from reaching the short grass below, although this is not essential.

When the time comes to move the vegie garden to a new area (every two years), mow the grass short and chop it up fine with a lawn mower in order to make tilling easier, spread a full dose of COF and then rotary cultivate. Do this early in autumn. Next spring spread another full dose of COF, rotary cultivate and start growing vegies. A few years ago I turned under some old grass such as I described here and had a soil test done the next spring. The organic matter content was 8 percent. My garden's normal soil organic matter level is 7 percent. I consider that a very good result for four years growing grass without any removals! After two years in vegetables that plot's organic matter level will drop enough that it is time to rotate back into grass.

If starting with infertile land (most likely the case), then the best thing to do is remineralize the entire area in the very beginning and to sow the reserve to an intentional mixture of grasses, broad leaf herbs and legumes that maximizes biomass production. To learn more about the benefits from growing complex mixtures do a websearch for "regenerative agriculture."

Mow whenever the grass starts forming seeds and for sure mow before those seeds could ripen as the straw dries out. At Grindelwald I had to mow two- and in a rainy summer, three times between October and February. So you'll need a strong lawnmower or a weedwacker—or you'll have to become skilful with a scythe. For more information see Robert Elliott's *The Clifton Park System of Farming*.*

I can not locate seeds in Australia for some of the broad leaf herbs used by Robert Elliott; in my experience importing seeds when Quarantine is involved brings forth dangerous emotions I'd rather not have to control. So I use this simple mixture that can be conveniently sourced from local farm suppliers. These amounts generously sow 100 square metres:

1 kilogram cocksfoot (orchard grass)
250 grams perennial rye grass
100 grams red clover

Perennial rye grass serves as a "nurse crop" because it quickly establishes a ground cover. Get any rye variety the local seed merchant has on offer. By the following summer cocksfoot will overwhelm the rye. Cocksfoot is very coarse (livestock eat it last) and makes a deep, strong root system (good) and huge stools that resist being tilled in a few years later (not so good).

Yes, gardens newly won from old sod are weedy, but if in recent years the plot was mowed before any grass makes seed then the new garden won't be all that weedy. If you use a sharp hoe and generous interplant spacing then weeding will not be difficult. If you crowd the plants or don't have a properly sharp hoe—you'll probably curse me.

Chapter 4

Garden Planning

The strip system [a farming method widely-used during the Middle Ages that steadily lowered soil fertility] *has also been adopted for the allotments round our towns and cities without any provision whatsoever on the part of the authorities to maintain the land in good heart by such obvious and simple expedients as subsoiling, followed by a rest under grass grazed by sheep or cattle, ploughing up, and sheet composting the vegetable residue. Land underallotments should not be under vegetables or more than five years at a time: this should be followed by a similar period under grass and livestock.*

Sir Albert Howard, ***Farming and Gardening For Health or Disease****, 1947

At age 65 I built my retirement home on a vacant quarter-acre suburban block even though I prefer rural living. I chose that block for its deep stoneless red soil, the most productive kind of Tasmanian agricultural soil. I chose a back block so that I could position the house in the far southeast corner where it would shade the least possible amount of land. I intended to grow food on every bit of my urban farm that was not covered with a structure—there would not be any lawn. Less than a year later I married Annie, who also is an avid gardener; together we bought an adjoining still-vacant quarter-acre block. The house block then became Annie's (mostly) flower and fruit garden; I grew vegetables on the other block.

None of my neighbours appreciated this marvellous soil. Their food comes from the supermarket. When I went into the garden seed business (1979) the average American backyard garden was 100 square metres. I wish every Tassie backyard would include a small food garden like that so the family discovers how good vegetables can taste and gets some perceptible and undeniable health benefits from eating nutrient-dense vegetables. Then that family might convert most of the rest of their yard to growing vegetables. And prioritise a larger building block with decent soil in a sunny position the next time they move house.

Managing 100 square metres of vegie garden does not place big demands on a family's time. A small garden like that leaves room in the shadier parts of the backyard for the kids and pets. That much garden can, in summer, produce what seems like a huge overabundance to people that deep down consider vegies to be an insubstantial garnish on the plate whilst *real* food consists of meat, potatoes and bread.

Your engineered garden

I thought it would be helpful, especially to novices, if together we plan a 100 square metre year-round food garden. I'll provide coaching; you provide desire.

Start out by listing those vegetables you and your family eat. If that's a long list just write down the ones you eat the most of. Then consider my list on the next page. It balances several factors—what each vegetable costs at the supermarket in the season you could grow it; potential yield per square metre; how long the vegetable will occupy valuable space before you can plant something else there; difficulty of cultivation. I urge novices to avoid everything from cauliflower to the bottom of the list. True, value is not only measured in dollars; how can one measure the dollar value of eating an ear of raw sweet corn seconds after tearing it off the stalk. That incredible taste might be worth more to you than a few kilos of potatoes or three big lettuces that could come from the same space.

The greatest economic return comes from growing salad greens and herbs. Uncrowded lettuce produces ten magnificent heads per square metre that, depending on variety, are harvested between 60 and 80 days after sowing. It's not just high economic benefit from greens—freshness makes a huge difference in how salads taste; and there are non-commercial lettuce varieties so delicious they'll make you choose to eat salad by the bellyfull.

Fresh herbs are very spendy from the shop and taste infinitely better than dried herbs. And the garden produces vine-ripe tomatoes the likes of which not even the super-rich can buy.

Harvest fresh vegetables twelve months a year

It is a good thing that Mainlanders think Tasmania has bad weather most of the year. To them it doesn't seem likely that harvesting a broad assortment of fresh vegetables is possible every month of the year here. Actually it is more possible here than in QLD. But enjoying this blessing only happens by following a plan. That is why I put a complete planting calendar in the first pages of Chapter 9.

The calendar combined with the vegetable by vegetable growing information in Chapter 9 suggests that broccoli, cabbage and cauliflower may be harvested from early September to the end of November if they were started the previous February, March, April—and overwintered. Without that foresight the first broccoli, cabbage and cauliflower of the season will be eaten in December or January. The calendar shows that a broad range of vegetables may be harvested during autumn and winter, but only if they were started between Christmas and mid-March.

Heat-loving vegetables must be transplanted out or sown during a short window of opportunity that opens as soon as there is no more frost danger and closes about one month later. That single planting slot establishes the entire summer's supply of tomato, pepper, eggplant, potato, melon, cucumber, pumpkin, zucchini and corn. These heat loving species are what most people imagine a garden is all about. Consequently, novices plant nearly their entire garden to heat loving crops. They harvest an abundance in January, cope with an absolute glut during February and most of March, followed by scarcity.

Achieving a year-round vegie abundance only happens with a plan. So why not make one right now! Get a large sheet of paper, a pencil, a rubber and a ruler. Draw a fairly accurate map of your existing or proposed garden space. If you're landless at the moment then imagine a 100 square metre garden.

Economic Value for the Space Required

Value lessens going from top to bottom.

fresh herbs: (basil, oregano, thyme, sage, rosemary, etc)
parsley
carrot
beetroot
parsnip
loose leaf lettuce
most other leafy salad greens
spring onion
bulbing onion*
English spinach (for salad)
kale
silverbeet
leeks
kohlrabi
potatoes
broccoli
swede
zucchini and other bush summer squash
tomato
cucumber
pepper (capsicum and chilli)*
French & climbing bean; runner bean
cauliflower*
cabbage
Brussels sprout
pumpkin
sweet corn
eggplant*
cantaloupe and muskmelon
watermelon

** Difficult; should be avoided by novices*

Imaginary practice garden plan

Please, you novices, don't think you can garden effectively without a detailed plan. I started vegie gardening in 1974 and only ten years ago did I get skillful enough to garden without first making a plan on paper. I'd work out next year's garden plan early in winter while that year's mistakes were still fresh in my mind and then I'd use my plan to limit my lust for buying seeds. By the time the tomato seedlings went out my much-besmudged plan mostly stayed in my seed box because by then I pretty much memorized it.

Suppose your imaginary garden is 10 metres by 10 metres. Divide that square into six beds, each bed is 1,200 mm wide and 10 metres long, with (narrow) footpaths between them.

Now reconsider and simplify your list of vegetable preferences because almost no one has all the space, time, interest or energy to grow everything they might want. At this step many gardeners err by practicing crowding rather than prioritisation. Crowding is the main ruin for people whose entire hobby garden consists of a few metal-sided above-ground bins filled with imported growing medium.

If you are new to food gardening—even if you own acres of good land and have more water than you know what to do with—please do not use more than 100 square metres the first year. You have so much to learn that if you take on more land you'll likely get discouraged.

Everything you attempt in the first year will be far more difficult than it ever will be again. Accept in advance that you will make errors . . . but you can limit them in advance to small scale errors.

Now, with a list in hand of what you're intending to grow, read in Chapter 9 about the vegetable you ranked number one on your list. Make your best guess about how much space it'll take to produce as much as you imagine that you'll want. Consult the planting calendar on page 120 and note when it'll be planted; maybe also consult some seed catalogues and make your best guess about when the harvest will happen. Then pencil in space on the garden plan for this vegetable and write in the sowing- and anticipated harvest date.

Almost certainly, before you get half way through your wish list the imaginary garden beds will be completely occupied—but there's actually more space than the plan shows because gardening is a four dimensional process that you're mapping in two dimensions. And one of those dimensions is time.

Successions

Suppose you're like me, addicted to huge green salads mostly consisting of the semi-blanched hearts of leaf lettuce. Most varieties of looseleaf lettuce take seven to eight weeks from sowing to achieving supermarket size, then the head remains in prime condition for one to two weeks and then it becomes bitter. Instead of planting my favourite variety every two weeks I sow a mixture of varieties that mature in succession over four weeks. I sow this mix once a month from spring through February. After mid-February vegetative growth slows ever more with each passing week so my late summer and early autumn lettuce sowings have fewer weeks between them.

Pencil that into your own garden plan as though you were going to do the same thing! Ten full sized lettuce plants barely compete when given one square metre of growing space. In order to harvest one full-sized head, two days out of three during as much of the year it is possible to do so, start a two square metre patch of mixed lettuce varieties on September 1, October 1, November 1, December 1, January 1, February 1, February 20, March 5, March 20, April 5. Lettuce arranged that way, will occupy at least two out of the six beds in our imaginary 100 square metre garden and most of space assigned to lettuce will be empty most of the growing season.

However, the area planted September 1 will be harvested and empty within 80 days. What to plant then? Root crops for autumn harvest; broccoli or cabbage. More lettuce. There's lots of options.

Now view the plan backwards. We've already decided to sow to lettuce during February. No sense having this area empty from September through January. On that space we could plant an early crop that would leave the bed empty by mid-January. Peas? Broccoli? And incidentally, the April 10 lettuce sowing overwinters as small plants; it will be harvested in September and early October.

The possibilities are so many that you'd best draw your plan with soft pencil and have a rubber handy.

Here are a few successions I rely on:

Beds that grew the winter harvest are growing weeds by early spring. These areas often get sown to shelling peas even if the peas would be far in excess of our requirement, in which case I consider excess peas to be green manure crops.

To grow vegetables excellently require

Free-draining soil at least 600 mm deep.

In order to develop full size and peak flavour, all fruit-making crops need direct sunlight from 10 am until 4 pm. If you have to choose between early morning or late afternoon sun then chose the more intense afternoon light. Root crops and brassicas will do fairly well with only four hours of direct sun during those six optimum hours. Leafy greens grow acceptably well in bright shade between October and April, but they do far better in full sun.

Country gardens need

Wildlife (and wandering livestock) fencing

Protection from strong winds

A dependable and hopefully adequate water supply (see Chapter 5)

Hillsides

Land sloping to the south at three percent (3 metres of fall in 100 metres of run) grows crops as though it was located a few hundred kilometres closer to the South Pole. Land sloping to the north at three percent grows crops like it was located a few hundred kilometres closer to the Equator. The warmest slope of all faces north-by-northwest. And that's where the very best wine grapes are grown.

Land sloping more than three percent must be terraced or else you'll soon lose the soil. My reading of history says whenever people terrace any land sloping more than three percent they eventually lose the soil. The civilization and its terracing may endure for several thousand years, but eventually political/social chaos arrives. When this happens the terraces get neglected, soon the whole hillside washes away. See Carter and Dale's *Topsoil and Civilization** and J. Russell Smith's *Tree Crops: a Permanent Agriculture.**

All the peas will be harvested and all the vines moved to the compost area before Christmas. These ex-pea beds then produce the large brassicas such as savoy cabbage, broccoli, kale, swedes or brussels sprouts. If I need a planting space in November or December, then some green manure peas may be terminated before they yield anything. Pea vines are nitrogen-rich. They make strong compost. And better, pea roots leave the bed loose, fine textured and ready to welcome the next crop.

Here's a succession lasting two years: After digging the main crop of spuds early in April immediately plant garlic, which will be harvested before mid-December; then brussels sprouts and other autumn-harvest coles go into the same area. Spuds, garlic, brassicas—three long growing crops on the same bed during two years.

Ten square metres of spring sown bulbing onions provides our kitchen for a full year. These onions will be harvested late in January. Crops intended for autumn/winter harvest can be sown immediately after.

Rotations

It is not smart farming to grow the same crop on the same land year after year. Crop rotation reduces insect problems *on the farm* because the areas involved are greater than some kinds of insects travel and because the farmer can remember what crops grew in which field for quite a few years back. Farm rotations can completely eliminate host plants from a large enough area that crop diseases fade away. Rotating cropping land into intelligently-managed grazing for several years increases soil organic matter and fertility. Traditional farm rotations make sure that the following crop is one that can handle the root exudates left by the proceeding crop. Before herbicides were commonly used crop rotation was the weed control method for growing small grains. *Most of this farming wisdom does not apply to the food garden* even though it gets uncritically repeated in garden books. Still, gardeners should rotate crops because some vegetables feed from the topsoil whilst others primarily feed from the subsoil. Some crops withdraw much potassium; others take little potassium. Rotating helps the soil rebalance itself.

The simplest rotation I have used divides the garden into equal halves. One part grows frost-sensitive summer crops that start in October in the milder parts of Tasmania. November is a more appropriate starting time for harsher districts. The remains of these crops should be cleared as soon as possible after summer ends and the space immediately sown to green manures that get cleared early the following spring. Frost hardy spring crops follow the green manures and following those come the crops for late summer, autumn and winter.

The other half of the garden grows spring-sown crops that finish by or soon after Christmas. These are followed by autumn/winter crops. After the winter crops have been harvested these beds are prepared in spring for heat lovers. Round and round. This pattern makes it highly unlikely that the same species will grow in the same spot two years in a row.

> I set out to produce at least half again more than I expect to need. Then I don't stress when insects or disease cause losses. If the weather doesn't cooperate I can still gift vegies to friends.

Here's a rotation involving only summer crops. Assign one large area to tomato, pepper, eggplant, zucchini and cucumber. Another area of equal size grows rambling pumpkin vines. Come autumn, promptly clear the crop remains and sow cereal rye over both areas (seed is obtained from the health food shop where its sold for grinding into flour). By mid-spring the rye will be chest high with seed heads appearing. As soon as seed is just starting to form in those heads mow the rye close to the ground, let the straw dry in the sun for a few days and then rake it up. The timing works out nicely; it's now time to plant heat lovers. Each year switch which area grows pumpkin and which grows tomato, pepper, zucchini and cucumber.

I use this rye straw for insulating compost heaps or for mulch. Enough very strong long straw is produced on two equal-sized areas to thickly mulch the one that grows pumpkins (which keeps pumpkin skins unblemished). After the pumpkin crop has been brought in the straw may still be still stiff enough to rake up and use to insulate the end of summer compost heap.

Seed box

The airtight containers holding my seed packets function like a sowing appointment calendar. During winter I organise all carried over seed packets into rubber-banded bundles that are labelled for the month that they'll be sown the first time. As I do this I am reminded of which new seeds I must buy. Anytime that I'm in doubt about what crop needs sowing this week/month I look at which seed packets are waiting for me in this month's bundle. Some packets will be sown more than once; after sowing the first time these packets are transferred to the appropriate bundle. Any packet that germinated weakly or slowly (but still germinates) is tagged for discard as soon as its last planting of that season is done.

Plant spacing

Plant spacing is an extremely important choice with many consequences. The amount of root zone provided for each cauliflower or cabbage determines how large the head will be every bit as much as soil fertility and soil moisture do. Plant spacing determines how many side-shoots a broccoli plant makes and influences how large they will be; how long root crops can hold in the ground before losing quality; if lettuce will form proper hearts; and when the largest harvest happens from tomato and zucchini. Plant spacing strongly influences how I often I must irrigate and how I control weeds.

The currently fashionable method is called *intensive* because plants are positioned very close together. I prefer the old-fashioned now-politically-incorrect extensive method wherein each plant is given much more growing space. This is how people grew vegetables before the mid-1970s, before John Jeavons, an aspiring garden guru, introduced Americans to the intensive method with his book *How To Grow More Vegetables.* Within a few years of its publication nearly every new gardening book, magazine article and government agricultural bulletin in the USA and Canada was pushing Jeavons' system. I hope you're aware that the Powers That Be try to control our thinking; I hope you wonder why Jeavons was so strongly promoted.

The way I see it, both methods have advantages and disadvantages. Intensive concentrates the harvest period; if it is a cut-once-and-done crop like cabbage, cauliflower or head lettuce or if it's a root crop, then intensive gives you more (smaller-sized) units from the amount of land involved and you might harvest them a few days sooner. Spinning the narrative this way can make it seem that intensive yields more. But concerning crops that could provide an ongoing harvest over several months—like tomatoes, peppers, eggplant, climbing French beans, broccoli side-shoots, cucumber and zucchini—the amount harvested from an intensive bed (and the quality of that harvest) declines greatly after a short initial burst. Providing more space between plants means less yield per square metre *at the beginning* but the amount harvested steadily increases because the plant has unoccupied rootzone to grow into. Ultimately, extensive yields more over a longer harvest period.

Suppose a cabbage variety could yield either 12 medium-sized heads on close spacing or six larger ones from the same space by giving each plant twice as much growing room. The six big heads combined will weigh more than the dozen smaller ones but the smaller ones may mature a few days sooner. Not much difference unless you're selling to supermarkets that will not buy large cabbages.

But see what happens from putting either four or twelve broccoli plants into the same space? The crowded bed yields a dozen small heads followed by a few small side-shoots. Then it seems sensible to pull these non-productive crowded plants and make room for something else. The same area sustaining only four broccoli plants yields four enormous heads that combined, significantly outweigh the 12 smaller ones, followed by six weeks of large side shoots. With some varieties the side shoots will as large as the main flowers from crowded plants. Larger, fast-developing broccoli flowers also taste better.

Tomato, pepper, eggplant, cucumber and zucchini yield less after their growing bed has been covered with leaves, which is also when root zone expansion starts being severely constrained. But these same crops will steadily increase their yield when the plants are far enough apart to experience no root zone competition. With generous growing space these vegetables ultimately yield far more. The plants get huge!

Intensively spaced gardens demand almost daily irrigation in hot weather; on many soil types extensive plantings allow you to enjoy a week's summer vacation without concern. Intensive demands bent-over or kneeling by-hand-with-fingers weeding; extensive allows most weeding to be done with a hoe, which is quicker and takes less effort. Ultra intensive requires ongoing transplant raising so that there's always a seedling ready to plug into any opening. Extensive allows you the ease of direct seeding most crops.

The intensive method fails outright when a bed is badly overcrowded. Pack a dozen broccoli plants into two square metres, something I am frequently shown, and you'll harvest main heads only five centimetres in diameter followed by a few tiny woody side shoots. Crowd cabbages like that and most plants fail to form proper heads. Iceberg and semi-hearting lettuces such as cos and butterhead do not head properly when overcrowded, nor will cramped carrots make smooth roots. The majority of overcrowded radish plants fail to make edible roots. Crowded bush beans make a slightly larger overall yield when gauged by weight but you'll harvest smaller pods that take a lot more time to pick and will be unnecessarily tedious to top and tail.

I know how unusual my spacing suggestions seem. But please don't discount them for that reason. In my 40-plus years of food gardening I've used seven quite different soils in two quite different climates. I've tried everything from the closest intensive interplant spacing to dry-gardening with extremely wide interplant spacing. I do not advocate what I only read about. No matter what you have been told or what you may have done in previous years, please try my spacing (and fertilizing) recommendations at least once.

> **This Principle Applies to Most Vegetables**
>
> If adjoining broccoli plants touch before you harvest their first set of side shoots—they were positioned too close together.
>
> If you provide a broccoli bed with all the growing room this book calls for and by the time you finish harvesting the first set of side shoots there remain gaps between plants—have a good think about soil conditions. Most likely you did not give the crop enough fertilizer. But it could be soil moisture was lacking or perhaps the useful root zone isn't deep enough.

My plant spacing suggestions may be adjusted according to your location. Chapter 9 calls for capsicum and chilli on stations 600 mm x 600 mm (0.36 square metre of root zone per plant). This layout works great in the warmer parts of northern Tasmania. A skillful East Coast gardener could usefully provide peppers with 750 mm x 750 mm (0.56 square metre per plant). But pepper plants grown outdoors around Hobart need only 500 mm x 500 mm (0.25 square metre).

Lovers of giant beets can increase my recommended spacing by as much as one-third. The same is true if you want very large heads of cabbage, cauliflower or broccoli or very large onions. However, unnecessarily wide plant spacing makes useless gaps unless you are dry-gardening. I'll discuss dry-gardening in the next Chapter.

Plants given the interplant spacing I suggest in soil that generously holds moisture should be irrigated every five to seven days in summer. If it's been very hot and breezy with low humidity, after four days. Crops on sand or light loam need watering more often. Crowded crops, especially on shallow soil, may need water every two days—or every day in hot weather There is a table at the end of Chapter 5 that shows how often irrigation will be required with various spacing arrangements.

Novices and gardeners who are currently using intensive arrangements should fertilize with COF and try the layouts Chapter 9 recommends. Or try them on a gradient scale: If your plants completely fill the bed this year then next year increase interplant spacing by 25 percent. See what happens. For example, if you used 600 x 600 (0.36 m^2 per plant) last time, increase that to 0.45 m^2 per plant (750 mm x 600 mm). Reassess this annually until the ever-larger plants get too big to suit you. I mean, a head of broccoli broader than a dinner plate is impressive but it may be too large for practical purposes. Take my word for it; a broccoli that big can taste just as good or better than one that is supermarket size.

Rows, raised beds, etc

I acknowledge that vegetables can be produced in stock watering tanks filled with landscape yard compost, in ditches that concentrate and trap rainfall, on mounds of decaying organic matter (similar to ABC TV's "lasagne garden"), in rows running north to south or in rows running east to west. Or with rows in concentric circles. Vegies can grow successfully in complex mixtures of companionable species or grow well (I think better) in small sections of monocropping. I confess to being a self-teaching individualist who is rebellious by nature so my book suggests only what I currently consider the most efficient and practical ways. I understand that my preferred gardening style is not the only way to produce a lot of food. I accept that some people garden with much less organization than I like and others are so organized they could be accused of having OCD.

To to make the best use of my book the reader should correctly visualize what I describe and try to understand why I do as I do. Best that novices do exactly what I suggest for at least one gardening year. And after that, do whatever suits.

All but a few of my beds are 1,200 millimetres wide and 8 metres long—a scant 10 square metres each. I grow small plants like lettuce, kohlrabi, beetroot and carrot in rows that are 1,200 mm long, arranged across the bed with 400 mm isles between the rows. Big brassicas like broccoli, cauliflower, brussels sprouts, and autumn/winter cabbages usually are on stations 600 mm x 600 mm (bigger varieties 750 mm x 600 mm) on a bed 1,200 mm wide.

Sprawling plants like tomato, zucchini and cucumber could be crowded into positions 1,200 mm apart down the centre of a 1,200 mm wide bed but these crops do much much better when they are given more space than that. For these crops I may temporarily combine two beds into one by fertilizing and digging up the path between them, thus making a bed 3 metres wide by 8 metres long. In order to fully pollinate, corn patches should be at least three rows wide; corn is more productive when it gets 750 mm isles between rows. Corn does much better on a double-wide bed holding three rows eight metres long, the plants 300 mm apart in the row, the rows 1 metre apart. You'll irrigate the corn patch less frequently if you make the rows 900 mm apart. You'll probably harvest just as much corn because given that much opportunity, some varieties will make two ears per plant instead of just one.

Unnecessarily broad paths waste potential growing room so I make them only 600 mm wide, which is just wide enough to allow a large wheelbarrow. Beds made less than 1,200 wide give over a larger proportion of the garden to paths. Beds wider than 1,200 would make more efficient use of space but the best compromise seems 1,200 mm because if they were wider I couldn't touch the bed's centre without stepping on it. They're 8 metres long because almost no crop needs more than 10 square metres to yield all we want and because I can, with a shovel, accurately toss compost half the bed's length from a wheelbarrow located on a crosspath. I also find it convenient to mix batches of complete organic fertilizer for areas of $10m^2$.

My growing beds are raised about 50 mm, which is just enough to distinguish them from the paths. I think this is enough raising unless the gardener can not no longer squat or touch their toes. Beds on slopes should form low terraces more or less on the contour lines; if the slope is less than 3% (three metres of fall per 100 metres of run) the beds do not need a retaining wall on their low side. The easiest way to make raised beds is to rotary cultivate the entire area and then transfer 25 mm of soil from what will be the path atop what will be the bed. Now the bed will stand nicely proud of the path with its edges flowing down to the path at a gentle-enough angle that rain or irrigation won't cause soil movement. When preparing beds on a slope always move soil uphill. Soil inevitably moves downhill when raking seedbeds, when making furrows and when hoeing weeds. So every time the bed or a section of the bed is prepared for the next crop, some soil should again be shovelled upwards from the path.

Enclosed raised beds

In my opinion, constraining the sides of raised beds with planks, blocks or with recycled whatever often creates unnecessary work. Here are some examples: It can be very difficult to remove clumps of grass when their roots attach themselves to the irregularities in a plank or concrete block. Retaining walls restrict hoeing; they force the gardener into laborious hand weeding. Raking easily combs lumps and clods out of the seedbed, they lodge on the path—if there are no retaining boards. Side walls also make the bed too permanent; they prevent temporarily merging beds.

Beds without retaining walls are easier to prepare for the next crop, no digging needed. First, clear the remains of the previous crop and then spread soil amendments. Then, a few millimetres of soil that inevitably moved down off the bed is tossed back up. Over all that spread a thin layer of compost. Next the bed is shallowly and finely chopped with a common garden hoe or else a stirrup hoe glides back and forth through the surface inch without digging in deeper until the surface 30 mm has become a loose, super fertile seed sprouting medium.

Before sowing seeds, lumps of compost and lumps of soil located close to the surface that didn't break up from hoeing are raked over the edge of the bed to a surrounding path. Raking also levels the seedbed. Raking turns the surface inch into a highly-effective seed germination medium. Your shoes then crush and mix lumps of compost and clods that raking deposited on the path. They become fine, humusy soil that gets tossed back up atop the bed when you next prepare it. Everything works together; you work less.

Spiritual gardening & companion planting

I have long been uncertain about vegetable friendships and dislikes, or as these phenomena are more accurately termed, "companionate effects." The idea is that some plant species grow better in close association with certain other species; some combinations are said to be antagonistic. Interplanting supposedly deters or confuses harmful insects that hunt by smell. Therefore we should arrange vegetables in complex, compatible mixtures even though doing that greatly increases gardening hours.

One of the first garden books I read was called *Companion plants: and how to use them* by Helen Philbrick and Richard B. Gregg. The first edition came out about 1943; it was much revised and reprinted by Philbrick and is often regurgitated by other garden writers. The original information came from painstaking garden experiments that Philbrick and Gregg did. Philbrick asserted that onions repel damaging insects and thus can protect all sorts of crops. So early on in my gardening career I sowed alternating rows of bush beans and onions across a 1,200 mm wide raised bed. The onions grew well; the bush beans were badly stunted. That same year everything else in my garden grew well no matter what it was next to, including another patch of bush beans that grew fine. And it's been that way ever since. Almost everything I plant grows well no matter what is growing close by. Perhaps I have not observed any other companionate effects because my soil provides intense balanced fertility. Whatever my experiences have been I am sure other gardeners actually do encounter what they believe to be companionate effects.

I'll explain this with some woo-woo; I hope you won't be offended. You've probably heard that marigolds deter unwanted insects. I'm sure they do! When I interplanted marigolds I had little problem with insects. But when I didn't interplant marigolds I also had little problem with insects. So maybe marigolds actually will chase away bugs *if you believe they will.* And I'll soon relate my own mystical method that works even better than marigolds.

Now maybe you love marigolds as much as you love vegetables—or even more. In that case you *should* interplant marigolds. Some believe garlic works better than marigolds. I suppose you could plant a garlic clove in every nook, cranny and gap in the garden and then work around this slow-growing allium no matter how many extra hours it takes. If you believe in garlic please don't take offense. Many things happen in the garden because the gardener believes. We are, after all, spiritual beings with a connection to God. We believe something is so and so it is. Creation by belief happens constantly—only most humans prefer to pretend they're the victim of the situation they've been asking for rather than take responsibility for it. I believe the actual force at work is God, who answers prayers that the person doesn't realize they are making.

I believe insects and diseases are entitled to their tithe. After all my garden is in their space. Because I am so generous the bugs and diseases take less than five percent. Really. I do not interfere with minor annoyances; I do care when insects or birds try to take way more than their share. Which isn't often. So I don't create the inconvenience of interplanting in order to avoid a problem that needn't exist in the first place. However I also believe—without reservation or doubt—that creating truly fertile balanced soil eliminates almost all problems with insects and/or disease. I believe foliar feeding balanced *chelated* plant nutrients as come from liquid fish and kelp or NTS 10-10-10 and/or spraying aerated compost tea *in addition to* soil remineralization will eliminate most insect/disease problems.

You may think all this is too fanciful. Well, let me share a couple of real life examples from the years I ran Territorial Seed Company.

An Oregon bushie wrote me a letter insisting that I recommend his organic remedy that stops cabbage root maggots from infesting radishes. (The root maggot is a fearsome pest unknown to us lucky Tasmanians. It is a fly larvae that eats brassica roots to the point the plant wilts and dies, it tunnels through radish and turnip leaving frass trails behind, it collapses and rots entire Chinese cabbages that are close to harvest.) This guy dissolved one tablespoonful of unadulterated completely genuine sea salt into four litres of distilled water (has to be *real* sea salt, not mined salt, has to be *distilled water* or rainwater or it wouldn't work). When his radishes got large enough to begin forming bulbs (which also alerts the cabbage fly to lay her fast-hatching eggs on the soil next to the just-about-to-appear food supply), this man drenched his rows with slightly sea-salty water. The result: no root maggots—unless he failed to harvest soon enough. Eventually, he admitted, this deterrent stops working and larger unpicked radishes do get maggoty. His result is identical to what happened in my radish patch if I harvested soon enough—but I didn't use slightly salty water.

I thanked him for sharing, told him I would try it out and tell others. And I am. Right now. I am sure his method works. I mean, if you really believe slightly salty water will do something good for your garden, then it might.

During the years I was running Territorial Seed Company I paid close attention to what Dr. James Baggett was up to. Jim was a highly regarded plant breeder on the faculty of Oregon State University at Corvallis; at the time it considered was one of America's best agricultural schools. Baggett's assignment was to forward Oregon's industrial agriculture. There is absolutely no commercial potential in growing eggplant in Cascadia; at very best the earliest hybrid varieties barely cope with the climate and produce a few fruit. No matter, Baggett, a serious home gardener himself, trialled a dozen supposedly early hybrid eggplant varieties every summer—and would inevitably include one heat-loving heirloom called Black Beauty. This variety always grew an entirely fruitless bush in western Oregon. I once asked Dr. Baggett why he wasted space on Black Beauty; Jim replied that if a summer ever proved so warm that Black Beauty did set fruit then he would disregard all the eggplant results from that atypical summer.

It was wintertime; I had spare time. So I was presenting in Seattle. A lady in the audience asked why my book *Growing Vegetables West of the Cascades* (similar to this one but for Cascadia) made such negative comments about Black Beauty. She'd had fine results with it! She had recently moved to chilly Seattle from semi-tropical East Texas. She had brought along treasured Black Beauty seeds that had been saved in her family over generations. The previous summer she transplanted a few Black Beauty seedlings next to a sun-facing white wall. In that position the variety grew fine and yielded well. She antagonistically pointed out that open pollinated Black Beauty seed is cheap, the gardener can save their own seeds; the hybrid eggplant seeds I recommended (that Territorial Seed Company sold) were pricey and then some. So why didn't I sell Black Beauty?!

I confess in that moment I allowed a mean-spirited impulse to run my mouth. After all, at that time I was widely regarded as the Gardener-Laureate of Cascadia, so with all the authority I could muster I informed her of Dr. Baggett's trials with Black Beauty and about similar results in my own eggplant trials. Then I felt ashamed that I had unnecessarily invalidated this woman so I added a qualifier—since she had such a good result with the family heirloom she should continue to grow it in that protected spot. But I wouldn't be at all surprised, her confidence shaken, she no longer got any fruit.

Root exudates

Roots exude sugars, fats and other substances. Making root exudates is so important to the plant that they can amount to about 25 percent of the plant's above ground weight. Root exudates do more than influence which microbes inhabit the area immediately around the plant's roots. They also help the plant win its struggle for light, water and nutrients by chemically suppressing competing species—much like herbicides do. Exudates from one species can damage another species. Some exudates can be positive for another species; this is often seen in native forests. And this is the physical basis of companionate effects.

Gardeners practicing companion planting have their focus upon what is happening *during the time* different species are growing in close proximity but companionate effects continue after the crop has finished. Sometimes long after. I already mentioned how onions interplanted with beans made beans grow poorly. Soil that is growing onions ends up rich in onion root exudates. If an overwintered onion crop that gets lifted late in November should be followed by bush beans sown in December, then the beans won't grow well. But brassicas would grow fine there.

The effect of root exudates can go on for more than a few months. If you harvest storage onions in February, follow them with autumn/winter leafy- or brassica crops and then plant French beans on that spot the following summer, the beans still may not grow so well. A farmer remembers that a whole field was in onions last year or even two years past. As you would expect, traditional farm rotations allow for long lasting exudate effects. But I can't recall where things were in my garden last year, and as I said earlier, I no longer make a detailed garden plan so I don't have the previous years' plans to refer to.

One way to limit these disappointments is to not grow vegetables for more than a few years on a plot, field or garden. Sir Albert Howard suggested the same thing in the quotation introducing this chapter. And keep in mind that Howard's use of the term "allotment" refers to a large rented garden plot whose *minimum size* (about 275 square metres) was specified by law. To the British of that era an allotment was intended to produce an important economic result. It was not one smallish bed in a contemporary community garden whose main purpose is to create community.

Positioning perennials

Fruit trees and smaller perennials like raspberries, currants and asparagus don't fit into rotations. Ideally, locate perennials in an area of their own.

Strawberry, globe artichoke and rhubarb are all perennials that shouldn't be grown for more than two years without being dug, divided and moved to another position, or in the case of a two year old strawberry patch, replaced with new, virus free plants if you can. These crops do fit in vegie garden beds although globe artichoke may be too tall for comfort in most positions.

Cloches and cold frames

We moved from Grindelwald to Chudleigh where it is much colder in winter and not nearly as warm during summer. It was November, 2020. I would soon erect a large polytunnel so we could enjoy higher quality salad radishes, more succulent lettuce, tender spinach and tastier cool-season greens during winter; harvest snap peas early in spring. Greens and winter radishes that are started mid-February do survive winter outdoors here but taste much better when they grow faster under plastic; they will be tender because there is no damage from wind or pounding rain and they experience no frost. Soon after spring bulbs flower outside I plant zucchini, cucumber and capsicum, chilli, eggplant and tomato. Under plastic they are safe from summer frosts—which are not unusual around Chudleigh—and the extra heat makes larger better-tasting fruit appear much sooner.

If I were short of funds I could choose an easy and inexpensive alternative, which is what I actually did when I lived in Oregon, where, incidentally, winter conditions are considerably harsher than they are close up against the Great Western Tiers. Cloches and cold frames inconveniently grow crops as well or better than structures you can walk into. I speculate that on really cold nights a tight cloche might be a degree warmer than an unheated polytunnel.

For low-growing frost-hardy greens, I suggest making crude rectangles of 10 x 2 planks—best to use expensive rot resistant hardwood for this purpose. The frame should be no more than three metres long so that it can be carried (awkwardly) on the shoulder of one strong person. Frames should be the same width as the recycled windows you found to cover them with. The frames would last many years longer if you'll get them out of direct contact with the earth when they're not being used. Wood frames can be protected by periodic treatment with a non-phytotoxic wood preservative.

I once used copper napthanate for this purpose but this substance has been banned. Deck oil helps. People once used dirty engine oil to preserve wood. I urge you to not use treated pine; the poison leaches into soil where it inhibits the soil ecology and may contaminate vegetables.

When the cloche is shut tight the glass should slope enough that rainwater runs off. But I'm not a skilled builder, so instead of constructing sloping frames I use a rake to slope the bed before the frame is put down on it such that the sun-facing edge is 5 cm lower than the south-facing side. Opened lights are prevented from sliding off the frame by small pieces of 2 x 1 screwed on to the north-facing side. The windows are propped open by a 150 mm long block of 100 x 100 (more likely 90 x 90 these days), with a chunk sawn out of it so the air gap it makes can be either 50, 100 or 150 mm. On cloudless winter days prop the windows open to the full 150 mm. When frost threatens, close the glass an hour or two before the sun sets. Keep a glass partly open to prevent rot during rainy periods with milder nights. There is no weather stripping, no crosspieces to plug a narrow gap between sashes, no attempt whatsoever to seal cracks. But these rough frames do allow plenty of light in. More advanced construction makes little difference in outcome.

I lived for eight years near a tiny village called Lorane, Oregon. It has a climate similar to Mole Creek, Tasmania but winters at Lorane are another thick blanket colder than at Mole Creek. There I routinely used four such frames. (For your convenience I'm translating the dates I used in Oregon into Tasmanian terms.) I sowed two frames to salad greens early in April and two more in the first two weeks of May. The April sowing was harvested mid-winter; the May sowing got much less light at first so it sized up in early spring. After being eaten bare during winter, the first two frames were immediately resown to another lot of mixed salad greens very early in spring that I intended to eat mid spring. It's that simple to produce tender sweet loose-leaf lettuce and spinach, mild young rocket and not-too-bitter-to-enjoy escarole/endive, salad radish and other low-growing cool-season vegetables.

A simple cold frame

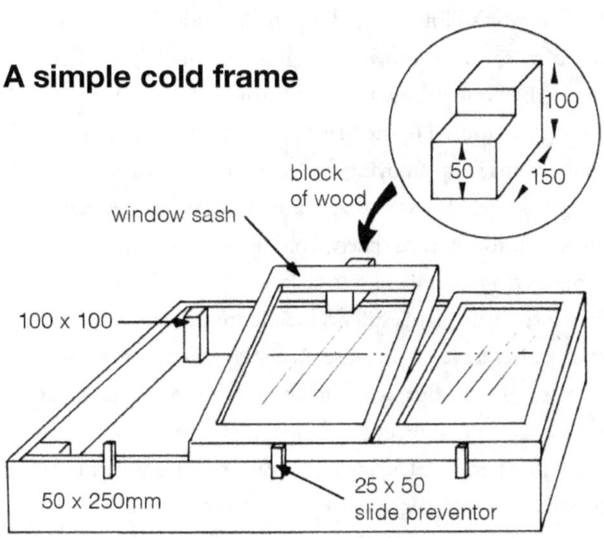

The tunnel cloche—a sheet of clear polythene stretched over supporting hoops to make a long low half-cylinder—is simpler to make than a low wooden box but is less convenient to use. The edges of the plastic may be held down with soil, or in a sheltered position by placing recycled 4 x 4s on them. One or both of the cloche's ends may be left open for air circulation or both of them closed against frost. I seal the ends by draping enough polythene over the last hoop to reach the soil line and then some. I anchor the end with lengths of 90 mm x 90 mm. The extra plastic at one or both ends can be folded back and temporarily anchored at the bottom with those same blocks.

Tunnel cloches can be squat narrow tubes only 400 mm high that are supported by stiff galvanized wire hoops that are ziptied to short wooden garden stakes. They can be metre high hoops made of black plastic irrigation pipe slid over garden stakes or lengths of rebar pounded into the soil. If you go this way I suggest finding more construction ideas on the net. Redpath (www.redpath.com.au) is a Down Under company specializing in high quality greenhouses. They also make cloche hoops ranging in size from 600 mm wide to 1,500 mm wide. Their hoops use a unique design that facilitates raising/lowering the side-walls to control ventilation. Their minimum purchase is a bundle of 25 hoops. Redpath also sells best quality long lasting clear plastic sheeting.

Polytunnels provide enough frost protection that-sensitive summer crops may be put outdoors up to one month before frost danger ends. If frost threatens, even if the forecast low is only 4°C, close both ends in late afternoon (or if you use Redpath hoops, lower the side walls). When there is no threat of frost the end flaps can be left open all night. At the moment the sun comes up the temperature under the plastic will still be a degree or two warmer than outside. This little difference can make a very big difference.

To achieve earlier ripe tomatoes try transplanting already blooming seedlings of a compact determinate variety down the centre of a tunnel cloche; do this a few weeks before the last usual frost date. In Oregon, in order to keep a 1,200 mm width tunnel cloche free of weeds a younger Steve crawled through on hands and knees a couple of times before the plants got too big. Alternatively you can remove the plastic, tidy up the bed and then re-anchor the plastic. (Redpath tunnels are much easier to manage.) To water a short tunnel spray from the ends with hose and nozzle or far better, when the cloche is erected use zipties to attach a 13 mm polypipe to the top of the each hoop and insert micro sprinklers in it. By the end of November determinate tomato vines could be ripening fruit and pushing against the plastic. That's a lot better than growing them without plastic and praying for the first ripe tomato by Christmas. Which has actually happened a couple of times since 1998. Chitted zucchini seeds will germinate in a tunnel cloche a week before the last usual frost (see Chapter 6/chitting and Chapter 9/cucurbits). These will start yielding much sooner than unprotected plants. Remove the cloche when plants begin pushing against the sides or when the harvest begins. Plant pepper seedlings under a cloche when your neighbours transplant tomato seedlings outdoors. Keep them under plastic until the cloche gets too hot on sunny days; the first ripe fruit will arrive weeks earlier.

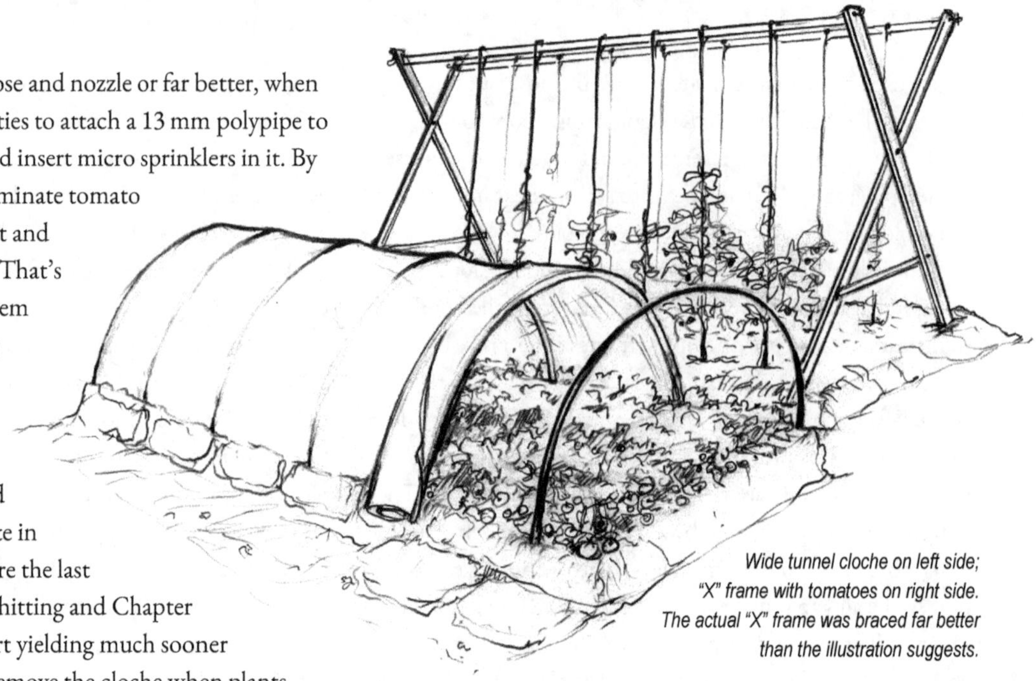

Wide tunnel cloche on left side; "X" frame with tomatoes on right side. The actual "X" frame was braced far better than the illustration suggests.

Even with both ends wide open, a tunnel cloche may get too hot in late spring. Either remove it at this point or else if this plastic is very cheap stuff or at the end of its useful life, cut several 300 mm diameter holes in the top to vent the heat.

Melons and cucumbers, being low growing vines, get a faster start in low wood-box cold frames similar to the ones I suggest for winter greens. However, on sunny days an unvented low cold frame can reach solar-hot-water-heater temperatures. To avoid frying the plants the sashes may have to be removed entirely on warm sunny days and then put back on the frames late in the afternoon. When the vines reach the cloche walls the weather should have settled enough that is safe to entirely remove the cloche and let the vines run.

The need to vent excess heat brings to mind one large plus from having a walk-in polytunnel. In every solar heated enclosure the air temperature at the top is higher than it is at the bottom. During a mild sunny December afternoon an inadequately vented greenhouse or walk-in polytunnel can be 30°C at the soil line, 40°C in the middle and over 50°C at the top. Most vegetables get severely stressed by temperatures approaching 40°C. No matter that you have a 900 mm high tunnel cloche, a box cloche with 250 mm side walls, or a 2.4 metre high greenhouse, top to bottom the temperature extremes will be similar. A 900 mm high tunnel will be too hot for comfort about 450 mm above the soil line; in this cloche low-growing determinate tomato plants spread out just below the hot zone. The lower the cloche is, the more attention must be paid to controlling the temperature. And the higher the cloche (or greenhouse) is the easier it is to keep destructively high temperatures above the level of the plants.

The opposite prevails at night when heat rising from the earth keeps the smaller air space of a low cloche warmer than an unheated greenhouse. This makes low cloches advantageous in winter.

Winter gardening

Unprotected locations close to the West Coast are too rainy and too windy in winter to grow vegetables without a (very stout) polytunnel. Similar story around the Central Highlands lakes where people have fishing shacks. Most other Tasmanian locations below 500 metres elevation do allow a productive unprotected winter garden. I've done soil consulting for a family gardening at over 500 metres elevation on Quamby's Bluff overlooking the Meander Valley. That position is warmer on winter nights and much less often frosty than it is around the nearby town of Meander at 300 metres elevation. I opine that the only thing stopping most Tasmanians from enjoying fresh garden food year-round is lack of desire. Or else perhaps discouragement after having failed previously, most likely from using poorly adapted varieties from mainland seed sellers.

Frost-hardy plants still find winter to be stressful. Harsh rain bruises leaves. Plants use up energy to resist humidity-induced diseases but weak sun and low temperatures greatly reduces sugar manufacture. Adjusting to frost consumes a lot of plant energy. During long overcast periods plants can't produce as much sugar as they must use to stay alive—much less grow—so they draw from their reserves. Endive is a good example of how this works. Endive passes unscathed through a colder than average winter with lower than average rainfall. Frequent sunny winter days provide the opportunity to rebuild food reserves, dry off, maybe even grow a little. Unprotected endive is often worth its bed space in a year like that. However, when the winter has been especially rainy and we don't see the sun for a great many days endive is forced to survive on stored sugar; this lowers its disease resistance. At the same time, moisture is constantly trapped in the dense rosette of thin leaves. The ever-weakening rosette of leaves slowly rots back. That's why endive/escarole make excellent cold-frame candidates. English spinach is similar.

Some varieties of cabbage survive winter because they are wrapped with several layers of extraordinarily tough outer leaves that shed water and protect the head from frost. Besides, it doesn't really matter to the gardener if the outer leaves you strip off anyway show a bit of damage. Kale survives very severe frosts because the cell walls are thick and strong.

Many species prevent their cells from bursting in subfreezing conditions by releasing sugar into their sap and cellular protoplasm. That's why brassicas and chicories taste sweeter after they've been well-frosted a few times. Breeding influences cold tolerance. Salad cabbages are tender because they have thin soft cell walls that easily burst when you chew them. Logically you'd expect freeze-hardy cabbage varieties to be chewy—and they are. As is kale.

In Tasmania it rains a lot most winters; and some winters it just rains and rains and then it rains some more. Most vegetable species die when their roots remain waterlogged for days. The only farm crops I know of that tolerate both waterlogged roots and severe frost are flax and paddock grasses. If the ground has any slope then poor winter drainage can be improved by making raised beds which encourages paths to carry away runoff. Some difficult situations can be fixed with a French drain, which is a narrow slightly sloping ditch up to one metre deep if possible, with a perforated field drain pipe along the bottom. The ditch is filled with drain metal. A French drain can help soggy soil quite a few metres to either side but only if there is somewhere downhill to direct the water.

Winter Salad Cloche & Cold Frame Calendar

Planting date	Harvest Period
Mid April	
looseleaf lettuce mustard greens spinach endive	June/July/Aug
Mid-late May	
looseleaf lettuce mustard greens spinach endive	Aug to Oct
August	
looseleaf lettuce mustard greens spinach bush peas	October
September	
lettuce mustard greens kohhlrabi English spinach broccoli cauliflower cabbage beetroot silverbeet carrots	November

Areas exposed to strong winds can be difficult, winter or summer. Shadecloth windbreaks and/or living windbreaks raise winter temperature considerably and may permit plants to make more growth. The locals call Grindelwald, a hilltop suburb, "windywald" When I lived there I got a lot better result from heat lovers by surrounding their patch with a metre-high barrier made of 900 mm wide 50% shade cloth stapled to strong 1,200 mm long wooden garden stakes. That way my zucchini leaves were not shredded, fruit-laden pepper plants did not have so many branches break, etc.

Winter yield

The fact that light fuels plants explains why a small garden can fully supply the kitchen from November through March. Given enough growing room, only two zucchini plants can overwhelm the household for over two months. And every few days we pick one or two kilos of climbing French beans from three metres of row. Three indeterminate tomato vines cover the laundry bench with ripening fruit during February and March. In fact, unless a lot of summer food is to be preserved or the family is extremely fond of space-hogging pumpkin or sweet corn, only 100 square metres of fertile soil provides a summertime overabundance and fills the freezer and/or a lot of canning jars.

Neither the cold-season vegetables nor the weeds grow much during winter. The winter garden mostly requires harvesting. Winter crops are sown mid- to late summer, grow fast during February and March and continue growing slowly through April. Whatever has pretty much reached full size by May is what gets eaten until spring. Each winter we go through about 10 square metres each of carrot and swede and 2 square metre patches of parsnip, kale and endive. At Grindelwald I always grew 10 square metres of leek; these days we use bulbing onions. I grow 8 brussels sprout plants (3.5 square metres) and a lot of space is assigned to winter cauliflower (10 m^2). We'll eat at least 10 big savoy cabbages (5 m^2) but I try to find room for 15 of them. One hundred heads of loose-leaf lettuce are barely enough between May and September (10 m^2). Add in miscellaneous items like rocket, French sorrel, parsley, Chinese celery, silverbeet and so on, and my winter garden requires 100 square metres of actual growing bed in addition to the land already growing the summer garden. And that's just for two vegetableatarian oldies and their giftees.

Winter gardening techniques

Constant humidity, low light levels, cold and frost weaken plants and make them susceptible to disease. Plants resist winter diseases better when they do not touch each other. Then air moves freely between them, drying them off. When loose-leaf lettuce encounters an unusually warm autumn and *grows too much too soon,* its inner leaves wrap themselves into semi-heads that trap humidity. This is why I see more damage, more rot spots and more decaying leaves during rainy mild winters than in dryish frosty ones. And that's why I sow lettuce every two weeks from mid-March through April; at least some of those sowings will do well. The April sowings might not look like much during winter but I patiently keep the weeds under control, side dress the rows when they start growing again in August and they provide tender salads in spring.

Practicing careful hygiene helps the winter garden avoid diseases and reduces the number of snails and slugs. Promptly transfer all trim, stumps and decaying materials to the compost area. Thin winter crops carefully so as to increase airflow around them and try to keep as yet unharvested areas thoroughly weeded.

Plants that haven't been pushed to grow extremely fast tolerate winter conditions better. Don't side-dress winter crops after mid-March so that the level of available nutrients drops by mid-May. Kelp meal is included in COF; it contains hormones and phytamins that make a plant more cold-tolerant. If you can afford the cost it is smart to mix in twice the amount of kelpmeal the recipe calls for when blending complete organic fertilizer for winter crops. Some gardeners spray liquid kelp every few weeks during autumn and continue to spray kelp during sunny spells in winter.

Winter varieties

Some lettuce varieties survive several degrees more frost than others. Some handle high humidity and moisture-induced diseases better. All brassicas tolerate mild frost; a few brassica varieties bred for English and Dutch winters can survive –14°C. I once trialled a brussels sprout variety in Oregon with an extraordinarily high fibre content; it survived one –15°C night but it tasted like cardboard.

The biggest obstacle to succeeding with winter crops arises from using seed sourced from mainland suppliers. Only a few mainlanders gardening at high elevations have reason to seek maximally frost hardy winter varieties. There are many reasons for English and Cascadian growers to want them. Chapter 6, "Seeds." has much to say about this. And Chapter 9 will mention specific winter varieties. If the variety is not available in Australia then the overseas source will be mentioned.

Chapter 5

Water

Drouth is said to be the arch enemy of the dry-farmer, but few agree upon its meaning. For [the purpose of]. . . *this volume, drouth may be defined as a condition under which crops fail to mature because of an insufficient supply of water. Providence has generally been charged with causing drouths, but under the above definition, man is usually the cause. Occasionally, relatively dry years occur, but they are seldom dry enough to cause crop failures if proper methods of farming have been practised. There are four chief causes of drouth: (1) Improper or careless preparation of the soil; (2) failure to store the natural precipitation in the soil; (3) failure to apply proper cultural methods for keeping the moisture in the soil until needed by plants, and (4) sowing too much seed for the available soil-moisture.*

John A. Widtsoe, ***Dry Farming**** (emphasis by Steve Solomon)

This chapter explains how the plant population density that you choose determines how often irrigation must be done. An extensive garden on deep soil that has some clay in it may need a thorough watering only once a week. An intensive garden might yield more from the space involved but it requires watering almost every day in summer. On deep moisture-retentive heavy loam or clay you can dry garden, a method requiring very little irrigation or none at all. However, dry gardening yields less per square metre. This chapter also explains how to construct an irrigation *system* that conveniently spreads water and does it uniformly.

A gardener's textbook of sprinkler irrigation

When it rains hard or when the irrigation system spreads water as fast as or faster than the soil can assimilate it then the soil's pore spaces temporarily fill up with water. Air is temporarily driven out of them. That's a good thing when airlessness only lasts a short time because soil air contains less oxygen and more carbon dioxide than the air does above ground. This CO_2 was exhaled by the microecology and plant roots. When the moisture inflow stops, excess water drains from the pore spaces and fresh oxygen-rich air gets pulled back in. Then plants grow better for awhile because oxygen in the soil acts like fertilizer.

Not all the moisture drains away; much of it *adheres* to soil particles in much the same way a balloon charged with static electricity sticks on a wall. To see adhesion at work dip a stone into water and then remove it. A few drops may fall off and then the wet rock stops dripping. If this rock were a soil particle then the amount of water adhering to its surface at the moment dripping ceases is its *full capacity* to hold water.

Plant roots extract moisture with very little effort when the soil is at full capacity. As soil dries the film of water adhering to its particles gets thinner, and as the water film thins it takes more energy for plants to extract that moisture. I call this plant effort *moisture stress.* Moisture stress slows growth; moisture stress is something the gardener wants to minimize. Strong moisture stress makes lettuce taste bitter. If a moisture-stressed cauliflower manages to form a good head then it will be harsh-tasting and lack crispness. Water-short zucchini become dry, pithy and sometimes bitter; moisture stressed cucumbers often are bitter. Moisture-stressed pumpkin vines don't set as many fruit and they'll be smaller and much less tasty. Radishes become pungent, dry and pithy.

Most kinds of vegetables wilt when they fail to extract enough soil moisture to keep up with the amount being lost in strong sunshine. Wilting is a self protective action that reduces moisture loss because drooping leaves no longer catch as much sunlight. The plants restore themselves after the day cools down or if the sun goes behind clouds; they may look okay the next morning. Actually, temporary wilting is a huge stress that slows future growth, maybe permanently.

Some crops store water in a fleshy root—lettuce, endive, parsley, radish, rocket, silverbeet, beetroot, parsnip, carrot and coriander. The allium family stores a lot of water in thick juicy leaves. By drawing from reserves these species may pass through a moisture deficit without wilting—but carrot and radish soon become tough and bitter; parsley stops making new leaves, onion stops growing, etc. No wonder gardeners quickly learn to fear dry soil.

If the garden is important to your family's health and economy then it is crucial to minimize moisture stress by irrigating it. But an irrigation *system* suitable for market gardening is not necessary if you discover with a simple test how fast and how uniformly ordinary lawn and garden sprinklers spread water.

Systematic watering

Wetting down the garden with hose and nozzle works quite well if you always enjoy the task. But if you don't relish the occasion then it is likely the garden gets watered too briefly. Even if the garden is watered every day—but always too briefly—starting 100 millimetres below the damp surface layer the bed may have been sucked bone dry. The plants never actually wilt because they're sustained by surface moisture but bone-dry soil below is not useful root zone. The gardener wonders why they grow so slowly and look stunted.

To avoid this possibility, John Jeavons recommends repeatedly directing the nozzle's spray back and forth across several square metres of bed (area A) until the entire surface sparkles, becomes shiny wet. The shine persists until most of the moisture has flowed deeper. Spreading even more water before the surface pore spaces drain would only have it run off the bed. Rather than wasting water and risk washing away topsoil, move on to the next few square metres (area B) and continue on B until that section gets sparkly and then return to A until the shine reappears on A, and then back to B until the shine reappears, repeating this pattern until the sparkling shine lasts long enough. The first shine may only last a second or so but as moisture percolates in deeper the shine appears sooner and lasts longer. How long do you want the shine to persist?

Jeavons suggests initially trying different shiny times combined with digging some test holes to see how deeply the soil had become saturated. Without this check, gross overwatering or underwatering could be the result. The desired shiny time only has to be determined once. It will be from one second to ten seconds depending on soil type.

Clayey soil holds a great deal of moisture but assimilates it slowly. So clay can show a sparkly surface for many seconds whilst still being quite dry 10 centimetres down. On the other hand, *coarse* sands take in water so rapidly it can be difficult to get a shine to appear on one no matter how fast water is put down—but sand gets leached when water passes through it. Tasmanian *fine* sands repel water when they get dry on the surface. I'll soon explain how to irrigate hydrophobic soils.

In my first year of backyard gardening I hand watered exactly as Jeavons suggested. It worked well enough but I have always grown a large garden and at that time I had a business to manage. So I switched to a sprinkler system that achieved a similar result without consuming my time.

Available moisture (mm of water per 30 cm of soil)*

Soil type	Available moisture
Sandy	8 mm to 30 mm
Medium (loam)	30 mm to 60 mm
Clayey	60 mm to 90 mm

** After the soil has delivered its available moisture, it has dried to the permanent wilting point. Vegetables experience moisture stress well before the soil has dried to the point plants die because there is no more available moisture.*

A wet to dry scale

	Soil moisture remaining
Totally dry	0%
Permanent wilting point	20-33%
Temporary wilting point	50%
Minimum moisture for intensive vegetable beds	70%
Field capacity	100%

Amount of water needed to bring 30 cm of soil from 70 percent to full capacity

Soil type	Irrigation in mm
Sandy	4 mm to 15 mm
Medium (loam)	15 mm to 30 mm
Clayey	30 mm to 45 mm

Summertime soil moisture loss*

Type of climate	Loss per day
Cool climate (Tasmania, sunny, under 25°)	4 mm
Cool climate (Tasmania, sunny, over 25°)	6 mm
Hot humid climate (Brisbane)	8 mm
Hot dry climate (Hobart, +40°, breezy)	11 mm

** Assuming the soil is covered by a dense leaf canopy*

How much water?

Sprinkler irrigation became the usual thing in the early Twentieth Century. Moisture stress became conveniently preventable. In response, plant breeders redesigned vegetables to grow quicker above ground at the expense of root development. This brings about larger harvests sooner—as long as the soil is kept moist. That's why many modern vegetable varieties, be they hybrids or open-pollinated, only grow well when soil is comfortably moist. So be guided by this vegie gardening principle: *once the topsoil has dried to about 70 percent of its total capacity to hold moisture it should be brought back to capacity again.* I'll soon explain how to gauge that conveniently.

Moisture in the top 600 mm of an average sand soil that is supporting a full leaf canopy can go from full capacity to 70 percent of capacity in two mild sunny summer days. A garden on sand may need topping up after only one hot breezy day. A clayey soil similarly covered with a crop canopy loses the same amount of moisture every day but this garden could be watered every seven days, and you'd spread much more water with each irrigation.

Small seedlings feed in the top 15 cm. For these, when moisture in the surface 15 cm has dropped to 70 percent of capacity, then spread half the amount of water recommended in the table called "Amount of water needed to bring a 30 cm layer of soil from 70 percent of capacity to full capacity." When the crop is two months old (after one month if the vegetable makes a tap root) the root system can reach down 60 cm, even deeper if subsoil conditions permit. Before two months pass the crop should form a dense leaf canopy that transpires a lot of moisture. At this stage replace about 10 percent more than the "Summertime soil moisture loss" according to the table on the previous page.

Soil moisture should be measured 100 mm below the surface by using the ready-to-till test. Squeeze a small handful of soil into a ball. If the ball feels wet, gooey, or sticks together solidly then the soil moisture is well over 70 percent, unless it is sand; sand won't form a ball no matter how hard you squeeze. If the ball sticks together firmly but breaks apart easily in your hand by pressing it with a thumb then moisture is around 70 percent. If a solid ball won't form then moisture is below 65 percent.

Daily moisture loss varies with the season. How much loss depends upon light intensity, temperature, wind speed, humidity and the amount of leaf cover. The scientific name for this loss is "evapotranspiration;" the word means evaporation from the soil's surface plus transpiration from leaves. Much more moisture transpires from the leaves of a half-grown crop than evaporates from bare soil.

A Tasmanian soil that is covered by growing plants loses 25 mm to 30 mm of moisture through evapotranspiration each average sunny week during December. During January and much of February, water loss ranges from 30 mm to 40 mm per week. Moisture loss can exceed 8 mm in one hot day with low humidity and a bit of breeze. In late February and the first half of March moisture losses slows to 20 mm to 25 mm per week. By April the loss is so small that the surface may remain moist for a few days after being irrigated.

I usually determine when and how much to irrigate without actually testing soil moisture. I assume moisture loss is about what the table on the previous page says it will be and periodically spread 10 percent more than that amount, less any rain received since the last irrigation. I also assume that on overcast days the soil loses about half as much moisture as when the sun shines.

The Bottom Line

Sandy soil supporting advanced crops should be given 12 mm of water every two days in average sunny summer weather. Sandy soil growing young plants (with shallow root systems) should be given 6 mm every morning if the previous day had been warm and sunny.

Clayey soils supporting advanced crops can accept up to 40 mm of water without being leached. This much every five or six days in summer is enough, except when outback mainland dust blows across the Bass Strait or when it goes over 40 degrees.

Some parts of the garden require almost daily light irrigation in hot sunny weather. This includes beds germinating seeds or growing small seedlings and beds growing species with unusually high moisture requirements such as radishes and celery. These extra needs are best supplied with hose and nozzle.

Designing systems

Lawn sprinklers spread water thick and fast because sod facilitates rapid moisture penetration. And quick seems convenient. But how *uniformly* do lawn sprinklers spread water? And how much time does your sprinkler have to run in order to spread a predetermined amount? Before irrigating a vegie garden with a lawn sprinkler please discover its application rate and uniformity of distribution. Position a few irrigation rate measuring gauges—empty tin cans or straight-sided drinking glasses—in the sprinkler's coverage area and operate the sprinkler for exactly one hour when the wind is light to non-existent. Position a gauge one metre from the sprinkler, put another one metre inside the far limit of its throw and a couple more in between. After the hour has finished measure the depth of water in each container, average those amounts and you know the sprinkler's *application rate per hour.*

In my experience, lawn sprinklers that cover a large circle spread more than 25 mm per hour. Some oscillating sprinklers, the sort that cover a rectangle, spread moisture at least that fast and others spread half that much per hour. Spot sprinklers and perforated hoses that spray water a metre or two high and to both sides usually put out an even higher rate. Have you ever seen water flowing down the street because a suburbanite has been overwatering their lawn? How much leaching do you suppose happens to a food garden when this sort of sprinkler runs longer than necessary?

The tin can test reveals how uniformly the sprinkler spreads water. Are all the containers filled equally, or typically, are the ones closer to the sprinkler holding considerably more water than those at the outer third of its coverage?

The most uniform distribution comes from agricultural sprinklers and especially from turbine-driven sprinklers designed for lawns and surrounds of commercial and institutional buildings. These initially cost more than consumer stuff but durability makes them less costly in the long haul. Find this kind of gear at an irrigation supplier; Tasmania has more than a few. The few privately owned hardware shops that are still in business and the big box home supply centres all sell impact sprinklers *resembling* the ones used by farmers but these usually have high application rates and low durability. I suggest you buy agricultural crop sprinklers from an irrigation supplier that can provide optional nozzle sizes and a range of sprinkler sizes. I'll soon explain why for vegie crops you'll want small sprinklers and small bore nozzles.

Every sprinkler is designed to operate at a limited range of water pressures. There are very small sprinklers with very small nozzles that work at 70 kpa (10 psi). They don't throw water more than a few metres. You can put one of these under each tree when establishing seedling fruit trees. These aren't for vegie gardens. Low output crop sprinklers suited to home gardens and smaller market gardens require 140 kpa (20 psi) to 200 kpa (30 psi). Farm-sized ones usually need at least 200 kpa and do better with more pressure than that. To roughly check the water pressure at the garden tap, see how far a common adjustable hose nozzle set to make a strong smooth jet can throw water. It should exceed 10 metres in a windless moment if your water pressure is around 200 kpa.

A sprinkler nozzle best suited for vegetable gardens should emit between four and eight litres per minute. To discover how many sprinklers a tap can supply at one time, measure how many seconds it takes to fill a 20 litre bucket through a full length of garden hose with an adjustable nozzle on it putting out its strongest, longest-throwing stream. The hose nozzle mimics the back pressure from an array of sprinkler nozzles. Before building a system that requires the entire amount the tap puts out, first see if the flow rate lessens greatly when someone in the house uses water while the bucket is filling. Maybe the irrigation system should be designed so as to not require the entire flow. Or perhaps it is possible organize a larger water supply.

Agricultural sprinklers usually accept a range of nozzle sizes. Farmer-sized sprinkler nozzles typically throw water 20 metres. Some *really* big sprinklers with a firehose nozzle can spray dairy manure slurry over a circle 50 metres and more in radius. Sprinklers suitable for vegetable crops use nozzles between 1.0 mm and 3.0 mm. A 1.5 mm nozzle can be expected to throw around 7 metres; a 3 mm nozzle throws 10 metres. Small nozzles like that are better for growing vegies because (1) they put out finer droplets that cause less soil compaction, and (2) a shorter throw radius helps keep the water off adjoining buildings and out of the neighbour's yard. Please avoid big sprinklers! The large droplets they throw hit the ground with enough impact to break up soil crumbs. Then silt and clay float to the surface where they form a smooth crust; this happens much the same way

Application rates from various nozzle sizes

Nozzle bore in mm	Operating pressure in PSI	Discharge in litres/minute	Throw in metres	Spacing in metres	Application in mm per hour
1.7	30	4	7	6 x 6	3
1.7	60	6	8	6 x 6	5
2.5	30	7.5	10	6 x 6	12
2.5	60	11	11	6 x 6	15
5	30	27	12	7 x 8	25
5	60	38	14	7 x 8	32
8	30	75	18	12 x 18	18
8	60	105	22	12 x 18	25

screeding concrete lifts the fines to form a smooth skin. Crust formation is the last thing you want; it blocks germinating seeds and stops air exchange. Crusts rarely form on sand but sandy soil is easy to overwater when the application rate is high. Use small nozzles!

Application rates ranging from 6 mm per hour to 15 mm per hour are ideal for food gardens. The best way to achieve that for a large garden is by having several uniformly spaced small nozzles running at the same time. Small nozzles have downpoints. Wind, especially when there also is strong sunlight, can evaporate much of a thin water stream before it hits the ground. This means that small nozzles should be used early in the morning.

A clay soil could be watered from bedtime to breakfast without leaching the root zone if the application rate is 3 mm per hour. Watering at night is reputed to cause disease. Actually, watering *all night* prevents disease by continuously washing bacteria and fungus spores off the plants before they can germinate. This principle is well understood by nurseries that root cuttings by frequent misting them. What *can* harm plants is to stop watering around nightfall. This makes plants damp all night—ideal conditions for the multiplication of disease organisms.

For sand or light loam soils, design a system that spreads 4 mm to 6 mm per hour so that the previous two day's moisture loss can be restored in the morning before the sun gets strong and the wind comes up. For hydrophobic soils an application rate of 4 mm per hour will not make water run off the surface.

Oscillating lawn sprinklers with a rectangular pattern usually spread water less uniformly than most circular-pattern sprinklers. I suspect the reason is that the device that pivots the spray arm pauses when reversing, putting too much water at the ends of its pattern and too little above the sprinkler itself. Own one already? You can find out for yourself what it does with a few empty tin cans and 60 minutes.

It is impossible to design an impact sprinkler that spreads water *uniformly* over an entire circle because to achieve that it must deposit nine times more water over the farther part of its throw than near the centre. And every point in between must get a different amount. To fully appreciate that please study the caption below the illustration on this page. Another reason the impact sprinkler doesn't spread water uniformly is that the rocker arm interrupting the water jet deposits a lot of water close to the sprinkler. Some consumer-grade impact sprinklers come with a diffuser flap or an adjustable screw to shorten the throw radius by diffusing the spray. But diffusing the nozzle's stream makes it throw even less water to the fringes and even more water close in. The more the stream is interfered with the worse this effect becomes. Agricultural impulse sprinklers do not have diffusers; they come with precision nozzles that if operated within the designed pressure range put down only twice as much water near the centre.

Market gardeners obtain uniform coverage from impact sprinklers by positioning them in an overlapping pattern—sometimes in a square pattern, sometimes hexagonal. Overlapping sprinklers even out water distribution because the heavily watered area near one sprinkler is also covered by the lightly watered area of other sprinklers. The hex arrangement distributes water slightly more uniformly but the square pattern works better in a backyard when the garden is close to buildings or where the sprinklers could throw water on the neighbour's property.

High-angle sprinklers throw a greater distance. These should be positioned no farther apart than 65 percent (2/3) of their throw radius. This allows for (light) wind blowing the spray. Low-angle sprinklers are less affected by wind. These can be positioned at 75 percent of their throw radius. The liability from using closer than recommended spacing is buying more sprinklers; the positive side of this is achieving a higher application rate without larger droplets.

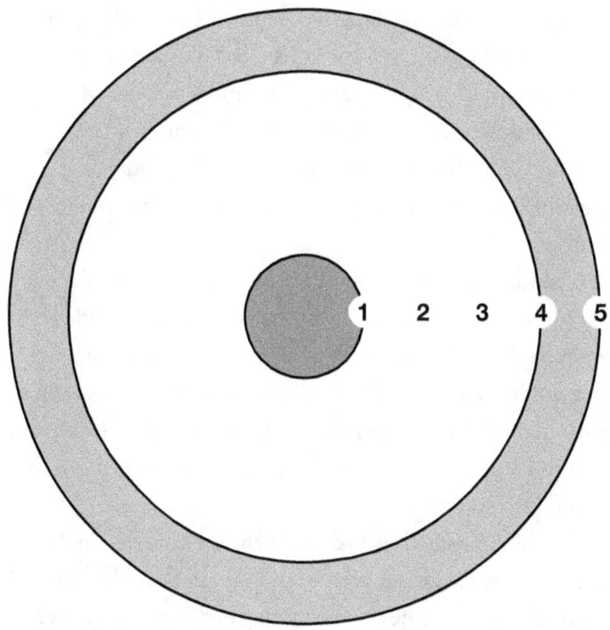

The formula to calculate the area of a circle is: Area = 3.14 x radius². Please imagine that water is being spread by a sprinkler having a 5 metre throw radius. The one metre radius circle located at the centre of the sprinkler pattern has an area of 3.14 square metres (3.14 x 1 x 1). The area of a one-metre-wide ring at the limit of coverage is around 28 square metres, calculated this way: the area of the full circle [3.14 x 5 x 5] minus the area in the inner 4 metres of the pattern [3.14 x 4 x 4]. Thus the nozzle must deposit roughly nine times as much water over the outermost metre of the pattern to end up with the same thickness of coverage as it spreads near the centre.

Any multiple sprinkler pattern still leaves a dryish fringe where fewer overlaps occur. On the farm, throwing some water beyond the field is unimportant; in the backyard it may be essential to keep all the water within your own yard and/or off your own windows.

Farm-sized impulse sprinklers usually point the water stream about 12° above horizontal to achieve a greater throw distance. These high-angle sprinklers normally have substantial nozzles so they're less affected by wind. High-angle sprinklers with small nozzles can produce a very low rate of application that allows a clay soil to be irrigated all night. I'll soon tell you about when I had to do that.

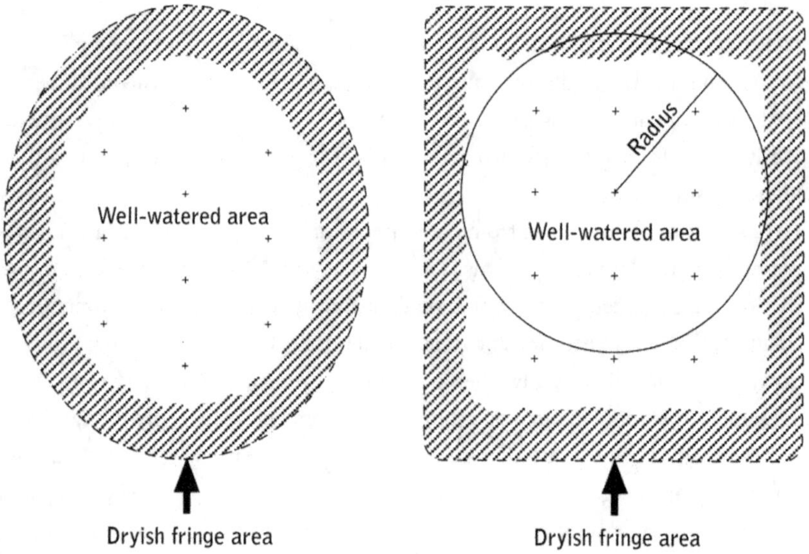

Using several correctly spaced sprinklers creates overlapping water patterns, permitting uniform coverage. The optimal spacing between sprinklers is about 60-70 percent of the sprinkler's throw radius. (Left side) Sprinklers arranged in triangular patterns. (Right side) Sprinklers correctly overlapped, arranged in square patterns.

Some gardeners avoid spreading water outside the garden by using part-circle impact sprinklers. I disagree for several reasons. Cutting an impact sprinkler's arc in half doubles its rate of application; cutting it to a quarter-circle quadruples the rate of application. Impact sprinklers spread water even less uniformly in part-circle mode because the rocker-arm's rapid reversing action drops a great deal of water closer to the sprinkler. Part circle impact sprinklers come with another downside: actuating the reversing mechanism requires considerable force; this means a large-bore nozzle putting out a powerful stream with high application rates and larger droplets.

Another way to reduce the arc of a full-circle sprinkler is to position a shield attached to a garden stake pounded in immediately behind it. The shield can be made from a cut-out tin can or half of a small plastic bucket. This method does not increase the application rate nor lessen uniformity of distribution—except that all the water it intercepts is dumped behind the sprinkler.

Turbine powered sprinklers are an advanced design. I think they spread water as uniformly as can be achieved from a single sprinkler. The slowly rotating nozzle head is powered by an internal propeller. Multiple water jets emerge from one rotating head. One jet points high so it covers the outermost part; other jets spread water closer in. Some emitter holes diffuse their stream; others make a rather smooth stream. The end result is uniform coverage. I think the best turbine sprinkler for vegie gardening is Nelson's "MP Rotator." It allows adjustment of the throw angle (distance thrown). The sprinkler also can be adjusted to spread over a full circle or part of a circle without increasing the precipitation rate the way part circle impact sprinklers do.

Agricultural sprinklers only distribute water properly when they are operated at a specific range of pressures. If water pressure is too low then the nozzle emits a very clean smooth stream that puts down too little water in the mid-zone. If operated at excess pressure the water jet becomes too turbulent which actually shortens the throw while greatly increasing the amount laid down close to the sprinkler. This makes the fringes too dry. Overpressure also shortens the sprinkler's life.

I urge all gardeners to visit an irrigation shop, spend some time; handle the bits sold there; study the charts and tables and see if all the pieces don't fall into place.

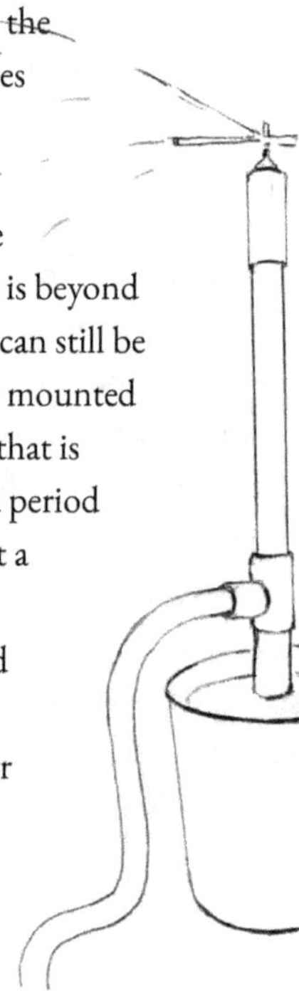

If a permanent multi-element sprinkler system that waters the entire garden or a large part of it at one time is beyond your budget, then uniform irrigation can still be accomplished with only one sprinkler mounted on a one-metre-tall homemade stand that is supplied by a hose. It is run for a fixed period in each position you'd would have put a dozen sprinklers had you been able to afford them. I watered Territorial Seed Company's trials ground this way for the first few years. I made the sprinkler stand with one sack of concrete, a 20 litre plastic bucket, 13 mm galvanized iron pipe and fittings.

Drip

From 1980 through 1986 I had to supply my house, irrigate a half-acre variety trials ground and water the family's 500 square metre kitchen garden—all from a 12 litre per minute bore. Twelve litres per minute can't supply even one sprinkler nozzle large enough to be used when the sun is hot and a breeze is blowing. So as soon as I could afford to I switched the trials ground to drip tapes—lightweight plastic hoses with a pinhole emitter every 300 mm. I'll soon tell you more about that disappointing bore and the lessons it taught me.

I came to know way too much about drip—and here's the downsides. Drip tapes are expensive even when purchased in farm-sized spools but at that time I did not mind how much my trials ground cost to operate—it was producing priceless information that made everyone's garden grow better. There were more downpoints. I'd accidentally cut driplines whilst hoeing. Then I'd have to replace the line with a crop already growing over it, not so easy to accomplish sometimes. All the emitter holes must face upward or they may become plugged but drip tape twists and rotates as it expands and contracts with changes in temperature. To minimize rotation and keep the water on young seedlings the drip tapes must be pinned firmly to the earth every few metres of run; and even so, many of the fine vertical streams of water still point to the side as much as straight up. Although I filtered the water supply to remove any particle that could plug an emitter hole, every emitter on every line still had to be checked each and every time a line was turned on because an emitter could be blocked by soil that was sucked back into the opening when the water was last shut off.

Drip tapes, individual drip emitters and soaker hoses do not suit sand because in sand most of the water goes straight down rather than wicking out horizontally which leaves areas of dry soil. The only way around this on sand is to lay parallel drip lines 300 mm apart with emitters 300 mm apart; doing that is costly and interferes with hoeing. If the soil is a medium loam or clay then water wicks out horizontally as much as 600 mm to either side of the drip line. Highly UV-resistant (long-lasting) driplines might be useful for permanent plantings such as raspberries, but given a large enough water supply I'd always choose sprinklers.

Microirrigation is a hybrid system supplied by black flexible poly pipes (like drip). The sprinklers are supported on inexpensive plastic spikes. The miniature sprinklers throw two metres at best with emission rates of a few litres per hour from each nozzle, not a few litres per minute. They are designed to operate at 70 kpa (10 psi). Microirrigation provides an inexpensive way to establish orchards, vineyards, and for watering narrow ornamental beds around houses. I mentioned already that I have used them in tunnel cloches. Microirrigation parts are bubble packed by the tens or dozens at garden centres and big box shops but you'll find a broader range at irrigation shops. If you're considering microirrigation don't assume the rate of application is low. Each micro sprinkler emits very little water but the nozzle doesn't throw far. And use an effective line filter! The nozzles are miniscule.

Gardening without much water: dry gardening

Irrigation makes all garden vegetables grow better. Radish, celery and Chinese cabbage and most cauliflower varieties only thrive in always-moist soil. Irrigation increases yield and often increases quality. Irrigation always makes the outcome more certain.

But many country Tasmanians depend upon rain water capture tanks or irrigate with dam water and must ration water in summer. These folks could practice "dry gardening."

How I got interested in dry-gardening

It was a few weeks before planting out tomato seedlings. My age was 36. I had just settled on a five acre Oregon homestead near Lorane, a community similar to Golden Valley, Tasmania—similar in population density, similar in distance from shops, similar in climate and similar in spirit. We'd come there by way of Los Angeles where I had spent the previous seven years saving up barely enough money to get settled free-and-clear. We moved on to the property early in May (Northern Hemisphere mid-spring). In that month the Lorane Valley is covered with green grass punctuated by liquid sunshine and rainbows. New to a territory reputed for rainy weather, I thought the grass would stay green all summer. I was wrong.

I intended to produce as much of my own food as possible, raise some kind of as-yet-to-be-determined (legal) crop to pay the bills, live simply so as to need less cash. Because I had horticultural ambitions my offer to purchase was subject to first drilling a bore delivering at least 1 litre per second. The fourth drilling attempt (and what I vowed would be the final attempt at finding a good yielding bore because I was paying) brought in slightly more than my minimum required flow. But—I was drilling in spring; I didn't appreciate the implications of that.

I finalized the purchase, returned to Los Angeles to sell up and pack, we returned, moved into a large tent, spread crushed rock on the driveway, put in septic tank, power pole and soon hauled in a new single-wide mobile home—not the rustic dream home we'd wanted but this oversized caravan was instant free-and-clear shelter. I immediately built a tool/firewood shed with space for a workbench. We had enough money left to live for two years if nothing major went wrong.

My first priority was establishing a 500 square metre food garden. I hadn't yet been properly educated about soil fertility so I spread sawdusty horse manure, aglime and cottonseedmeal, hired a neighbour who did custom tilling, erected a wildlife fence (many many deer around Lorane) and assembled an excessively permanent irrigation system using ten small agricultural all brass impulse sprinklers with 1.7 mm nozzles; each one emitted a bit under 4 litres per minute, arranged in a pattern that uniformly spread about 5 mm per hour over the entire garden.

I expected that 60 litre per minute bore would supply those ten sprinklers and allow minor household use at the same time. So all ten sprinklers were turned on and off by one valve. I used galvanized pipes for supply lines and risers because I expected I would be living there for the rest of my life. Wrong again!

Summer arrived. Those lush green paddocks quickly browned off. It hadn't rained a drop for two weeks. I didn't yet realize that Oregon summer normally means warm sunny days and zero rain for the next three months. My garden needed irrigating for the first time. So I twisted the valve and stood outside the garden gate admiring ten little impact sprinklers bouncing out crisscrossing streams, psit, psit, psit. But after a few minutes the pump shut down. Not yet knowing much about Oregon Coast Range bores and how they typically declined (and sometimes completely dried up) in summer, I spent a few hours repeatedly repriming and restarting the pump before I realized that the pump kept shutting off because the bore's static level was being sucked down below the intake point. My 60 litre per minute bore now produced under 40 litres per minute.

In response, I ran fewer sprinkler heads at one time. I was profoundly fretting—was I drawing from an underground stream that diminished in summer like most above-ground streams but would not disappear—or would it dry up altogether? Would my horticultural ambitions be thwarted? Had we purchased a property that could not even feed us? By mid summer the bore could supply only three sprinklers. Fortunately, that was its minimum output. By running three sprinklers all night I could cover the entire garden in three nights. Pfew!

Two years later that pitiful bore was called upon to also supply Territorial Seed Company's half acre trials ground. Initially I watered the trials with a single high-angle 10 litre per-minute impact sprinkler mounted on a home-made stand fed by a hose, just like the stand illustrated on page 78. I'd start up the sprinkler about 8 pm, wake by alarm clock at 2 am, stumble barefoot down the cold dewy path, move the sprinkler to its next regular position, wipe off my wet feet, go back to bed, awaken at first light and shut the system down at 8:00 am so the household could have morning showers. This happened four to five nights a week; on the remaining summer nights the water went to the kitchen garden. No wonder when the seed business could afford drip I started using it. With drip I could irrigate the trials in the daytime and generously water the kitchen garden at night.

A few years after starting Territorial Seeds I had to replace the bore pump. Those kinds of things often happen at the worst possible moment; the bore pump failed during the hottest part of summer; it took more than one week to get my water system working again. After just a few days without water our John Jeavons style intensive kitchen garden began to suffer. The widely spaced plants in the trials ground showed no sign of moisture stress after one week. That experience forced me to confront how tenuous my food production system actually was. I became curious: how did the Oregon Territory's early settlers manage to grow gardens in a climate where most summers meant no rain during the entire frost-free growing season?

Garden books written before the 1970s prescribed arranging vegetable crops single file in long rows, the row centres 900 mm to 1,200 mm apart with narrow foot paths between rows. Pre-World War II gardeners in many Tasmanian towns did not have reticulated water and expected to go through long rainless periods by depending upon rainwater capture tanks—and in those days household water tanks were smaller than they are now. So irrigation was doled out. Even dirty dishwater grew vegetables. Blessedly, drought does not necessarily start after a few weeks without rain. John Widtsoe, whose wise words begin this chapter, defines drought as beginning when the crop is severely damaged. The onset of drought has little to do with how much time elapses between rains; it has everything to do with how much water the soil naturally makes available to plants and upon how wisely the grower manages that moisture.

Back to Oregon: I discovered an old guy growing unirrigated carrots on deep alluvial sandy loam in the hottest part of southern Oregon; this is also the district with the least annual rainfall and absolutely no hope of summer rain, like how Bothwell relates to the rest of Tasmania. He sowed carrot seed in spring when the topsoil was still moist enough to germinate it. He soon thinned to 30 cm apart in the row; the rows were 1,200 mm apart. He gave his carrots no irrigation but they grew to enormous sizes, remained quite edible all summer, and the overall yield per area occupied by the crop was not as low as you might expect.

I found further hints in a book by Gary Nabahan called *The Desert Smells Like Rain,* which describes Native Americans growing unirrigated desert gardens (very hot climate) in positions where deep loamy soil soaks up runoff from a brief period of reliable seasonal rains. They used extraordinarily wide interplant spacing. I read about how native South Americans in the Andean highlands grow food crops in a cool, low-humidity environment that gets only 300 mm of annual rain. And I discovered John Widstoe. His book is in the Soil and Health Library for free download.

My first unirrigated summertime vegetable happened by accident—or was I being Guided? I had sold Territorial Seed Company and moved to 16 acres of Oregon's best riverside alluvial silty clay loam located near Elkton, which is a small town in the area possessing Oregon's best climate. I had plant breeding in mind. My first project was to make a productive open-pollinated late savoy cabbage variety out of a hybrid because savoy cabbage was our family staple but the only remaining open-pollinated variety, Chieftain Savoy, had hugely degenerated.

I knew that rain on seed crops that are drying down lowered seed germination and vigour. So during winter I dug up six fully-headed Savoy King hybrid cabbages which is a productive variety similar to Chieftain in most respects and transplanted them into a bed located well beyond my sprinkler system's reach. Big savoys are usually grown on positions 60 cm x 60 cm, sometimes 60 cm x 75 cm if you want really large heads, but for seed making I spaced them 120 cm x 120 cm because blooming brassicas make huge sprays of flower stalks. I did not intend to water these plants at all because cabbage seed forms during late spring while the soil is still naturally moist.

Seeds developed, it all went as I'd hoped, but one plant did something I didn't anticipate—it started forming a new cabbage among its seed stalks. I watched this unwatered cabbage enlarge steadily through the hottest and driest summer I had yet experienced in Oregon. I felt I was being shown something important so I gave the plant no water for the rest of the summer although I did eliminate all weeds after I removed the seed stalks. At maturity the full-sized head was as sweet and as tender as any other of its type when given all the water it could use.

Because Nabahan's book emphasized the extreme plant spacing used by desert gardeners and because I knew about those dry farmed carrots, that unwatered cabbage Spoke! Next spring I dry gardened a pair of 30 metre long rows with 1,500 mm between the row centres and even more bare land than that to either side. Early in spring the rows had been fertilized with COF that was rotary cultivated into them. In-the-row spacing was extreme. I tried an assortment of vegetables that I hoped could cope. I pretended it was the year 1866; that I had settled on a homestead without a spring uphill of the garden. I'd try to garden with absolutely no irrigation; I'd start everything in spring whilst there was still enough soil moisture to germinate the seeds.

I grew olraecea kale, Savoy King cabbage, purple sprouting broccoli, carrot, beetroot, parsnip, parsley, swede endive, shelling beans, potato, French sorrel, and sweet corn. I also transplanted one compact determinate bush tomato plant and one sprawling indeterminate tomato plant. (Each tomato seedling did get one cup of water when transplanted.) The tomatoes produced extraordinarily good tasting fruit until the end of summer although they were smaller than their usual size and had thicker skins. Kale, Savoy King cabbage and parsley grew fine. Purple Sprouting broccoli looked gnarly and stressed at summer's end but it grew lushly once the rains returned in autumn, got enormous during winter and produced abundantly the next spring. The potatoes yielded half their usual amount, with thicker than usual skins that stored better. They also had a richer flavour. I found out later that potatoes grown dry often have more protein. The enormous carrots were chewy but tasted fine. There was a semi-failure—the swedes (intended as winter food) had too much growing time. They were huge by mid-summer and became inedible before autumn.

The following year I grew two complete gardens side by side, each garden occupied 700 square metres. The insurance garden was irrigated so that no matter what came of my dry-gardening experiments we would still have plenty to eat. The dry garden received the absolute minimum of water. Since I was living by a small river, I'd direct my pioneer spirit to transport 200 litres per day—seven trips to and from the river every day using a shoulder yoke holding two buckets. That seemed barely doable. So I made that yoke and actually carried those two heavy water buckets—a few times. But it wasn't really Armageddon and hauling water that way took a lot of time and energy so I henceforth I allowed the dry garden no more than 200 litres of borewater per day.

By midsummer some unirrigated vegies were severely moisture-stressed. I recalled reading a report of an 1882 dry farming experiment wherein it took 1,100 pounds of water to grow one pound of dry plant matter on poor soil but only 575 pounds of water to produce that same amount of plant matter on fertile land. I wondered if my plants might need less moisture if they had better nutrition. So I tried foliar-feeding a broad-spectrum chemical fertilizer (similar to Miracle Gro). Within days I could see it helped a lot. I reasoned that the fertilized topsoil had become too dry to feed the plants; the still moist subsoil in this new garden plot was still extremely short of plant nutrients. So I improvised a subsoil fertigator. Next to some of the plants (and not others) I placed a 20 litre white plastic bucket with one- 6 mm diameter hole drilled in its side just above the bottom. The bucket was filled with the same solution that I had foliar sprayed. After the bucket had emptied there was a dessert plate sized wet spot on the surface. The fertigation mostly went straight down. I gave the lucky plants another such drink three weeks later. Most mornings that summer I filled ten fertigation buckets in the dry garden.

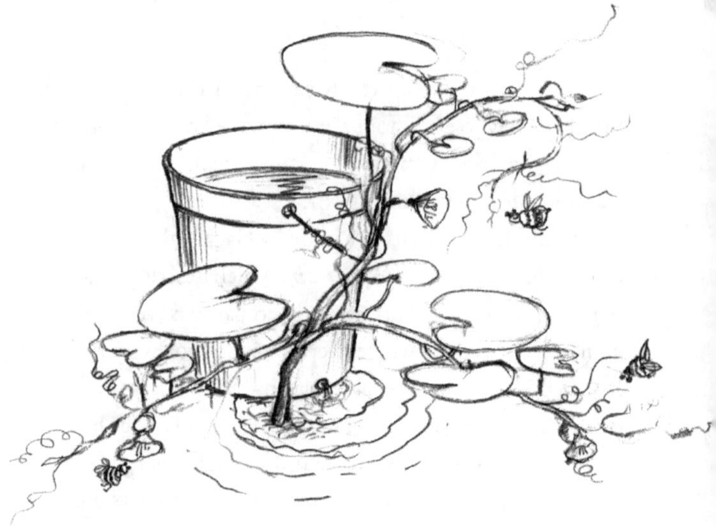

Unfertigated pumpkin vines looked moisture stressed all summer. Each unfertigated hill yielded about 7 kg of very average-tasting food. The vines given two fertigations extended twice as far as those given none and yielded over 25 kg per hill. And the fertigated pumpkins tasted much better.

Some plants got fertigated with a mixture of seaweed extract and fish-emulsion. Others got soluble chemicals with trace elements, like Miracle Gro. Both approaches worked but the chemicals worked better. At that time I opined that was because chemical fertilizers provide far more phosphorus. Now I understand that soluble chemical fertilizers with trace elements *and* significant amounts of phosphorus in them are far closer to being in balance than any combination of fish and kelp.

The following year I integrated everything into one garden. There were entirely unirrigated areas, unirrigated areas with some fertigation, half moist areas on the fringe of the sprinkler's pattern and fully sprinkler irrigated beds (see illustration). Water-demanding vegies like lettuce, Chinese cabbage, celery, onions, and leeks grew in a parallel pair of sprinkler irrigated raised beds that were 1,200 mm wide and 30 metres long. These two beds occupied around 20 percent of the garden. Beyond those two raised beds the short-throw low-angle sprinklers I was using threw much less water. In this area I put a pair of long single rows that were 1,200 mm apart centre to centre. Entirely beyond the sprinkler's throw I practiced absolute dry gardening or else fertigated. Everything worked! Many species grew surprisingly well when given small amounts of water—or none at all. At the end of that summer I wrote a little labour of love about these experiments called *Water-Wise Vegetables*.* There is no need for you to download a free copy because the book in your hands provides better information than *Water-Wise* did.

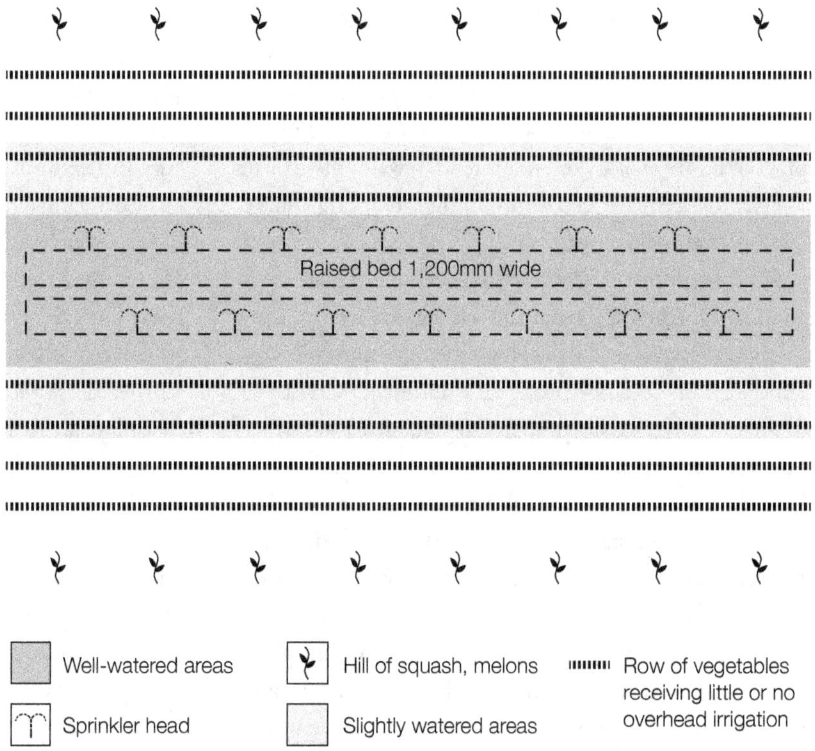

Dry-gardening is possible because plants can be sustained by subsoil moisture. Humid-climate subsoils are too leached of nutrients to adequately feed vegetables but they do hold a lot of moisture after a rainy winter. Even if that subsoil is so airless or chemically so hostile that vegetable roots can not survive in it, the moisture in it still rises up slowly and replaces water lost from the topsoil. Fertigation increases subsoil fertility and supplements that moisture.

How soil loses moisture

Suppose winter had, as usual, delivered plenty of rain. In August the subsoil would be at full moisture capacity as far down as it went. Imagine keeping 100 square metres of that land entirely bare by repeatedly and thoroughly hoeing the surface from early spring through the end of summer. The hot sun beats down on that bare earth all summer. It totally dries out—or seems to.

Summer rain is scant in Tasmania; when it happens it usually comes in insignificant amounts. A summer that provides so much rainfall that the paddocks remain green after being hayed is extremely unusual. Most people opine that at summer's end the topsoil and the subsoil will be dry.

But that is not what has to happen. The hot sun does dry out the surface but if we dug past 150 mm in high summer we would encounter dampness. Dig a little deeper and there will be even more moisture. The reason is that when the surface inches are kept loose by hoeing they act like a mulch. Dry farmers called this a dust mulch. Without growing plants to suck moisture up from deeper, the subsoil moisture remains—like money in the bank at call.

I suggest you do a quick study of the root system drawings in Weaver's *Root Development of Vegetable Crops**. Some of them are reproduced in miniature in Chapter 9. This downloadable free book shows that most kinds of vegetables form a root system that can extend as broadly as the plant is tall and more broadly than that with some species. Weaver's drawings show how spacing corn plants on a 1,200 mm x 1,200 mm grid provides each plant with sole access to all the moisture in a 1,200 x 1,200 space—all the way down. You'll also see that in the prairie soils of eastern Nebraska (where Weaver did this research), roots of many vegetable species penetrate 1,200 mm (and deeper). And maybe you'll agree that subsoil moisture could sustain vegetables.

The moisture-supplying ability of any position depends on soil depth, on the subsoil's moisture-holding capacity and to a lesser extent upon how much root penetration that soil permits. To find out for sure if your land can support a dry-garden you can try it on a small plot. I assure you there will be useful moisture when there is more than one metre of subsoil, especially so when the subsoil contains a fair bit of clay. Gardens with less than one metre of soil beneath them and gardens on deep sand that holds very little moisture can still be managed so as to reduce the frequency of irrigation by increasing the amount of space between plants.

Subsoil moisture can sustain uncrowded plants. Moisture is pulled up from the subsoil to replace moisture being lost closer to the surface. The physical process at work is called capillary flow. Trees lift water to their tops through tiny tubes without using any energy. The same thing happens in soil because openings between soil particles form interconnected microtubes that draw up moisture against the force of gravity. Even in the best circumstances the upward movement of subsoil moisture is too slow to fully support high density vegetable crops. I suppose that's why intensive gardening gurus and industrial vegetable producers completely ignore the possibility. However, many kinds of vegetables can forage enough moisture to support themselves through months without rain or irrigation when plant population density is low.

Mulching dry gardens

It *seems* that mulched soil loses less moisture. I suspect soil mulched with any form of loose vegetation like straw or wood chips actually loses slightly more moisture than a dust-mulched soil—not that the small difference matters much. When dry gardening I speculate it is best to spread a *thin* mulch *after the soil warms up*. The mulch should be removed by the end of April. Keeping the furrowslice moister in summer means the plants can feed where the most available plant nutrients reside. As I have already pointed out, keeping mulch in place over the winter breeds trouble.

There have been catastrophic dust storms in districts practicing dry *farming*. These happened during droughts lasting several consecutive years. The dust storms also happened because depleted farm soils lacked organic matter. When garden soil receives compost and develops a strong crumb structure there's little risk of significant wind erosion. In most of Tasmania there is very little risk of several consecutive years of extremely low rainfall.

Low plant density

The amount of water a crop transpires is determined by the amount of leaf cover. The loss is amplified by wind and sun. In this respect the crop functions like an automobile radiator. With radiators, the larger the metal surfaces, the colder the air and the higher the wind speed passing over the cooling fins then the better the radiator works. In the garden, the more leaf surfaces, the faster, warmer and drier the wind, the brighter the sunlight, then the more water is transpired. Where there are no plants growing at all and a dust mulch has been created, then soil moisture is lost only very slowly. If a complete mature leaf canopy is present, then the rate of water loss will approximate what this chapter recommends should be added through irrigation.

A crop with a dense leaf canopy that is growing on sand can experience moisture stress two days after being irrigated, even sooner than that if it has been hot, sunny, breezy and the humidity has been low. On a deep clay soil that same crop could comfortably grow through one week of such conditions without irrigation. But if plants on heavier ground are given more than enough growing space this apparent waste would result in a much slower rate of soil moisture depletion and allow the plants to make broader root systems. Under these conditions the amount of moisture rising by capillarity may be sufficient to support the crop. This is dry-gardening in a nutshell. And this is how to garden without having to irrigate so frequently in the same nutshell.

Can you dry-garden?

Absolute dry gardening requires very deep open moisture-retentive soil but anyone standing on more than 600 mm of soil can usefully increase the amount of time between irrigations by lowering plant density.

I suggest digging a metre-deep hole in the garden. Evaluate what you discover against the table in the first part of this chapter, "Available Moisture per foot of soil." If you discover a plow pan it should be broken up by deeply digging the entire garden. Otherwise your plants will be forced to form roots in the topsoil only. If the topsoil is sandy and doesn't hold a lot of moisture but upon reaching 400 mm you discover airless clay that is exhausting to dig into then I can't advise you for sure other than to not wear yourself out trying to dig further. This position might work for dry-gardening if you got plants well established when the topsoil was still naturally moist or could irrigate them for their first six weeks. After that moisture uplift might support a spread-out garden through the entire summer. Attempting to dry garden a few plants is the way to find out for sure.

Vegetables that aren't suited to dry gardening

Bulbing onions (spring sown)	Lettuce (for summer harvest)
Cauliflower (except overwintering types)	Radish (spring radishes will grow on rainfall)
Celery / Celeriac	Spring onions (for summer harvest)
Chinese cabbage	English spinach (summer varieties)

Plant spacing possibilities in relation to irrigation

Soil depth (in centimetres)	30	60	90-120	120-180	over 180
Frequency of irrigation needed	2 days	4 - 7 days	10 - 14 days	3-4 weeks	uncertain
Broad bean, autumn sown	20 x 45	20 x 60	30 x 75	30 x 90	30 x 90
Bean, bush, French	15 x 45	20 x 60	30 x 90	40 x 120	45 x 120
Beetroot	8 x 45	10 x 45	10 x 60	15 x 75	30 x 120
Cabbage, autumn/winter	60 x 60	60 x 75	60 x 90	90 x 120	90 x 120
Carrots	2 x 30	2 x 45	2[-]3 x 60	10 x 90	30 x 120
Corn	20 x 90	20 x 90	30 x 105	60 x 120	120 x 120
Cucumber	90 x 120	105 x 120	120 x 120	150 x 150	150 x 150
Endive (chicories)	30 x 45	30 x 45	45 x 60	60 x 90	60 x 120
Kale	45 x 60	60 x 60	75 x 75	90 x 120	120 x 150
Parsley	15 x 45	15 x 45	15 x 60	20 x 75	30 x 90
Parsnip	not possible	10 x 45	15 x 45	15 x 60	----------
Peppers	45 x 60	60 x 60	75 x 90	90 x 120	90 x 120
Potatoes	20 x 105	30 x 105	30 x 120	45 x 120	45 x 150
Swede	15 x 60	20 x 60	30 x 75	45 x 90	45 x 120
Squash, bush (zucchini)	75 x 90	90 x 105	105 x 120	120 x 150	150 x 180
Silverbeet	30 x 45	30 x 60	40 x 75	45 x 90	60 x 120
Tomato, indeterminate	60 x 90	90 x 120	120 x 120	150 x 150	180 x 180
Pumpkin	120 x 120	210 x 210	240 x 240	300 x 300	300 x 360

Chapter 6

Seeds

Caveat emptor. [Let the buyer beware.]

—Ancient Roman saying

You can sell the home gardener the sweepings off the seedroom floor.

—An agribusiness suit telling novice seedsman Steve Solomon why he should buy his company's cheap garden seed, 1979

The two pests that most degrade garden performance are AQIS and Quarantine Tasmania

Steve Solomon, garden writer and seedsman

I feel blessed to live in Tasmania. Tassie's climate allows me to eat a diverse range of vegetables fresh from the garden all year. Tassie may be remote but I still can buy almost any *thing* I can afford. Thanks to Tassie's agricultural economy I can conveniently access a broad range of soil amendments. One essential thing I can't buy here is the best possible seeds for the full range of vegetables that Tassie could produce. I can't buy these seeds because Quarantine stops me. That makes me cranky.

Tasmania really is another country when it comes to food gardening. A vegetable variety that does well in NSW all too often does not work here. Some heat lovers that thrive in Victoria do sort of okay in Tassie. Victoria's cool season varieties often don't cope with our winter. Varieties that are crucially important to eating well during winter and spring are not available. Yes, Tasmanian vegetable farmers grow winter vegetables in the mildest districts; they use high quality seeds from the world's finest primary growers but gardeners can't access them. Chapter 9 mentions little-known winter vegies that Tassie's commercial growers do not produce, varieties that tolerate much harsher weather than happens close to the Bass Strait. Tasmanians in the island's interior would benefit.

If there were far fewer import restrictions a Tasmanian garden seed business like Southern Harvest could easily source from regions with similar climates—like England and western Oregon/Washington/coastal British Columbia (a bioregion named Cascadia). But Biosecurity makes overseas purchases daunting, sometimes prohibitively costly and all too often outright impossible—unless the import concerns large scale production. Then the hassles become a minor irritation relative to the potential profits. Tasmanian garden seed sellers are inevitably tiny businesses because of our small population. They do not buy thousands of dollars worth of seeds for only one variety so they can not afford to jump over biosecurity hurdles. Quarantine justifies their restrictions by frightening us about the next English sparrow or preventing some biological nightmare. Actually Quarantine's main activity is not about protecting us. It is about forwarding Tasmanian agribusiness. Quarantine's seed import restrictions allow Tasmanian farmers and commercial vegetable seed growers to certify that their exports are free of a certain pest or disease but these same restrictions encourage ethically-challenged garden seed sellers to offer low quality seeds and inappropriate varieties.

High quality seeds, low quality seeds? Grow a variety trial yourself and the difference becomes obvious. I could try to explain in words but there's an easier way. Please mouse-around a few online seed catalogues. The most appropriate *mainland* seed seller for Tasmanian gardeners I know of is Mr. Fothergill's'. Compare their prices and depth of choice with Territorial Seeds in Oregon or Johnny's Selected Seeds in Maine or Moles in the UK. The main reason these foreign seed sellers can offer so many varieties and almost all of them of the highest commercial quality—is population. Territorial Seeds focuses on the Cascadia bioregion; their climate is like Tasmania but Cascadia has eight million people in it. Another reason these companies do a better job is that the US imposes very few restrictions on importing vegetable seeds. And why does that matter to us? Because a great many commercial-quality vegetable varieties that best suit Tasmania or Cascadia originate from Dutch and English seed growers.

Buying effective seeds

I published the first version of this book in 2002. Then I started being asked to give talks, often about seed saving. When I presented in those days no matter what my main topic I always mentioned that Tasmania needed a quality-minded regionally-focused garden seed business. It needed someone ethical, not lazy, passionately motivated to sell strongly germinating seeds of varieties that actually produce in Tasmania. I said that someone willing to responsibly create such a business could earn enough from our small population to maintain a modest lifestyle. That assertion has been proved correct. I said it could be a relatively simple business—but I was wrong about that because I did not yet appreciate how the rapidly expanding global biosecurity system would harm the interests of Tasmanian gardeners. I said that some of the high quality varieties appropriate to Tasmanian gardens could come from mainland distributors that sell to market gardeners and vegetable farmers. A trials ground could quickly sort out which of those varieties were appropriate on Tassie. This was correct. I said a Tasmanian garden seed business could also buy from large high quality ethically responsible seed businesses operating in North America and England. It would not be necessary to even do variety trials with anything from Territorial—because everything that company sold to Cascadians would be well adapted to Tasmania's climate, suit home garden conditions and would taste good. In reality, buying abroad isn't so easy.

It took a few years of repetition but now we have Sam Bayley's Southern Harvest Seeds. Sam is a Tasmania-focused garden seed seller that I can recommend. Southern Harvest should have had an easy task, repackaging seeds bought wholesale in bulk from Territorial and a few other ethical companies in North America and England. Thanks to Tas Quarantine Sam too often couldn't.

I wish all Tasmanians could conveniently buy high quality seeds for vegetable varieties that sustain health and are a pleasure to eat in all seasons. The internet makes it easy to buy seeds from any country in any currency. But BiosecurityTas makes importing seeds into a stressful experience. Not just home gardeners get daunted—Quarantine discourages garden seed merchants. One such person (who, to avoid bringing them trouble shall remain nameless) told me in private conversation that he experienced dealing with Quarantine as torture, like "death by a thousand cuts." But major Australian farm seed importers and overseas primary seed growers that produce seeds in Tasmania do not experience Biosecurity as painful; they pay someone to deal with the forms and submissions and procedures, they cheerfully pay the fees—because Quarantine's procedures also function like protective tariffs that increase their profits. In real fact, almost every Quarantine restriction is imposed to increase someone's profits at someone else's expense.

Editions of this book issued before the year 2010 accurately listed the few vegetable species that Quarantine was restricting at the moment. I uncertainly recall that it was five restricted species. Seeds for most kinds of vegetable entered without difficulty. After 2010 more restrictions were imposed. Then even more. These days a seed importer never knows what new rule will appear during the time their overseas purchase is in process. If Solomon were king of Tasmania I'd levy against the exporters of onions, glasshouse tomato and capsicum, carrot seed or whatever other farming industry Quarantine is making more profitable. I'd use that levy to eliminate fees for non-commercial seed imports and to make them convenient. I'd have someone who is gardener-friendly available on Quarantine's telephone ready to help out the little guy.

Picture-packet seed racks

Picture-packet seeds are sold at garden centres and big box shops. Many (most?) packets show mouthwatering generic images (rarely of the actual variety being sold) and promise success all over Australia. Casual gardeners assume what's offered are proper vegetable seeds.

But mainland picture-packet companies too often sell varieties in Tasmania that do not grow so well in Tasmania. Many of their packets contain cheaply produced non-productive varieties. Too often the seeds germinate weakly—or not at all. Picture packet quality can be this low because casual gardeners never realize that the seeds they planted are the reason things didn't go so well. When the seeds fail to come up or they grow poorly gardeners usually reckon it is their own lack of knowledge or skill. They never suspect that cheap broccoli varieties like DeCicco, Green Sprouting and Waltham 29 *always* make small, coarsely budded, poor-tasting main flowers and small woody side shoots; that Long Island Improved brussels sprout *always* forms loose clusters of cabbagey-looking leaves where the sprouts are supposed to be. And makes no sprouts. When carrot, silverbeet or onions go to seed a few months after sowing it's actually caused by lack of supervision from a skilled breeder. It is poor genetics; it is not the gardener's fault. But unethical primary seed producers know that gardeners will blame their own fertilizing or watering or the weather that season. A plainer-than-the-usual speaking executive in this business once put it to me this way: "The gardener is an uncritical trade. You can sell the gardener the sweepings off the seedroom floor." However, there are *some* decent seeds on seedracks.

Mr. Fothergill's: I've *almost* always enjoyed effective germination and tasty vegetables from their packets. Because Fothergill's is a British company most of their varieties perform well in Tassie's climate but many varieties we could use from England are not on their rack. Fothergill also has an online shop.

Contact: http://www.mrfothergills.com.au

Yeats: I have discovered a few productive varieties on Yeats seed rack, especially their Shogun broccoli and Sun n Snow bicolour sweet corn Yeats once sold Sweet Grey hybrid pumpkin which has long been popular with Tasmanians. They now sell a different variety that looks the same but is not long-keeping like Sweet Grey.

Hollander Imports provides an in-shop seedrack with generous packets that are often used by small market gardeners. Also find interesting tools from Holland.

Contact: 87 Brooker Highway, Hobart
Telephone (03) 6234 5799

Southern Harvest has a few seed racks in garden centres around Hobart and at least one in Victoria.

Catalogue seed merchants

I mentored, encouraged and still support Southern Harvest. I also advised and encouraged the owner of Birdland Seeds in southern Victoria. Both fully understand that their mission is to provide us with all the varieties we need in order to produce every type of vegetable that is possible to grow in Tasmania in every season it is possible to do so, and also to provide seeds that actually come up and perform as described. Birdland's focus is on southern Victoria.

Birdland sells only certified organic seeds and aims to have them be of commercial quality. Many of their varieties are produced by Ben Cohen on a farm in southern Victoria. Seeds for some varieties are imported. Ben maintains a high standard by regularly growing out much of his catalogue. He responsibly tests germination. Ben is becoming a skilled breeder who improves and refines what he produces himself. I admire his ethics.

Contact: http://www.birdlandseeds.com

Southern Harvest Seeds, Sam Bayley operates from a homestead near Kingston where he does variety trials and also produces seeds. Southern Harvest sells commercial quality seeds bought from mainland distributors and also imports important varieties. Largely thanks to Quarantine's ever-expanding import restrictions SH is developing a network of local seed growers, including Steve Solomon. Sam regularly germ tests his inventory.

Contact: http://www.southernharvest.com.au/

Activevista. Long doing business as Langley Organics, near Kingston, this company now provides, amongst other interesting items, a limited range of commercial quality vegetable seeds for serious gardeners and market gardeners. Their smallest size packet usually provides enough for several years in a home garden.

Contact: http://www.activevista.com.au

Importing

I just praised Southern Harvest and Birdland but I dislike their small packet sizes and limited choices. It is not their fault. Tasmania is a very small country; the Bureau of Statistics says there are about 200,000 households but I guess no more than 25,000 of them grow a food garden and most of these are small gardens. Which is why Southern Harvest and Birdland sell a limited range of varieties, mostly in tiny packets.

Before 2010 this book urged Tasmanians to buy many sorts of vegetable seeds from quality-oriented foreign sellers. Importing was simpler then. Lower prices in genuinely competitive markets overseas balanced out the exchange rate handicap and shipping costs. On arrival, the parcel was automatically routed to Quarantine because the customs declaration said "seeds." If the packets in your order were labelled with Latin species names and didn't contain a few restricted species—beans, peas, corn, sunflower, or solanums—all the seeds were immediately released.

However, in 2009 Tasmania Quarantine began requiring a single-page "declaration of intent to import," be lodged with them at the same time the seeds were ordered. Since Customs already diverts anything containing seeds to Quarantine I can't see any point in lodging a permit application except that the requirement discourages people. The last time I checked the declaration was downloadable from Tas Quarantine's website. Last time I checked no fee was charged for clearing non-commercial imports.

With enough determination Quarantine can be dealt with. If more of us gardeners did start importing then the road might be smoothed. A steady stream of gardeners engaging with Quarantine might even make importing easier for our small seed merchants.

Buying garden seed from abroad doesn't guarantee getting productive strongly germinating seeds. I wrote a lengthy article for *Harrowsmith* magazine (Canadian) in the early 1990s evaluating individual North American garden seed sellers. First I sent a brief questionnaire to every substantial North American catalogue seller offering them an opportunity to be mentioned in my forthcoming article. Their answers (and the many non-responses) showed me that the majority of vegetable garden seed sellers did not conduct useful variety trials. Nor did they insure quality by performing grow-outs of seeds they purchase and repackage. Nor did most of them routinely germ test their carried over inventory. In this respect many North American seed vendors operate as irresponsibly as many Australian garden seed vendors do.

Here is my short list of recommended overseas suppliers offering high quality varieties that suit Tasmania and who still are willing to do business with us despite the paperwork hassles it creates for them:

Adaptive Seeds is a strictly-organic Oregon homestead-based business that on the surface seems similar to Australia's Eden and Greenpatch. But their level of quality and professionalism is far higher. The bright, hard-working young couple creating Adaptive produce close-to-commercial quality open pollinated seeds. Their heat lovers are terrific here! Their winter varieties thrive in conditions that are more severe than anywhere in Tassie below 500 metres. In recent years I have used quite a few of Adaptive's varieties; all their seeds germinated well; they grew productive plants.

Contact: http://www.adaptiveseeds.com

Johnny's Selected Seeds focuses on serving gardeners in the northern United States and southern Canada. When buying from Johnny's keep in mind that their trials ground is located where summer days resemble Tasmania, their autumn is short and quickly leads into a harsh winter that ends the garden. Johnny's spring and summer varieties work for us; many of their autumn varieties last out our winter. Johnny's supplies the same high quality seeds to home gardeners that they provide to farmers. Many of Johnny's customers are certified-organic market gardeners using certified-organic grown seeds of commercial quality. Johnny's breeds and produces an ever-increasing number of its own varieties and does that to a very high standard. Johnny's runs a large trials ground. Their catalogue is truly without overstatement or sales puffery, describing precisely how each variety performs on their trials ground in Maine. Johnny's accepts orders from Australians although their overseas shipping fee may deter you.

Contact: http://www.johnnyseeds.com

Stokes Seeds: Before I went into the seed business myself I bought almost all my seed from Stokes. When writing the aforementioned *Harrowsmith* article I learned that the majority of serious gardeners in the northern USA and Canada buy from Stokes, whose average non-commercial order was double the amount of the garden seed industry average. Stokes has an extensive trials ground and is a major supplier to large vegetable growers in southern Canada and the northern U.S. Stokes provides the same high quality seeds to home gardeners. I've never been disappointed.

Contact: http://www.stokeseeds.com

Territorial Seed Company: When I started Territorial in 1979 I used Johnny's as my business model. Johnny's had already been in business for seven years. Because Johnny's does not provide many of the varieties that the Cascadia bioregion needs the owner of Johnny's, Rob Johnston, generously mentored me. In 1986 I sold Territorial to a local homesteading couple who are temperamentally better suited to doing business than I am. Territorial still follows the operating practices I established. It primarily sells commercial quality seeds. It stores its as yet unpacketed inventory at a stable 10°C and 50% RH. I'll soon have more to say about improving your own seed storage. Their entire seed inventory is germ tested twice a year. Territorial does extensive variety trials that are evaluated according to what the home garden needs. Territorial custom-grows some locally renowned or especially well-adapted non-commercial varieties. TSC is now organically producing an ever-broadening list of heirloom varieties and has been applying professional plant breeding to their restoration.

Contact: http://www.territorial-seed.com

Moles Seeds is a leading wholesale supplier of commercial quality flower and vegetable seeds throughout the UK. They are willing to ship to Tasmanians. Their main business involves market gardeners who buy more than a pinch at a time, but their smallest size packets will suit a serious gardener. Make sure to remind them that Quarantine requires all packets be labelled with the Latin botanical name.

Contact: https://www.wholesale.molesseeds.co.uk/

Succeed with seeds

The variety may score 9.8 out of a possible 10.0 for taste or maybe it produces the most or is the best for whatever trait but if the seeds didn't shoot then all that promise matters not. Many gardeners have had such poor results getting seeds to come up that they only use seeds for species that germinate powerfully, like peas and beans, or that can't be transplanted successfully, like carrot and parsnip. This inability forces the gardener to accept the limited range of seedlings offered at the garden centre. Seedlings also cost a great deal more than seeds. Far better to learn how to make seeds shoot and grow.

I may be repeating myself in this paragraph, which is considered to be bad form when writing books, but here I will state the reasons I think gardeners have poor results with sowing seeds. One, the seeds they buy are of low quality and lack vigour. This handicap can be overcome by sourcing elsewhere. Another reason direct seeding is avoided is that garden seed packets usually contain so few seeds that the user is almost forced to start seedlings with them because seeds that start out in sterile growing media at close to ideal temperature and moisture germinate more often. Outdoor conditions aren't sterile, nor are they stable; I must sow several seeds outdoors to establish one good plant. When the gardener only has weak seeds from a tiny packet that cost far too much then successfully direct seeding seems impossible. I can afford to direct seed because I can grow my own seeds for carrot, beetroot, parsnip, lettuce, silverbeet, kohlrabi, endive, escarole, bean, pea, bulbing onion and radish. And the seeds I grow are vigorous because I grow fresh ones every few years, I harvest and clean them gently so as to not damage a lot of embryos and mine are produced on remineralized soil which results in high vigour.

The germination lab I operated at Territorial Seed Company taught me a great deal about how to make seeds come up. Maybe it can teach you as well.

Vigour

My garden is essential to our health and it reduces inflationary stress at the supermarket. So I do whatever it takes to have a good result. So what happens if I start with weak seeds? After sowing there's a longer wait than there should be and often there eventually is a thinly populated row of spindly slow-growing seedlings. For the next few weeks there will be many mysterious disappearances. If these weaklings eventually do start growing right (and some never do) they ultimately produce less than strong seeds of the same variety would have done. Vigorous seeds emerge quickly and grow fast from the start. Vigorous seedlings have a low infant mortality rate.

In Territorial's germ lab I would test many varieties of the same kind of vegetable at the same time. Some seed lots made strong looking seedlings that appeared quickly. Others took days longer to emerge; these looked spindly and weak compared to the strong lots. The quicker to shoot lots also germinated at a far higher percentage and proceeded to grow faster from the get-go. That's vigour demonstrated.

A very high percentage of vigorous seeds shoot successfully in a germination laboratory *because* they are provided with ideal conditions. It isn't unusual to see a 90-plus percent result. Farmers understand that the lab germination percentage relates to field performance, but not exactly. Broccoli that achieves 90 percent lab germination can be expected to produce 50 percent field emergence of vigorous seedlings. Broccoli seed that scores 70 percent in the germ lab is tired old stuff that will probably fail to shoot in the field. Vigorous seed is denser when it is first put in the bag—the trade term for this is "fat." A given volume of fat seed weighs more. That's because vigorous seeds hold larger reserves of complete nutrition for the embryo within. It'll have a longer storage life too.

As you would expect, commercial seed growers do their best to achieve maximum vigour. They eliminate insects that might reduce parent plant health and use fungicides against any disease that could attack the forming seed, weaken the mother plant or if carried on the seed coat, harm the seedlings. Primary growers grow seed crops in districts where climate and soil conditions are near perfect for the species. Consequently much of the world's cabbage, beetroot and spinach seed is produced around Mount Vernon, Washington, USA. Seeds for Japanese broccoli varieties are produced in California's Imperial Valley; Dutch seedsmen grow brussels sprout seed in northern Italy. And lately, Bejo Zaden, probably the largest privately-owned international vegetable seed grower that hasn't yet been gobbled up by a great financial shark, started producing carrot seed in Tasmania. Not surprisingly, commercial seed productions usually arrive at the warehouse in vigorous condition.

Vigour and germination percentage decline during storage. I'll soon explain how to create excellent storage conditions at home that greatly lengthen seed life, save you money and prevent failures.

Germination is a dangerous passage. The embryo must grow itself into a fully functional seedling using nutrients and fuel reserved within its seed coat with very little help from what's in the soil. If the embryo gets stressed or slowed whilst sprouting then it consumes more of its reserves; they may become exhausted. If the nutrients in its reserve prove even marginally inadequate then the seedling is far more likely to be attacked by insect and disease. Dangerous: a clod above the seed can prevent emergence. Temperature outside a narrow range will kill it. Another reason vigorous seeds survive better is that they more quickly extend their roots, thereby reaching a reliable moisture supply before the surface inch dries out.

Most kinds of vegetable seeds initially put up simplified leaves called cotyledons (this sort of plant is termed a dicot). After that they proceed to make "true" leaves with their usual shape. Dicots can not photosynthesize enough sugar to fuel their own needs until the first pair of true leaves has at least half way developed. I'm not sure when monocots like corn and onion have made enough leaf to operate on the current account. If cold wet soil slows down sprouting or should compacted soil resist the seed's effort to move root and shoot through it then the vigorous seedling survives anyway and usually thrives when a weak seedling, if it emerges at all, does so with severely depleted reserves; it is more likely to succumb to environmental menaces and grows very slowly in its first weeks, ultimately yielding less.

Strong seed is highly prized in the seed trade but the word *vigour* is strongly avoided by seed sellers. The last thing a seedsman will promise is that any particular seed lot will actually come up and grow. There are just too many uncontrollable risks; there would be too many lawsuits. So seeds are evaluated according to their certified-laboratory-determined germination percentage and the fine print legalese on the back of the sales contract always says in essence:

> 'we guarantee that this bag of seeds contains real seeds that did germinate at a certified seed testing laboratory at a stated percentage on a specific date (within the last six months). And correctly labelled or not, whatever happens after sowing these seeds is not our responsibility. The purchaser agrees as a condition of this sale that any liability the seller may have is limited to the price of the seed itself.'

So, if the seeds fail to establish a crop then all the money spent on preparing and sowing that field and what contract lawyers call "lost opportunity" is not the seller's responsibility. Enforceable contracts can be based upon lab germination results. Divide a bag of seed amongst a dozen certified seed testing laboratories in a dozen different countries and every one of them will get almost identical test results.

The germination rate discovered in a laboratory only *predicts,* it can not guarantee what will happen when those seeds are sown in the field. Sow high germ seeds in decent field conditions and a large fraction of them will actually emerge and grow. Sow low germ seed and a few slow-growing seedlings might emerge. Smart seed distributors (who do not grow the seeds they resell) give the primary growers who supply them notice in advance that the seed they are ordering must meet or exceed a specific lab germination percentage or they do not want it. Smart farmers also ask about germination before buying. The minimum percentage demanded by knowledgeable users differs from species to species. For example, it will be over 85 percent for brassica seeds, carrot over 70 percent.

I hope you found all this interesting but the subject makes little difference when buying garden seed in Australia. Our garden seed packets are never labelled with the results of a recent germination test. Aussie gardeners must hope the seed merchant operates ethically. And by ethics, I mean that the merchant has their own germ lab and retests everything they have in storage at least once a year, better every six months. And when the germination drops below a commercially acceptable minimum for that species, that lot of seeds is discarded.

Getting the most out of seeds

The best an Australian gardener can do is to buy from a seed merchant with a good reputation and hope that almost all their packets contain seeds that will germinate if the seeds encounter satisfactory conditions. That's your job, improving the conditions.

Laboratory germ tests are done under ideal conditions for the species. Every certified lab in the world creates exactly the same species-specific sprouting environment as it is prescribed in the International Seed Testing Association's manual. The test is conducted inside a cabinet that maintains the ideal temperature (or an ideal daily range of temperatures that imitate the day/night cycle) and the cabinet provides light (or not) as needed for that species. The germination medium always is sterile and ideally moist at all times. Soil in the garden is not sterile, not stably warm and not ideally moist at all times.

Because outdoor soil may contain harmful microorganisms that reduce germination, seeds sold to farmers are often coated with fungicide. Garden seeds are rarely treated. If I had strong reasons to grow out an old weak seed packet—suppose these seeds might be the last of an otherwise extinct variety I wanted to conserve—then I would sprout them at an ideal temperature that I held as stable as possible in a home environment. Sterile fine-textured germination medium would be put into a sterile, never before used seedling container; the medium would already been brought to the ideal moisture content with distilled (sterile) water. The seeds would be placed barely beneath the surface. The container would then be sealed in an air-tight poly bag until shoots emerged.

Moisture, but not too much

Most kinds of seeds germinate less well when moisture is steadily lost from their sprouting medium and then is replaced every day. That's because watering lowers soil temperature until the sun warms it back up. Watering sprouting seeds temporarily increases the moisture saturation around them to 100 percent. But cold, wet soil conditions are ideal for the development of damping-off, a disease that attacks seedlings before or soon after they emerge. Damping-off continues to knock off seedlings until their stems have formed a protective skin. You can recognize damping-off when a newly-emerged seedling suddenly falls over because a scaly collar forms at ground level and pinches off circulation. Damping-off doesn't thrive in warm soil that is at 70 percent of total moisture capacity; in that degree of dampness most kinds of seeds germinate their very best.

Gardeners are often surprised when I tell them that seeds sprout far better in soil that is moist but not wet. Seed testing labs obtain the highest possible germination percentage by placing seeds for most species atop a sheet of sterile blotting paper that was brought to the correct moisture by immersing it in sterile water and then squeezing it hard in tight fist to remove as much moisture as possible. You can conveniently feel something at the perfect dampness by strongly squeezing a wet dishrag in your fist until water stops dripping out.

A few vegetable species germinate better in actual soil than on blotting paper. For testing these seed labs use sterilized light loam soil. Usually water is slowly added to oven-sterilized dry soil until a handful squeezed into a ball will stick together in a ball yet it will easily crumble with thumb pressure. (The same procedure determines when to till.)

When I ran Territorial Seed Company I intentionally germ tested in *unsterilized* soil straight from the trials ground. The soil moisture was brought to 75-80 percent of capacity, seeds were thinly sprinkled into furrows which were the same depth they would be in the field and then the tray was sealed with a transparent plastic lid. I was not interested in determining a specific percentage of germination; I did hope to see crowded rows of vigorous seedlings emerging quickly from a medium matching what they would actually encounter in a garden. If I didn't see this indication of good vigour from a variety then I might count out 100 seeds and do a sterile test on blotter paper before deciding what to do with that seed lot.

ISTA germination tests are done in airtight containers that stably maintain ideal moisture. When I first did germ tests my seedling trays were not covered, they had to be remoistened daily; in this case about half as many seedlings emerged. Most gardeners think they must water seedbeds every day but there are ways to slow drying out so that seedbed watering may be done less often. And there is a best time of day to water.

Sowing

An emerging celery or cabbage shoot can't push past a pebble or a lump of hard earth. Small seeds like these must start in a finely textured loose seedbed. Commercial seedling growers use a lightweight, loose growing medium that holds a lot of moisture and doesn't compact. Similarly, we gardeners should create seedbeds that are slow to dry out and remain loose.

Tiny seeds must be placed close to the surface. But the seed dies should the soil around it get too dry. The appearance of the shoot says the seedlings have put roots down far enough to survive one sunny day. Most species need no special watering after that. Before shoots appear you who must keep the seedbed moist. But watering lowers soil temperature and on some soils irrigation creates a crust that blocks emergence. So be mindful that there's rarely need to remoisten seedbeds on a cloudy day or early in the morning following a cloudy day. We can try to irrigate mid-morning so that the seedbed soon gets warm again. The worst thing would be to water sprouting seeds so late in the day that the bed can't heat back up until mid-morning the next day. If your soil forms crusts then try refilling the furrow with a light, loose, moisture-retentive medium similar to that used in greenhouse mixes. Doing this is not much trouble. Finely sifted compost or else a container growing medium as recommended in Chapter 7 are suitable. Only one litre of moist light loose material will fill lineal metres of furrow or cover dozens of positions.

The generally-accepted rule for sowing depth is three times the seed's largest dimension. In the cool of early spring the surface stays moist for several days after it rains; I sow very tiny seeds (French sorrel, celery, some herbs) then by scratching a very shallow "V" (only 6 mm deep) with the corner of a common hoe and sprinkling seeds into that furrow *without covering them.* Light watering with a fine spray moves some seeds into cracks and crannies and washes soil off the furrow's sides and over them. I get good emergence this way.

When sowing ordinary small seeds (cabbage family, carrot, lettuce), I place them in a furrow or depression 10 mm to

13 mm deep and cover them; huskier seeds (spinach, radish, Chinese cabbage) go in 15 mm deep; large seeds (squash, cucumber, melon, beans, corn, peas) 25 mm to 30 mm under the surface. Bush beans sown in summer's heat are placed 40 mm deep.

If the soil has been loosened recently you can reduce the rate at which the surface inch dries out by resettling the soil before sowing. I mentioned in the chapter on watering that fine soil pores act like microtubes that bring up subsurface moisture through a natural process called "capillary flow." Cultivation temporarily shatters that network. So if you're going to dig before sowing best to do that two weeks ahead so that capillarity has time to restore itself before seeds go in.

Have you ever seen this happen? One spring morning a garden is rotarycultivated into a fluffy damp carpet but the perfect smoothness of it is blemished by a few footprints. By late afternoon the surface has dried in the sun. Early the next morning the footprints are moist while the rest of the area remains dry on top. Foot pressure on those spots restored capillary uplift. However, the sun again shines on that moist footprint; it soon dries out. The next morning it won't be moist.

Suppose immediately after the footprint was made seeds were placed on top of it and covered with a mulch of loose fine moist soil or with an airy container mix that wouldn't crust over. The seeds rest on damp earth exactly like they do on damp blotter paper in a germination lab. Moisture under the seeds would be protected by the loose soil mulch. Unless conditions got hot and windy it would not be necessary to irrigate these positions for several days. To restore capillarity there's no need to compress soil as severely as happens when making a footprint. If you're planting on stations just make a fist and gently push it into loose just-spaded earth. Stop when you feel more than slight resistance. If the bed was shallowly hoed, not dug, it may be enough to press down with the flat of the thumb. Put seeds in that depression and cover them with loose soil.

Gardeners more often succeed with big seeds—beans and peas and corn—because they're planted deeply enough that the soil doesn't dry out so fast. But even for these it is wise to let capillarity restore itself first. Then you won't have to sow them quite so far down, they'll emerge faster and at a higher percentage.

Most gardeners, including me, make furrows with the corner of a common garden hoe. I can make a furrow of uniform depth that way because I have many many years of practice. When the depth of the furrow varies the less covered seeds may fail to sprout because they dry out and the ones buried too deeply may not make it to the surface. The most predictable result comes from a time consuming way; compress the furrow with the narrow edge of a 1,200 mm piece of 2 x 1 or else place a hoe handle flat on the bed and press it in whilst sliding the handle back and forth slightly. I mix compost into the surface inch with a hoe. That way the surface becomes a friable germination medium much like the potting mix delicate seedlings do best in.

When I start expensive hybrid brassica seeds in my excellent soil I usually do not dig the bed. Instead I spread COF and a thin maintenance-layer of compost, hoe them into the top 25 mm and then rake the bed so that it is level, lumpless and smooth. Then on positions where seeds are to go, I gently press down with a fist or my thumb until the spot slightly firms. Then four or five seeds are carefully placed in a knuckle dent or thumbprint and covered to the right depth with fine humusy earth. To keep track of where this position is until seedlings emerge, using one finger I boldly inscribe a 200 mm diameter circle in the soil around each position. The planting spot then looks like a target with seeds at the bullseye.

Progressive thinning

Inevitably, some seeds fail. Pests and soil diseases may kill or severely damage the weaker seedlings. After a seedling has been growing for two weeks it will probably survive to maturity. It has become what I term *well established.* That's why I sow three to five seeds for every plant desired and gradually thin out the extras that nature doesn't take out for me. When starting small seeds on positions (like 450 mm x 450 mm) I put four to six seeds at every station in a cluster the size of a 20 cent piece. When sowing large seeds like bean or a cucurbit, three seeds per position is usually enough to insure that two seedlings emerge. Then I gradually remove the less desirable seedlings until there remains only one strong plant.

Suppose you want 100 mm between plants in the row. To achieve that, place one seed every 25 mm. If you want to end up with one plant every 25 mm (salad radishes or small carrots for example), place one seed every 6 mm. Farmers do this with a precision sowing machine; when gardeners sow by hand some seedlings will emerge in clusters and the interplant spacing usually varies. Shortly after germination remove enough seedlings that none touches another. After growing for a week they'll probably be touching again, so thin again. Repeat this a few times; the row be properly spaced and there will be no empty spots.

Temperature

Most kinds of vegetable seeds will germinate when the soil's temperature is between 15°C and 30°C; between 20°C and 25°C produces a far higher germination percentage with most species. Some tropicals like pepper, eggplant and cucumber don't sprout at all below 20°C. A few species sprout far better at cool temperatures. Spinach can sprout at 7° but does best around 15°C. On a sunny summer afternoon bare soil may be so hot near the surface that it kills sprouting seeds. Spinach seed rots when soil temperature goes over 24°C; it ranges from unlikely to impossible to get spinach to germinate between mid-December and mid-February. Lettuce, silverbeet and beetroot also don't germinate in hot soil. So during high summer await a spell of cloudy, cooler weather before sowing these cool season vegetables.

Sowing according to soil temperature always works better in spring than doing it by the calendar. The main milestone is passed when the soil reaches 10°C early in the morning measured 25 mm below the surface. Ten degrees is the minimum germination temperature for most cold-tolerant species. Tasmanian soils are still too chilly to sow vegetables when the first daffodils emerge. Light loams warm up faster than moisture retentive clays. North facing slopes warm up the most rapidly. West-facing slopes will be a degree warmer than east-facing ones. South-facing slopes make for late gardens.

Novices should invest in a soil thermometer; their appreciation of soil temperature will be uplifted by it. However, the succession of spring flowers and of blooming fruit trees conveniently reveal the soil's temperature. Overwintering garlic and onions begin growing fast when early spring bulbs come up; then it is time to side-dress overwintering alliums. When Japanese plum varieties bloom it is time to sow radishes and spinach. Different apple varieties bloom over several weeks. I have read that when the middle-range of apple tree varieties are flowering it's safe to plant out tomatoes. When I lived at frosty Lorane, Oregon, after losing a lot of tomato seedlings to frost I learned that when the cow parsnips growing in the ditch across the road from my driveway entrance bloomed it *probably* was safe to plant out tomatoes.

Soil temperature changes rapidly near the surface. From mid August to mid-September when the air temperature is only 10°C the surface few centimetres of dark-coloured soils can exceed 21°C in the early afternoon when the sun shines. That night the soil temperature may drop below 10°C, pausing the sprouting process. But the soil warms up quickly if the sun comes out the next day. However, if the weather becomes cloudy, or worse, rainy, these same soils may stay cold until the weather improves. And germination fails.

Spring's unstable weather makes germination dicey. But not planting can result in a late harvest or none at all. That's the eternal dilemma when growing food. If we miss a window of opportunity there may not be another until next year. But at least we can plant something else in that spot. This reality also highlights why weak, unvigorous seeds can produce an even worse outcome than no-germ seeds because some do shoot and the gardener keeps on hoping they'll grow really well—which they often do not.

Chitting

Seeds germinate much better in soil when you partly sprout them before sowing. Pre-germinated seeds emerge more reliably in both summer's heat and in dicey spring conditions. Brits name this technique "chitting." To chit corn, pea, bean and other large-seeded legumes place the seeds in a jar, cover the jar with a square of plastic fly screen held on with a strong rubber band and then cover the seeds with tepid water for six to eight hours. Soak them in a warm place in the house. Do not submerge the seeds longer than eight hours. Then drain all free water and position the jar on its side so that the damp seeds get the best-possible air supply. Rinse with tepid water and immediately drain two or three times daily for the next few days. *Sow them as soon as the first root tips appear on some of the seeds.* Do not delay sowing because the fast-emerging roots are brittle, they break easily (that kills the seed) and soon the roots will become inseparably tangled. Gently stir barely sprouting seeds into finely divided damp compost or sieved garden soil and then uniformly distribute the mixture in the furrow.

With large-sized seeds, gently position each sprouting seed in the furrow one at a time with the emerging root pointed horizontally or in a downward direction. If the emerging root points up then it will immediately form a loop and head back down but the loop may ever after interfere with growth. You can count on nearly 100 percent emergence from sowing large seeds that were already beginning to sprout.

Chitted seeds require less frequent watering before they emerge. You'll use quite a bit less seed per length of row than you previously needed, you'll get a far higher percentage of emergence and save time thinning. Chitting also alerts the gardener before they sow a packet of hopelessly weak or dead seeds. Instead of waiting a few weeks to realize that seedlings will not emerge there may be enough time to obtain better seed or choose to grow something else.

In Chapter 9/Cucurbits, I have more to say about chitting squash, cucumber and melon because seeds in this family should not be soaked in water.

Filling the row

Gardeners can't help but be uncertain about how well any new seed packet will germinate so they sow thickly and often end up with an overcrowded row or position. If the gardener has any sense they promptly thin this overseeded row no matter much time doing that takes. Here's a simple time-saving seed-packet-stretching technique that works nearly as well as precision planting equipment farmers use and costs nothing. When growing small-sized vegetables in rows put a quarter- or a half-teaspoonful of dry (not chitted) seed into a litre or two of slightly damp finely sifted compost or soil and thoroughly blend the seed in. Then distribute this mixture in the furrow and cover to the appropriate depth. There'll be much less thinning.

A heaped ½ teaspoon kitchen measure of *strong* carrot seed that has been thoroughly mixed into a few litres of compost can establish one carrot roughly every 12 mm along 5 lineal metres of furrow. If the seed isn't strong it could take several times more seeds. After shoots appear thinning takes only moments. There will be very few seed clusters or gaps in the row exceeding 25 mm. There's no way for me to be specify exactly how much seed to use because the size of carrot seed varies from one lot to another and so does the percentage of seedlings that will emerge. One half teaspoon of strong lettuce seed might establish twice that length of row. Even if you sow too much seed for the length of row the thinning needed to correct it will prove far less work than had you sprinkled seed into that furrow by hand. The next subsection explains that you may anticipate by past performance how well a seed packet will germinate.

Saving money

Some gardeners expect that this year's seed packets will not germinate well next year. Some start every year with all new packets. I disagree. If the packet sprouted vigorously and grew well this year, if the variety pleased you enough to want to grow it again next year, if there's unused seed to carry over, then use this seed next season. Even if you've already had that packet for several years, if it still sprouts strongly it'll very likely carry over to next year. If the seed packet sprouted weakly this year, then discard any remaining seed before the next season comes around.

If there's a good chance you'll grow a variety more than once then buy a money-saving larger-sized packet when you can. If a $4.00 packet of some variety provides 1 gram of seed, then the next larger size probably contains 5 grams and costs $6.00. The only time you won't save much is with expensive hybrids because some species of hybrid seeds cost as much per gram as precious metal whilst the costs of packeting and distribution make up the smaller part of the price.

Vegetable seeds usually retain good vigour for a few years when they are stored in a cool part of the house where humidity is not high. I wish I could provide a chart of anticipated seed life by species but without the result of a recent germination test there is no way to guesstimate how intrinsically vigorous any garden seed packet is at the time of purchase, nor can we know how many years have passed between the date that seed was actually harvested and our purchase of it. Despite the uncertainty it still pays to buy enough to plant for several years. You won't discard nearly the value you'll use.

You can easily make seed last many years longer than it does when it is kept in a cardboard box in a closet, pantry, garage or garden shed. Assume that "normal" seed storage is in paper packets that are kept in a heated/airconditioned room in the house at a stable 20°C and 70 percent relative humidity (RH). Storage life doubles with each 10°C decrease in stable temperature combined with a reduction in humidity that lowers the seed's moisture content by one percent. In 70 percent RH air seed moisture stabilizes near 13 percent. Storing seed in an airtight container with at least as much weight of active silica gel as there is seed in the container lowers seed moisture by few percent. If you also lower the temperature to a stable 4°C (such as inside a fridge) then the storage life will be trebled or quadrupled. Strong cabbage family seeds may germinate after five years if kept in the closet of a normally unheated guest bedroom that isn't damp. But stored with an old sock half full of active silica gel in an airtight container in the fridge they may last 12 to 15 years. Silica gel comes from chemical suppliers in Melbourne if you're willing to buy 10 kg online—clubs and seed savers groups could do that. Amazon.com now sells it. Sometimes small bags of silica gel come free when you buy new electronic equipment and tiny sachets of it are found in vitamin bottles. I save and reuse every bit.

Silica gel takes moisture out of the air until it has saturated itself. Most silica gel crystals are dark blue when the material is very dry; they become light blue when partly saturated with moisture but are still capable of soaking up more. When the gel turns pinkish it has adsorbed all the moisture it can. I refresh pink silica gel by putting it in an oven at 100°C for a few hours; the gel crystals are spread out in a roasting pan. Beware: if the oven goes much over 100°C you'll destroy the gel; you'll know you did that because it'll come out of the oven black instead of blue. Some silica gel is orange when active and turns green when filled with moisture. Some is semi-transparent with no colour indicator.

To passively lower and somewhat stabilize storage temperature keep the airtight container in the crawlspace under the house or in the coldest room in the house. Or do as I do. I store seeds in a refrigerator that also keeps apples and overflow produce. The fridge is best by far; it's the coldest and the temperature is stable; temperature change hastens seed death.

Do not freeze vegetable seeds. Germination may be preserved for a century or more by freezing seeds but before freezing them the seeds must first be dried to a laboratory-determined moisture content or else freezing may kill them. The amount of moisture is usually around 7 percent but it varies from species to species. *I repeat: do not carelessly freeze vegetable seeds.*

Temperature above 20°C and relative humidity above 70 percent ages seed faster than normal. Keeping seed in paper packets under a greenhouse bench leads to dead seed almost as rapidly as putting the shipment of seeds you just picked up at the post office on the dashboard of a car with closed windows that is parked in full sunlight for several hours.

Grow your own

Vigorous seeds for most vegetable species can be raised in Tasmania. For me, the resilience I enjoy from growing my own is reason enough to do it. Also, I like it that my own seeds for swede, kale, kohlrabi, pea, bean, lettuce, frisée, beetroot, silverbeet, parsnip, parsley, tomato, pepper, etc. have virtually no cost. I like to be able to share my seeds with others. Interaction with Quarantine also inclines me to produce my own. Maybe you can too.

Chapter 9 provides specifics for producing seeds for each vegetable. This section provides a general overview that applies to most vegetable species.

There are two broad subtypes: dry seed and wet seed. Wet seeds form and mature inside a moist fruit. The seeds have to be dried after extraction. Here we're describing tomato, pepper, eggplant, asparagus, zucchini, pumpkin, cucumber and melon. To produce vigorous wet seeds allow each seed-producing fruit to get fully ripe or beyond fully ripe before harvesting it. The most vigorous wet seeds are harvested before the end of February when the sun's intensity is high. Dry seeds usually are attached to branches or form in pods or are retained in the flowers; they usually dry down in the field, often ripening as the plant dies. To produce vigorous dry seeds in most cases you must allow the majority of the seeds on each plant to have pretty much dried down before harvesting the whole plant, which also means you should avoid overhead watering as the seeds finish because maturing seeds that pick up moisture again before fully drying down have less vigour.

To end up with highly vigorous beans or pea seeds where the entire garden gets regular irrigation, hand harvest the pods one at a time when the stem end wilts, becomes floppy, when the pod has only started dried down; this indicates the seeds within are no longer drawing from the plant's vascular system. Allow these pods to dry fully indoors before removing the seeds. Hand picking a few nearly-mature pods to get next year's planting seed isn't much trouble.

Dry seed does not ripen all at once. The first seeds to finish may fall from the plant before the later ones are ripe. What is the best compromise? The home seed grower should delay harvesting dry seeds until about ten percent of them have detached by themselves and been lost. Species that mature dry seed at summer's end (corn, French- and runner beans) often experience dew and rain when the seed should be drying out. I repeat: partly drying down, then picking up moisture and then drying again lowers seed vigour. If weather conditions are too humid when the seeds are drying down then pull nearly finished plants from the earth, roots and all. Shake as much soil as possible from the roots and then fully dry the plants under cover, hanging upside down over a tarp or else spread out on one.

Raising your own seed inevitably means you are a plant breeder. There is no avoiding this responsibility. You must choose which plants to save seeds from. Even if you make seed from all the plants you started with that too is a choice and usually it is not the best choice. If you're serious about producing your own I recommend reading Susan Ashworth's *Seed To Seed* and Carol Deppe's *Breed Your Own Vegetable Varieties.* For the truly serious, John Navazio's *The Organic Seed Grower* is a compendium of professional seed production methods as they apply to organic farmers and market gardeners. Ashworth's book usefully describes small scale harvesting and seed processing techniques for many vegetable species. Deppe's book shows how to maintain uniformity and vigour. Gardeners currently providing nonperforming seeds to Eden, Greenpatch and the like should have *studied* Deppe and Navazio.

Pollination

Bean, pea, lettuce, tomato, pepper, eggplant, chicory—all resist outside assistance to pollinate their seeds. These vegetables almost never cross pollinate without being forced to do that by a plant breeder. Other species encourage bees or other insects to exchange pollen between plants or let wind do it.

Most gardeners think open pollinated varieties differ from hybrid varieties. Fundamentally they do not differ. All hybrid seeds come from flowers that have been cross pollinated. Open pollinated asparagus, beetroot and silverbeet, corn, all brassicas, all alliums, English spinach and all biennial root crops cross pollinate (hybridize) indiscriminately with every other blooming plant in the vicinity. Some species have gender: male plants only make pollen; females only develop seeds. Asparagus, cannabis (hemp) and English spinach reproduce this way. In this case every seed must, by definition, be a hybrid. Some species make flowers that contain both pollen and ovary. Each flower can either self pollinate or outcross. Some of the resulting seeds will be self pollinated and some will be hybrid.

Balanced remineralized soil, good weather and letting seed get completely ripe before harvesting it encourages *seed* vigour but the underlying source of *genetic* vigour is outcrossing—which means each of the seed's parents contribute different genes—this is called hybridization. Hybridization produces "hybrid vigour." The opposite of hybrid vigour is "inbred." Species making flowers that must self pollinate, like bush beans, usually grow less vigorously because they must be inbred.

Nature has a clever method that eliminates inbred seeds and increases genetic diversity in species whose flowers contain both ovary and pollen. These flowers produce more than a few self pollinated inbred seeds. Lacking hybrid vigour the self-pollinated seedlings often disappear by themselves. They get choked out by more vigorous seedlings, die from damping off or else you thin them out for being weak and slower growing.

Hybrid varieties are made by intentional crossing two highly inbred lines, both of which are weakly growing perfectly uniform varieties that have been repeated self pollinated. Each inbred generation ends up with less genetic diversity than the previous one and consequently grows even less vigorously but becomes more uniform. A hybrid *variety* is produced by intentionally crossing highly inbred lines. This produces a perfectly uniform row of highly vigorous plants, *but only in the first generation.*

Open pollinated varieties in normally outcrossing species are actually mixtures of similar hybrids that also includes some self-pollinated inbreds. Keep this in mind for what comes soon.

Self-pollinating plants very rarely cross even when they are grown in close proximity. Occasionally one flower produces a few outcrossed (hybrid) seeds because an unusually aggressive bee or a small insect managed to transfer pollen between plants. Then a whole bunch of new varieties are created. Plant breeders force crosses to occur between normally self-pollinating plants. Almost all modern open-pollinated varieties started as an intentional cross pollination.

With a strictly self-pollinated species like tomato, lettuce or French bean the gardener can save seeds from several varieties that are growing in a small garden at the same time. Ensuring genetic purity means keeping track of which plant produced which seeds. If an unwanted cross shows up it will be a very rare event. The greatest likelihood is that the cross will be recognizable in the first generation—treat it like a weed; there's no more problem. A few self-pollinating species occasionally outcross and need a few metres of isolation. These include peas, peppers, broad- and runner beans. (Chapter 9 is specific about isolation distances.) But an unanticipated cross might prove interesting, perhaps you'll wish to make it into a new variety. Refining an intentional or accidental cross into a uniform open pollinated variety can take several years. To learn how start with Carol Deppe's book.

It is not necessary to involve more than one plant when producing seeds for a self-pollinating species. A self-pollinating variety can have many generations of seeds saved from single plants without any loss of vigour. The backyard gardener *should* save their own seed from self pollinating species. I would buy seeds for self-pollinating species from alternative seed companies. Seed saving groups inevitably concentrate on self-pollinated annuals like bean and tomato.

Unfortunately, most bee- or wind-pollinated species that get reproduced in backyard gardens become more inbred with each generation; the variety loses ever more vigour with each seed increase. The technical term for this is "inbreeding depression of vigour." Inbreeding makes a variety become less productive within a few generations. Nonproductivity all too often accurately describes cabbage family varieties purchased from alternative seed sellers who hate hybrids.

Maintaining vigour and productivity in an outcrossing variety requires including many carefully chosen plants in each and every generation. The minimum number of individuals needed varies by the species. For some species it takes at least 100 plants in every generation to prevent loss of vigour. Or 300 plants. In every case a large amount of seed must be made in each production; the grower must be able to allocate enough land to do that.

With outcrossing species, the more uniform an open pollinated variety is made to become the less vigorous it also becomes. A vigorous open-pollinated variety is by definition a mixture of very similar hybrids that cross in each generation. The great majority of those crosses produce similar plants.

Wild plants were trained to be garden vegetables by saving seeds from the most pleasing individuals. This reduces variability in the genepool and leads to inbreeding. The more inbred the line becomes then the more uniform the row and the less vigorous the variety will be. Growing seeds for an unrefined outcrosser like kale is easier because kale is not that far away from the wild plant it started out as. You might maintain an open pollinated kale variety over a dozen generations by involving a dozen plants in each seed production. But with the highly inbred cauliflower, if you reduce the gene pool below 50 plants you'll soon see a complete breakdown. This wouldn't happen in a remote third world village where every garden in that community grows the same variety of pumpkin, onion or kale. Then each gardener could save their own seed from only a few best plants but pollen would be exchanged with a great many similar plants nearby.

Highly productive seeds for refined brassicas like cauliflower, broccoli, Brussels sprout, cabbage and possibly for sprawling cucurbits can only be produced by seed companies or market gardeners. Someone with a large backyard garden might do a good job producing seed for small-sized vegetables like kohlrabi, carrot or onion by involving 50+ plants in each seed production over quite a few generations. But accommodating 50 full grown cabbage plants making seed? That takes a minimum of 25 square metres and would do better if it were allowed 50 square metres. To find 50 close-to-perfect plants of an open pollinated cabbage probably requires growing several hundred to full size.

One last bit of advice. In order to produce seed from a outcrossing open pollinated variety, start by sowing a great many extra seeds and then thinning progressively to eliminate rogues (offtypes) at the same time. Once the row is a few weeks old and solidly established, remove the weakest plants; these are either inbreds or possess poorly adapted traits. Over the next few weeks rogue out tall poppies. These super vigorous individuals are that way because they have been endowed with the most genetic diversity; they have the most hybrid vigour; they would produce a highly variable result if used for parent plants. Aim at making seed from the middle-range of vigour. Until the desired plant density has been achieved continue roguing out plants that differ from what you desire. And if after that point a plant shows undesirable traits, harvest it or kill it even though it leaves a gap or space in the row or bed! Do not allow it to contribute pollen.

Hybrid vs. open-pollinated

The three following opinions have been used like propaganda. I do not agree with any of them. I smell profit-motivated hype wafting up from them:

- Hybrid varieties belong in the same immoral categories as do chemical fertilizers, synthetic herbicides and unnatural pesticides.
- It is not possible to grow your own seeds from hybrids. Once hybrids replace open-pollinated varieties we will no longer be able to grow our own seeds. Then we all will be slaves.
- Hybrid varieties are not nutritious, nor do they taste as good as the old fashioned sorts.

Territorial Seed Company's first catalogue (1980) offered only open-pollinated seeds because at that time I foolishly accepted all of the above beliefs: I though that hybrids were less nutritious, couldn't be used to save seed from and that the big seed companies pushed hybrids in order to discourage farmers from growing their own seeds. That same year I started conducting half an acre of variety trials. To populate the trials ground I asked primary growers for sample packets of their few remaining open-pollinated varieties; I completely ignored their many hybrids. But those sly Dutchmen slipped in a few unasked for hybrid seed packets. And finding space for them in my trials ground I grew out those packets.

I first discovered that hybrid seeds germinated faster and grew more vigorously from the get-go; some of the open-pollinated varieties barely came up. So I wondered: if a vendor would send me weak seed as a trial sample wouldn't I be a fool to put that variety into my catalogue? Inquiring, I was told those open-pollinated varieties "were no longer in commercial use; seeds for them were rarely produced which is why I was sent older, weaker seed. Hybrid seeds get produced frequently. Hybrid seed is always fresh." I was promised that I would always be sent vigorous, high-germination seed when I ordered hybrids. Actually, the phrase *rarely produced* probably meant old seed lots of obsolete varieties almost forgotten in the back corner of the warehouse that only an ignorant newbe like me would purchase.

The unasked for hybrids in my 1980 trials proved to be the most productive varieties and were excellent eating. The open-pollinated varieties I received did not do nearly as well. Ah, I realized, that's why farmers prefer hybrids. The higher seed cost is minor compared to the increased production.

I had read that traditional open-pollinated varieties

taste better and are more nutritious but what was revealed on my trials grounds was the opposite. Many of the hybrids had superior flavour. Not all of them; some varieties are bred for high fibre content so that the vegetable could be frozen without totally turning to mush, or are bred to appear ripe when it really is still unripe inside—and still firm enough to transport cheaply. This is often the case with supermarket tomatoes. This brings to mind a hybrid cabbage variety called Stonehead—compact pretty plant, perfectly round heads hard and dense as a rock and all exactly the same size, fast growing, maturity so uniform you can cut the whole field on the same day. Flavour? Like tough paper. Then why is there a Stonehead? Because Stonehead is ideal for making the kind of thinly sliced tinned sauerkraut preferred by Americans; the taste need not be in the cabbage, it develops from fermentation, salt and flavouring agents—but the kraut absolutely must be crunchy-crisp when it comes out of the can.

Another example: a plant breeder and I were cruising his small fruit trials. It was the beginning of summer, the main berry season; I was stuffing my face—raspberries, blackberries, marionberries. Then we got to a huge strawberry patch growing I don't know how many dozen varieties. We came to one that made enormous, huge, gigantic, plum-sized intensely red strawberries that were so hard I nearly broke a tooth. The taste was extremely sour. Why this variety, I asked? Oh, said the breeder, we're very proud of that one! He discerned my dismay so he went on about it. This variety is for freezing. The berries are still firm when you thaw out the package—as for sweet . . . it already has lots of tart, strawberry flavour. The processor simply adds sugar.

Hybrids can make useful seeds

I bred an open-pollinated carrot out of an unusual F_1 hybrid called Merida and an open-pollinated kohlrabi seeds from an excellent F_1 hybrid called Kolibri. Southern Harvest currently sells Kolibri F_1. The open-pollinated carrot came out quite similar to the hybrid I started with although the percentage of germination of the OP seed was rather low. My open-pollinated kohlrabi grows and tastes the same and is nearly as uniform as the hybrid.

The kohlrabi project was easy. Every plant in a F_1 hybrid variety has identical genes so there is no need to involve more than a few plants the first time seed is produced. Twelve Kolibri plants filled half a pillowslip with (F_2) seeds that grew a crop so uniform one might think Kolibri F_1 actually may be an open pollinated variety being sold at the high price of a hybrid. I used my own seed from that one production for many years.

However, getting seeds from Merida F_1 required Carol Deppe's help. Merida has a unique and useful characteristic. It overwinters as a small plant and forms a nice carrot in spring instead of going to seed right away. The parent lines used to make this variety had been so highly inbred that Merida F_1 is totally self-sterile. The first time I attempted to make seed not a single seed formed—exactly like the anti-hybrid propaganda claims would always happen. Carol suggested I cross Merida with another variety that looked more or less the same, it could be open pollinated or hybrid, it didn't matter which. I chose an OP called Armstrong and got lots of seed on Merida.

In the next generation I backcrossed [Merida x Armstrong] to Merida F_1 by growing a short row of the cross next to a short row of the original. This backcross produced plenty of seeds on the Merida F_1 plants. These seeds contained three-quarters Merida genes. The backcross retained considerable self-sterility but plenty of viable seeds also developed. Those seeds grow something so similar to Merida F_1 that I can't tell the difference. I've carried my open-pollinated version through several succeeding generations. It's not quite as uniform as the original Merida but it still works as an overwintering carrot, tastes great and is productive enough for the home garden.

Umpqua broccoli was developed by a self-taught Oregon breeder named Tim Peters. Tim ended up directing Territorial Seed Company's trials ground after I sold the business. Tim told me he started Umpqua with a popular hybrid called Green Valiant. He let it make seeds. Like many hybrids Green Valiant was highly self-sterile. So each plant produced only a few seeds but those seeds were viable. In the next generation most of the self sterility had selected itself out so the line set seeds like a normal open-pollinated variety. Then Tim refined Umpqua until it had become a uniform, productive variety that is far better than the raggedy so-called heirloom open-pollinated broccoli varieties remaining in the cheap end of the seed trade. It is currently produced by Adaptive Seeds in Oregon and also sold by Southern Harvest and Birdland.

Dr. Alan Kapuler, founder of Peace Seeds, Corvallis, Oregon gave me this bit of his wisdom in personal conversation. For thousands of years each agricultural family grew its own unique varieties. Some varieties were more nutrient dense, some less so. The children born to families whose varieties lacked nutrient-density more frequently died from childhood diseases. Thus less-nutritious varieties tended disappear along with the family that grew them. Thus, for thousands of years our food crops had been unintentionally selected for greater nutrient density.

After 1870 agriculture transformed. It was no longer about supporting a self-sufficient family that had a bit of surplus to sell; it became something mainly concerned with profit. The profit motive shaped most choices. The newly discovered Mendelian genetics was then used to accelerate the development of fruit that looks ripe when it really isn't; vegetables were redesigned hold up better when shipped long distances—and who cares what they taste like or how nutritious they are. I'm referring here to open-pollinated varieties bred after 1870. The names of the open pollinated varieties in general use around the Second World War are still well known to gardeners but they are not really heirlooms. They may or may not provide the level of nutrition than vegetables once had.

And now genetic engineering is being applied to achieve greater profit. Catering to pubic opinion, many garden seed merchants promise to never knowingly sell seed or plants which are genetically engineered. I see nothing *inherently* wrong with genetic engineering. GE is but a tool we can use to bend plants to the shape we wish them to be. If our goal would be to increase nutrient density, bring greater health and increase lifespan then genetic engineering could be useful. But at this time the main goal is selfish profit so GE accelerates the loss of nutrient-density in industrial foods. GE has been used to make crops contain toxic insecticidal substances. I have read reports of livestock not thriving on GE feed; about Indian farming villages getting sick (and some people dying) when toxic pollen released by nearby GE crops was blowing through their village.

The best reason to preserve genuine heirlooms is the possibility of using their genes to improve nutrient density in modern varieties. However, those seeking business profits by cultivating gardener's prejudices are often selling obsolete highly degenerated open-pollinated varieties that had been bred for industrial agriculture a long time ago. And what of the actual heirlooms? It may be possible to rescue some of them even after a century or more of inbreeding and poor selection by backyard seed savers. A few of the largest North American garden seed businesses that employ qualified plant breeders are working on that.

Chapter 7

Raising Seedlings

My well-beloved had a vineyard in a very fruitful hill;
And he digged it, and cleared it of stones,
And planted it with the choicest of vine,
And he looked that it should bring forth grapes,
And it brought forth wild grapes.

—5 Isaiah, ***The Holy Scriptures*** (Masoretic text)

Garden centres allocate far more space to seedlings than to seed packets. Some of their seedlings look like my home-grown; others are weak, likely to die soon after transplanting. The purchaser's challenge is evaluating the true nature of what's in front of you.

A healthy seedling looks sturdy—it is thick stemmed, stiff and stocky, not so delicate that a moderate breeze will tear it apart. Vegetable seedlings should have formed at least three completely developed (pairs) of dark green leaves (unless the variety is naturally purple or some other colour, or doesn't form leaves in pairs, like onion). The seedlings should be well rooted but not yet pot-bound. You should examine the roots! Place the stem between the second and third fingers, invert the pot and tap the bottom until the growing medium loosens and rests on the palm of your hand. Then ease the pot up and expose the growing medium. If only a few root tips can be seen (or none at all) then the medium probably will break apart during transplanting; many roots will be destroyed. Don't buy this one; slide it back into its pot and move on. Even if you manage to transplant it without damaging the roots that plant almost certainly will go into shock when put outside because seedlings that are large enough above ground to sell with inadequate roots got that way by being kept too warm and being feed too much nitrogen. If you must have this plant better to harden it off until its roots properly fill the container and it adjusts to lower temperatures. Then transplant it. I'll soon explain how to harden off seedlings.

If many roots have wrapped themselves around the outside of the growing medium the seedling has become pot-bound. This plant can look okay on the sales bench for up to two weeks after getting pot-bound if it is frequently fertigated. But that seedling has too much top and not enough bottom; it may be severely moisture stressed the first time it experiences direct sunlight with a bit of breeze. Any plant that gets stressed this way in the seedling stage will never grow as well as it might have done. It likely will wilt after transplanting unless you continue to water it every sunny day for at least a week. With fancy brassicas like cauliflower, cabbage and broccoli, becoming pot-bound in the seedling stage can lead to disappointment; these plants often head up when they still are small.

Pinching off the lowest pair of leaves when setting out potbound seedlings reduces the amount of water the roots have to supply and allows the root ball to be buried deeper where the soil doesn't dry out so rapidly. Even though you have removed some of its sugar-factory this seedling will grow better without having to cope with moisture stress. Still, losing leaves is a setback; better to start out with leaves and roots in balance. If you must have this plant, immediately pot it up one size and put it in bright shade for a few days. Then back in full sun until the larger container is well rooted before transplanting it.

If numerous root tips are visible with no more than a few beginning to wrap around the outside then the seedling is perfect for transplanting. The growing medium will hold together; the root system will continue expanding without interruption. This seedling needs nothing special except watering in when it is transplanted.

In seven days a containerized seedling can go from having barely enough root development to transplant without being damaged to being pot-bound. Buyers at garden shops: be alert. Garden centres often sell too-small seedlings with insufficient root development when terrific spring weather creates greater demand than had been anticipated. After the main planting season I find pot-bound seedlings on the sales bench that should have been marked down to fifty cents each.

Soft plants

You can easily inspect a potted seedling's root system. Evaluating robustness is not as straightforward.

The seedling you buy from a shop was almost certainly grown by a specialist nursery whose usual main motivation is profit. One way to increase earnings is to grow seedlings faster and reuse each precious square metre of bench space as often as possible. When all water given contains fertilizer and the growing medium is always comfortably moist with it; when the temperature is mild at night and pleasantly warm night and day; when there is never more than an intermittent slight breeze; then plants grow incredibly fast above ground by forming larger cells with thinner walls. These plants make too little root to replace what their overblown delicate leaves would lose in full sun unless the soil is made very moist. This plant is *lush* and *soft*.

Lush plants look gorgeous on a sales bench where they are almost certainly under shadecloth so they don't have to be watered so often but actually they are so fragile that a moderate breeze might rip their delicate leaves. Lush seedlings often wilt when first experiencing full-strength sun and wind. A soft seedling usually goes into shock when it is transplanted. This stops it from growing for a week or more. If it doesn't promptly die.

Plants growing in a cooler environment and given less nitrogen fertilizer form smaller tougher leaves on shorter, stockier stems and make larger root systems. Seedlings like this are much less likely to be damaged by handling, by winds, or by insects. Seedlings like this take longer to grow; the seedling nursery would have to charge a higher non-competitive price for them.

When a lush pepper seedling that never yet experienced a night below 15°C is put outdoors and then on its first night is exposed to 6°C it may not grow much for a few days after. Chilled again that strongly or moreso the following night it may become stunted. A pepper seedling from the shop that been hardened off by the gardener before being transplanted would not be severely stressed.

Cold hard rain a can be a severe shock to a hothouse plant. A light frost stuns a frost hardy brassica seedling that never before experienced temperatures below 10°C. Loss of root hairs, almost inevitable when transplanting, is also a shock. Visualize a greenhouse seedling coming from a almost sterile environment with ideal growing conditions that is suddenly exposed to wind, rain, root damage, unfiltered strong sunlight, low overnight temperatures, soil diseases and hungry insects—all at once.

I once wasted valuable space and my time by including both hard and soft tomato seedlings in a variety trial. This happened at Lorane, Oregon (275 metres elevation), a place where frost occurring after the last usual frost date is the usual thing. So I always grew extra tomato seedlings and held them in a cold frame, just in case. That year I transplanted on the date my neighbours considered safe. That year there was a frost 13 days later. I lacked enough reserve transplants to fully restore the trial so I filled the gaps with seedlings from the local garden centre. My own seedlings had formed strong dark green leaves and thick stiff stems in the cold frame; the garden centre seedlings were light green and delicate. My reserve seedlings were slightly pot bound but they started growing fast as soon as they discovered more root zone; the garden centre seedlings went into shock and were badly chewed by flea beetles. I had to spray them twice. My home-grown seedlings were not bothered by flea beetles. My seedlings ended up much larger and bore far more fruit.

How To Transplant

Make a hole about 100 mm deep and 200 mm across. Pour a ¼ cup of COF into that hole. Using a hoe, fingers or trowel, mix COF into the bottom. Then refill the hole and smooth the surface.

Now make a smaller diameter hole in the centre of the diggings. Make it slightly wider than the root ball and deep enough that the seedling's bottom leaves will be just above the soil line when the hole is refilled. Without damaging its roots, invert the pot, tap the seedling out into your hand and place it into that hole. Do not immediately refill the hole with soil.

From a bucket of tepid water containing liquid fertilizer or compost tea, scoop out half a litre and quickly pour it into the hole. Take care not to wash soil away from the transplant's roots.

Immediately, before the water soaks in, push enough loose soil back into the hole to form a muddy slurry that coats the root ball while pretty much filling in the cavity. Then completely refill the hole. The seedling has been mudded-in. It will not wilt and won't need any special watering after that.

I advise you to always harden off garden centre seedlings before transplanting them. I suggest immediately potting them up one size and growing them on until the larger pot has properly filled with roots. Usually that takes 7 to 10 days. On the first day, put seedlings outside in bright shade to become accustomed to mild breezes and indirect full spectrum light unfiltered by glass or plastic. Bring them indoors before sunset and keep them overnight in a cool part of the house. The next morning introduce them to direct morning and/or late-afternoon sun and bring them in at night. Then give them full sun (if there is any) and that night put them in an outbuilding or enclosed porch to experience lower night temperatures. Let them pass the night after that outside in a protected spot such as hard up against a north-facing wall—unless the low temperature is forecast to drop below 4°C for frost-tolerant species; below 7°C for tomatoes or pumpkin/zucchini; below 10°C for tender species like peppers, cucumber and eggplant. After a week on this routine they'll transplant with a much higher likelihood of thriving. By potting them up one more time into an even larger container you may protect them for several more weeks. Doing this can be useful in spring because the seedling will grow faster in a protected sunny position against the house or outbuilding than it would have done in the garden.

Garden centre transplants can disappoint for other reasons. Much like supermarket fruit that looks ripe when it really isn't, some vegetable varieties have been bred especially for nursery trade profit, not for the gardener's needs. They make a great visual appearance when small. They'll have thick stems and tolerate higher concentrations of fertilizer so they're large enough to sell a week sooner. The food quality these seedlings ultimately produce is of little concern. Beware: the seedling nursery may provide the shop with varieties that perform well in Victoria but not all that well in Tasmania. The brassica seedlings on offer may not suit the season. The seedling raiser may have not yet realized (or didn't care) that the (large) difference between how much hybrid seeds cost versus what open pollinated seeds cost will prove to be the least important difference.

Raising Your Own

These days I do not purchase seedlings—nor do I grow many. That's because raising seedlings uses far more of my precious time and attention than direct seeding does and in my experience direct seeded plants grow better. One allure of seedlings is that they are three- to four weeks old when you set them out. It therefore seems they will be harvested that much sooner than a directly seeded crop. But if the seedlings have not been hardened off, if their root systems are damaged while transplanting, if a lot of things, they usually end up being harvested only one week earlier than seeds sown on the same day. Except in the case of solanums—tomato, pepper and eggplant.

I got quite skilful at seedling raising when I did trials for Territorial Seed Company. How else could I look at tomato, pepper or eggplant varieties! Knowing no better in those days I also transplanted my own-grown brassica and celery seedlings. These days I only raise seedlings for tomato, pepper, eggplant and basil. The rest of my garden crops are directly seeded.

To grow great transplants you must control light, temperature and moisture; use an airy moisture-holding growing medium that doesn't compact; provide sufficient air movement and balanced complete fertility—not too weak but not too strong. Success will come only to the degree that each of these factors is properly managed. Direct seeding lets nature handle most of it.

Temperature

A compromise temperature is needed if you wish to grow many species at once. The matter is complex so before getting into the details I'll start with the take away: all the vegetable species we can grow in Tasmania thrive between 18°C to 21°C in the daytime and 10°C at night. Warmer than that makes lush weak plants; colder conditions make them grow too slowly, especially at first.

Seeds for melon, cucumber, pepper and eggplant barely sprout below 21°C. They germinate best at 25°. Most other vegetable seeds will shoot above 15° but do best between 20° and 25°. This temperature works for everything except parsley, celery, celeriac, spinach and lettuce, which don't sprout well at all above 21°C and do best around 18°C. I suggest that when germinating seeds indoors use an electric heat mat and aim for 24°C where the seeds are; to hit this target you may have to create an air gap between the heat pad and the bottom of the seedling tray.

Heat lovers—pepper, eggplant, melon, squash and cucumber—grow fast enough at temperatures between 18°C and 21°C in the daytime. Temperatures over 24°C make tropicals grow much faster but they get too soft and will go into severe shock when put outside. Tropicals grow too slowly below 18°C in the daytime. Ideal dark period temperatures for tropicals should be 15°C until they've developed one pair of true leaves; then you may teach them to be comfortable at 10°C during their dark period.

Cool-weather seedlings—the coles, celery, parsley, and lettuce—get spindly and weak when grown at temperatures tropicals would find ideal. All these (except celery) do best at 15°C to 18°C in the daytime and 7°C to 10°C at night.

All species benefit from dropping nighttime temperatures in their final week.

Growing medium

Seedling roots develop best in an airy, loose medium. Even if you have excellent garden soil in which seeds come up well and grow fast, it should not be used (as it is) as a container growing medium. The reason is that small containers in bright light must watered frequently. A half grown seedling in bright light needs water every other day. When soil is moistened, it swells. When it dries, it shrinks. Frequent swelling and shrinking causes the whole mass to tighten; there will be less soil air and less space for roots. A seedling that needs three to four weeks to reach the four leaf stage in a proper container growing medium takes a week or two longer to achieve the same size when the container is filled with straight garden soil. And soil is weighty. It takes strength to lift a flat of seedlings growing in soil.

Commercial producers raise seedlings in light weight materials that resemble soil but resist compaction and hold a lot of moisture. They blend sand, coir, sphagnum moss, vermiculite, perlite and compost. Seedling raising mixes sold in poly bags are similar, often they are pre-fertilized with chemicals and (if you're lucky) hold some aglime, but even when prefertilized, they contain only enough nutrients to sustain slow growing shade plants.

Here are two typical recipes for commercial seedling growing media. I'm not suggesting you use them. I am suggesting you consider the intention behind their formulation and then do something better. Both of them contain aglime because only a few two-part liquid fertilizers used for growing marijuana provide any calcium. Without available calcium plants shrivel and die; if calcium is in short supply they grow poorly.

University of California Mix

75 percent coarse sand
25 percent sphagnum (peat) moss
Add to each cubic metre of mix:
3 kg agricultural lime
1 kg dolomite lime
1.5 kg 10-20-10 chemical fertilizer

This growing mix, being mostly sand, is inexpensive but weighs a lot in the pot or flat and has little ability to hold on to nutrients so the chemical fertilizer is soon washed out. No trace elements are provided.

Cornell University "Peat-Lite"

½ cubic metre sphagnum moss
½ cubic metre horticultural-grade vermiculite and/or perlite
2 kg dolomite lime
½ kg superphosphate
2½ kg 5-10-5 chemical fertilizer

A lightweight mix like this reduces the amount of strength needed and fatigue generated when handling a great many plant trays. Vermiculite also adds buffering capacity, to be explained shortly. No trace elements are provided.

My own seedling raising medium

1 part by volume my best garden soil
½ part by volume compost
1 part by volume sphagnum moss
Blend into each 20 litres:
200 ml my complete organic fertilizer (1:100)

My mix is not sterile. I garden on a heavy loam. I use properly humified compost made by me. Every part of the mix provides buffering capacity.

If my garden soil was clay then I'd change the recipe to ¼ part by volume clay soil; ¼ part by volume compost; ¼ part by volume moss; and a generous ¼ part by volume perlite plus COF at 1:100.

Sphagnum moss is more expensive in Australia than coir is, probably because moss is shipped from high-wage Canada and coir comes from India. Moss is sterile and soaks up several times its weight in water. Moss provides almost no plant nutrients and has an acidic pH, about 3.5. It contains natural fungicidal substances that inhibit damping-off diseases. Sphagnum moss in compressed bales should be finely ground although it is often clumpy. Slow to take up water when completely dry, moss should be thoroughly remoistened before use. Drop any hard chunks into a bucket, cover with water and they will expand nicely in an hour or so. Then squeeze out or drain off excess moisture.

Vermiculite is made from mica, a naturally occurring volcanic mineral that expands like popcorn when roasted. Consequently vermiculite is sterile. Vermiculite is lightweight, has a pH of about 7.0 and is able to hold three to five times its own weight in water. Plant nutrients strongly adhere to vermiculite so it smooths out (buffers) the ups and downs in nutrient availability that fertigated container plants experience. One obstacle gardeners growing in sand have to overcome is that sand lacks buffering capacity. Consequently both nutrient availability and soil pH cycle up and down with crop extractions. This irregularity makes plants grow less well. Vermiculite remains loose after going through many wet-dry cycles. Vermiculite comes in four horticultural sizes: # 1 is too coarse for bedding plants; # 2 is the regular horticultural grade. The very fine #3 and #4 are used as germinating media for extremely small seeds.

Perlite is made from pumice, which is a lightweight volcanic rock that is crushed and then heated so it expands like popcorn. The coarse spongy bits are very lightweight. Perlite will hold three to four times its own weight in water. It has no ability to buffer plant nutrients, has a pH of about 7.0 and is used to lighten and aerate soil mixes. You probably won't find perlite or vermiculite at most garden centres but if you'll visit a hydro shop you'll find these lightweight bulky materials on offer in huge bags. Perlite has a downside: when dry it flies a long distance in a light breeze. So open the bag, add a litre or two of water and stir well before removing any.

Composts are highly variable; some commercial batches make seedlings grow noticeably better, some do little and some contain so much incompletely decomposed woody material that they interfere with growth. The humified compost you can make for yourself can hold many times its weight in water; landscape yard woody waste compost doesn't hold nearly as much. Compost resists compaction. Composts should be the opposite of sterile and that's a big plus point because seedlings are far healthier when they grow in a medium containing a complex microecology. That's one benefit I get from including garden soil in my growing medium. Some commercial composts are mostly semi-decomposed woody waste; this kind is okay as part of a growing medium for shade-tolerant house plants or for mulching ornamentals but having this stuff decomposing in a vegetable seedling's root zone slows its growth. Do not expect much from compost sold in airtight plastic bags because they provide very little microbial activity. Using balanced liquid fertilizer with trace elements covers a multitude of sins.

Coir is coconut husk fibre. It is slow to decompose, light, naturally fluffy. Coir holds an enormous quantity of moisture yet it remains airy when completely wet. Growing media with plenty of coir in them do not need watering as often. Coir is a renewable resource while sphagnum moss isn't. Coir is often sold in compressed dry bricks that must soak up water before use. While being rehydrated the brick crumbles by itself as it expands to several times its compressed volume. Coir contains few plant nutrients. So I suggest rehydrating it with compost tea or better, with a full strength dilution of liquid fertilizer. I rehydrate mine with NTS 10-10-10 at full strength—10 ml/litre. Coir is separated from coconut husks after first soaking them in water for an extended period. Cheaper grades of coir often originate as a third-world homestead product. Often the soak water was sea water and the resultant coir contains so much sodium it can damage plants. Make sure the coir brick you purchase is "low sodium" or is labelled "horticultural grade." At one time I recommended using coir over sphagnum moss but in the last years I've been sold coir bricks that were supposed to be horticulture grade but had not been properly leached of sodium. The seedlings I tried to grow in this stuff just would not grow well. *Caveat emptor!* Hydroponics shops sell already hydrated coir in large bags. This product is more reliable.

Watering

Confinement in a container forces the root system to have a greater density. The same sized plant growing in the garden would have ramified (occupied with roots) several times more soil volume, thereby giving it access to several times more moisture. That's why containerised seedlings that have grown close to transplanting size have to be watered frequently. This makes it essential to use a soil mix that holds a lot of moisture, that can rapidly reabsorb water after pretty much drying out and that doesn't shrink as it dries. When a growing medium shrinks it pulls away from the sides of the pot; then water may run down the sides and out the bottom without really wetting the contents. Once the surface tightens up water uptake may slow down so much that the soil looks saturated when a few centimetres down it actually is dry. Once sphagnum moss has fully dried it is difficult to remoisten. For that reason, I find that about 40% moss by total volume is the maximum safe level.

Tiny young seedlings in lightweight growing media can be uprooted unless you add water gently. The best small scale method I know is a 5 mm to 6 mm diameter clear plastic siphon tube draining a large jar, a 2 litre plastic milk container or a household sized pail located 30 to 60 centimetres above the seedlings. If you want to increase water flow rate then increase the reservoir's height above the seedlings. I suggest allowing the water to stand for a few hours to warm up before using it. This reservoir can be more than an irrigator, it can also be a fertigator.

Seedlings in a cold frame may be watered from a large plastic bucket using a similar siphon. I tie one end of the syphon tube to an old broom handle that allows me to conveniently move the hose around in my cold frame. To provide the right amount of water pressure while taking the stress off my arm and hand I stand the water supply bucket atop an inverted bucket next to the frame. If the flow rate seems too slow, raise the bucket higher or use a larger diameter tube (see page 107).

A bucket siphon system also serves to spot fertigate small plants in the garden. Carry the bucket in one hand and lash the outlet end of siphon to a broomstick held in the other hand. Place the outlet near the soil and siphon fertigation solution straight into the root zone of a small plant.

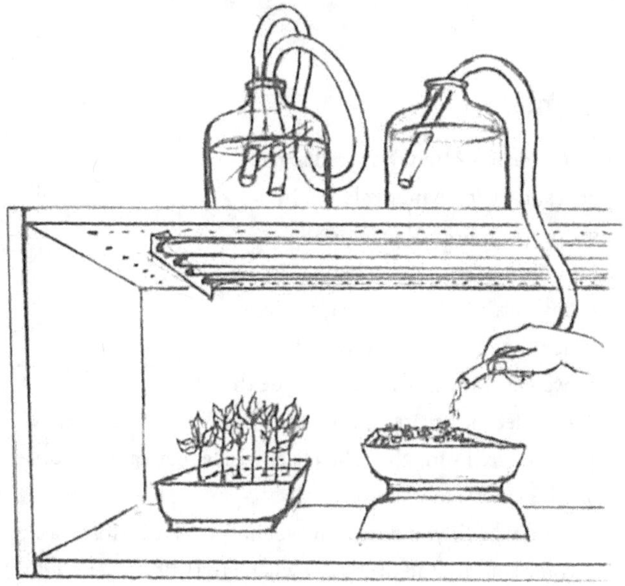

Containers

Commercial seedling raisers aim to profitably raise the largest possible number of seedlings from each precious climate-controlled square metre of bench so they use the smallest practical pot or cell size. They can make this work because it's their job; they can water or fertigate twice a day if necessary. The gardener can use containers providing at least twice as much soil volume per plant as the ones you see on a seedling sales bench. Doing this maintains a bigger moisture reserve, results in stronger seedlings and takes pressure off you.

I wish I could say one container size is best for all species but many factors influence the growth rate and ratio of top to root, including light level, temperature, species, variety and growing medium. Root mass normally increases at the same rate as above ground growth. If there isn't room in the container for that to happen, then the plant gets stunted unless it gets constant fertigation, and in that case it makes too much top for the size of its root system. A 75 mm diameter (or square) pot usually provides adequate root zone for small-seeded species to grow three pairs of leaves. Peppers, eggplants and tomatoes benefit from plenty of hardening off time so I start them in small containers and pot them up to 150 mm diameter containers. Then I can I delay transferring them to the garden until the weather improves. A 150 mm container is sufficiently lightweight that a tray holding five or six seedlings can be taken inside on cold nights.

Melon, cucumber, squash and bean seedlings get big quickly. These should be sown in 100 mm pots.

In the event seedlings of any type fill their pot before the season allows safe transplanting then pot them up one size up before they get the slightest root bound and hold them for another week or two before putting them out.

I've had poor results from compressed peat pots and expandable peat pellets. It is hard enough to keep a small container moist without also having it evaporate a lot of water through its sides. The sales pitch for these is that you can plant the pot along with the seedling and the roots will proceed to grow right through the pot. Sometimes the roots actually do that. And sometimes the pot strangles the seedling. So if you use peat pots be sure to tear off the bottom when transplanting. Compressed peat pellets do not allow mixing aglime into them. I have mentioned before that plants lacking calcium can not grow well. Only a few of the many two-part hydroponic systems sold at the hydroponics shop provide any calcium. Which is why having both gypsum and lime in COF so strongly improves container media.

Germination

The best way I know to germinate seeds in a container or cell tray is to first bring the growing medium to the ideal moisture level (70 percent of capacity) and then fill the containers with it. Do not pack growing medium tightly in a container; keep it loose. Poke a hole into the medium about 5 mm deep with the blunt end of a pencil, put a few seeds into that hole and flick a few bits of growing medium over them. If the soil mix is not sterile then put three or four small sized seeds in the hole and plan to thin gradually. Extra seedlings allow for losses from damping-off and elimination of weaker seedlings. I seal each individual pot in its own airtight poly freezer bag until the seedlings emerge. I fit a poly bag over the top, down the sides, gather the excess plastic at the bottom and put the container on top of the gathered plastic to keep it sealed. That way no watering is needed. When seedlings first begin to emerge, remove the poly bag.

Light

Gardeners often raise seedlings on a sun-facing window ledge. In my previous home I grew seedlings on a tiled concrete floor behind a sunny north-facing sliding glass door. When the weather was favourable I conveniently put them just outside the door to let the breeze exercise their leaves and stems as they got unfiltered sunlight. Then back inside they came at sunset or when it was too blowy.

And what if you don't have such a position? Most species become spindly and overly tall when given insufficient light. Seedlings with thin weak stems don't transplant well—you absolutely must provide very bright light.

A close together pair of *cool-white* fluorescent tubes provides barely enough light directly under them to grow seedlings to their four-leaf stage. Fluoro bulbs come in 600 mm and 1,200 mm lengths. A fixture holding from two or four parallel cool-white tubes suspended over the growing area can produce enough seedlings for a home garden. The minimum light intensity required to grow strong vegetable seedlings is the maximum light intensity fluorescents can create when the tubes are positioned close together and suspended only a few inches above the top leaves. As the seedlings grow the lamps must be either raised or else the height of the shelf holding the seedlings must be lowered or else individual plant containers must be on props that are gradually lowered as the seedlings grow. When I used fluoros I preferred the last option because at any one time I was growing a mix of seedlings. Fluorescents generate useful heat. If you'll put the lights in an unheated room where ambient daytime temperature is around 15°C, then the heat from the lights may create near perfect temperatures around the seedlings.

I now use a 315 watt ceramic metal halide (CMH) light to grow vegetable seedlings because it produces much greater light intensity and outputs more light from each expensive kilowatt hour. That means my seedlings grow more than twice as fast as they would under fluorescents and half again faster than they do indoors against a north-facing window. The higher light intensity makes my seedlings stockier and a lot stronger. And I spend less on hydro.

My cmH bulb is suspended over a 600 mm x 900 mm growing bench. I think this bulb could illuminate a 900 mm x 900 mm footprint. The bulb, its required ballast and a reflector to equalize light distribution, all of these items combined cost slightly more than one fixture holding four 40 watt fluorescents. But 160 watts of fluoros only illuminates an area 300 mm wide by 1,200 mm long and sustains plants only until they are about 150 mm tall. The cmH bulb can sustain plants that are 400 mm tall. What takes three weeks to develop under a cmH bulb takes six weeks and longer to accomplish under fluorescents. And now the hydro shop sells 200 watt LEDs that put out as much useful light as a 315W cmH while making less heat.

Plants grow faster when they have a dark period. Four hours of darkness and 20 hours of light makes the fastest growth. But after being pushed that hard some species will be shocked when suddenly experiencing a shorter outdoor light period. I suggest providing a stable 16 hour light period and 8 hours of darkness, controlled by a timer.

Configuring and using fluoros

No. of Tubes	Max Height Above Plants in mm	Width of Illuminated Area in mm	Period of Growth with Sufficient Light
2	50	150	4 weeks
4	75	225	6 weeks
6	100	300	8 weeks

Exercise

When seedlings develop in still air they become weaklings. When the leaves tremble in the breeze the plant builds stronger structure. So the seedlings on my lounge room floor were given outdoor exercise as often as possible. The first few times I make sure the day isn't windy. After being outside during a few pleasant afternoons the seedlings can take a fairly stiff breeze without damage. When growing seedlings entirely inside it smart to have an oscillating fan gently fluttering their leaves for at least a few hours every day.

Fertilizers

Whenever I've put enough COF into a soil mix to rapidly grow a seedling to transplanting size without any fertigation (two times as much as in my growing medium recipe, or 1:50) I've reduced and sometimes wrecked seed germination. The fix for this is putting moderate balanced fertility into the growing medium (1:100) and supplementing that with liquid fertilizer. But liquid *organic* fertilizer concentrates do not provide balanced plant nutrients. Liquid fish provides nitrogen but not nearly enough phosphorus and sometimes too much potassium if the raw fish was decomposed with potassium hydroxide. Liquid kelp has some potassium, (weak), trace elements and micronutrients (both very weak) but without a useful amount of nitrogen or phosphorus.

For organic believers I think the best compromise is one-half tablespoon of liquid seaweed concentrate and one-half tablespoon of fish emulsion per four litres, in all water given.

I've gotten good results using my own growing mix recipe (that supplies adequate calcium) and then fertigating with Miracle-Gro or Maxicrop Seaweed Plant Food Concentrate, either one included in all water given and diluted to one-third the concentration recommended on the package. Fertigation is synergistic in that the more the sun shines or the higher the light intensity then the more water plants transpire, the faster they'll grow and the faster they intake fertilizer. I dilute soluble concentrates this much because a richer solution results in tender leaves and spindly stems. An even richer mix overdoses seedlings, producing a yellow/brown fringe of poisoned cells on leaf margins. At the first hint of leaf margin browning immediately flush the pots with enough pure water that a considerable amount flows out the bottom and is discarded so it is not drawn back up and then reduce the fertilizer concentration to what I recommend.

Twenty years ago the garden centre nearest to my home opened an hydroponics section featuring a baffling display of liquid fertilizer concentrates and supplements. I felt compelled to investigate these products because, I reckoned, the very high profits obtained from illegal cannabis growing combined with the very high cost of electricity must have inspired those growers to use extremely effective fertilizers. However most of them are multi-part *hydroponics* fertilizers. I tried using such a product with my own soil-like medium (against the shop's advice) and sure enough, exactly as the shop had warned me, because my medium has a very high buffering capacity the plants soon begin to suffer from toxic imbalances.

Hydro shops now sells liquid concentrate systems designed for growing cannabis outdoors in soil. Tell them you want to raise the best possible vegetable seedlings using something way better than Miracle Gro. They'll probably conceal a smirk (thinking you're fibbing about the intended crop) and then will recommend something that'll significantly outperform Miracle Gro or MaxiCrop—and costs more. It likely will consist of several bottles that have to be carefully measured and mixed into a reservoir that can be fed to vegetable seedlings in all water given.

In the section on foliar feeding I recommended using Nutri-Tech 10-10-10. Here's an inexpensive fertigation recipe based on Triple Ten that grows very strong seedlings and costs much less than anything the hydro shop sells. In every 15 litres of water dissolve 1 kitchen measuring tablespoon (15 gm) of potassium sulfate and then add 35 ml of 10-10-10. Use this in all water given.

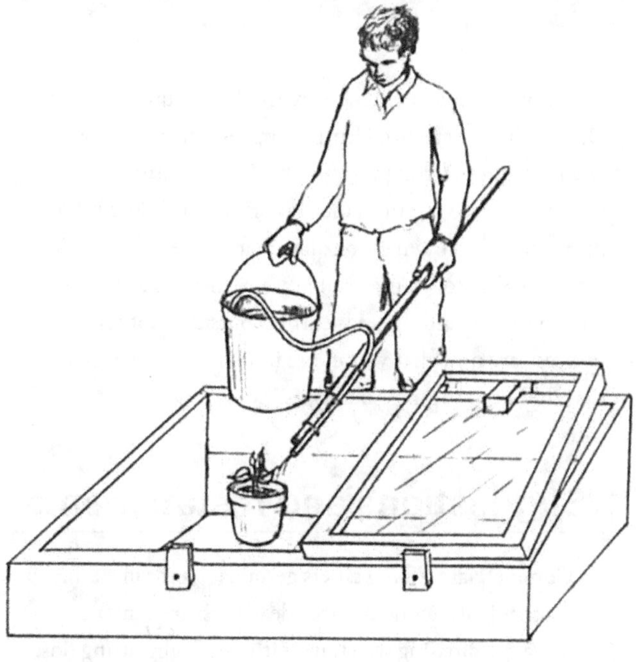

Cold Frames

After a seedling has produced two pairs of true leaves it can be moved to an inexpensive cold frame cobbled together from recycled materials. A cold frame 1.5 metres long by 1,000 mm wide, 450 mm tall at the back and 300 mm high at the front will hold all the vegetable seedlings a large family needs A frame with thick side walls and tightly fitted windows—all joints caulked, all gaps sealed—can hold nighttime temperatures five degrees warmer than the air outside. Even a hastily constructed drafty frame keeps nighttime temperatures a few degrees warmer. When a strong frost is predicted old blankets and/or tarps can be spread over the frame late in the afternoon.

Using an indoor grow light to start seedlings and a cold frame to harden them off works great. By the end of August the light level outside is high enough to produce rapid growth of frost-tolerant species. Daytime temperatures in the frame can be kept cooler than inside the house and night time temperatures will be considerably lower, making frame-grown seedlings much stockier. They'll harden off best with the glass entirely removed on days that aren't too windy.

By mid- to late-September frost tolerant vegetable seedlings will have been transplanted. Now the frame environment will be comfortable for tomato seedlings. If they already are three- to four weeks old around mid-September, pot them up a size and move them to the frame. Thoroughly hardened off tomato seedlings in 200 mm containers can have flowers (and maybe a fruit or two) on them when you transplant them out. Around the time tomato seedlings are planted out the cold frame becomes a benevolent environment for hardening off peppers, eggplants, melons, and cucumbers. These can wait in the frame for a few weeks until warmer weather arrives.

A hot frame is a cold frame with a heat source below it. During the Nineteenth Century frames were placed over pits filled with fresh strong manure that heated naturally. Now most people use thermostatically controlled electric cables buried in the soil. I made one like that in Oregon when I grew variety trials. Hot frames enable a gardener to germinate and grow heat-demanding seeds entirely outside. Hot frames are unnecessary now that we can use indoor growlights except that they keep the mess outdoors.

Suggestions and restatements

Commercial seedling raisers germinate seeds in sterile media that is always held at the ideal moisture content by covering germinating seed trays with clear tight-fitting lids. Trays are placed on heated benches and kept at optimum germination temperature until seedlings appear. There is no damping-off disease. The germination rate achieved will be very close to that of a seed testing laboratory. If (very expensive) super-high-germination hybrid seeds are used then the grower can have automatic seeding equipment place one seed in each cell, ending up with nearly every cell occupied and every perfect plant in the tray exactly the same size.

If a nonsterile growing medium and untreated seeds are used then the germination percentage will drop. If the variety is open-pollinated then some seedlings will not be vigorous or desirable. Consequently, the gardener should put three to five seeds in every container or cell and then gradually cull weak seedlings until only one remains.

Before sowing seed make sure that the planting mix is quite moist but not so wet your fist can squeeze water out of it. Then press a small hole with the blunt end of a pencil 5 mm to 6 mm deep and place three to five seeds in the hole. For big seeds like beans, cucurbits and corn put two or three seeds into a larger deeper hole. Trays and pots that are germinating seeds can be put above a fluorescent light array or below a cmH bulb where the heat generated by the lamp creates warm conditions. In fact, this can be a too warm. In that case, raise the bulb further from the trays or pots, or if the seeds are germinating above fluoros create a few centimetres of air space below the pots. The extreme end of the mantle over a fireplace insert may be a good spot to germinate seeds if it doesn't get too warm there. Inside a cookstove oven with the oven lamp on as the heat source also works as long as no one accidentally bakes the seeds. My oven temperature stays around 25°C with the oven light on but yours may be different. It depends on the size of the bulb and how well the oven is insulated. Atop the hot water tank once was a good spot but is no longer because hot water tanks are too well insulated these days. Garden centres sell electric heating pads to put under germinating seedlings.

Maintain the proper moisture level during germination by sealing the container in a clear plastic bag until the seedlings emerge. After germination, thin progressively. Don't let young seedlings direct their stems very far off vertical as they compete for light. Thinning is best done with small, sharp scissors. Thinning should have been completed by the time the seedlings have started their second pair of true leaves. Then they're about ready to be moved to a cold frame if you've got one.

Growing guide A to Z

All planting dates in this section work in the mid Tamar Valley. Gardeners close to the Bass Strait or near the East Coast might start seedlings two weeks earlier; gardeners in Southern Tasmania, the Midlands or inland at elevations over 100 metres might start seedlings a week or two later. In what comes I will unsubtly try to persuade you to not raise seedlings but instead to directly seed outdoors in most cases.

Beans: French, Lima and Runner. I would only go to the inconvenience of raising bean seedlings if my goal was to harvest two weeks earlier. And why bother with that when the peas finish about the same time direct seeded French beans first get harvested. Be that as it may . . . about two weeks before the last frost date, sow two seeds per individual 75 mm pot. Sprout at 21°C to 24°C. Thin promptly to one plant per pot. Grow under lights for about one week, and then harden them off in a cold frame until the first pair of true leaves has fully developed and the next pair is forming. Transplant outdoors about one week after bean seeds would normally be sown. An early start like this is essential to obtain any yield at all from lima beans. French beans start producing at best a week sooner if transplanted.

Beetroot. Grow a few transplants to achieve the earliest possible harvest; direct seed later plantings. Beet seeds are actually fruits containing several embryos. One very strong seed can produce a cluster of seedlings. It also can take two weak seeds to produce one seedling. In early September, sow three seeds per individual 75 mm pot or cell. Sprout at 21°C. Grow under lights for a few weeks; keep temperature below 24°C. If available, transfer to a cold frame soon after germination. Do not thin unless you end up with more than four plants per pot. Hold in a cold frame until the seedlings approach 75 mm tall. Do not allow beetroot seedlings to become pot-bound. Transplant clusters of three or four seedlings 200 mm apart, in rows 450 mm apart. Several plants on each position may seem crowded but with sufficient spacing between positions almost every seedling forms a root (although not perfectly round).

Broccoli. I suggest raising seedlings only to harvest the first broccoli of the year two weeks sooner than would be possible from a directly seeded crop. At best. And don't be too eager. Earliest broccoli is risky because seedlings that have been slowed by cold conditions may not make large flowers. Sow mid-August, three to five seeds per individual cell or 50 mm to 75 mm pot. Broccoli seeds sprout fast at 20°C. Thin pots/cells gradually to one seedling. Grow two to three weeks under lights with temperatures 18°C to 20°C daytime, above 6°C at night. Transfer at the two-leaf stage to a cold frame, if available. When seedlings have three fully developed true leaves (this usually happens five to six weeks after sowing if they are hardened off in a cold frame), they should be well rooted and ready to set out. Try to schedule transplanting during the earliest week you could direct seed broccoli. Maybe you gained a few week's head start. I prefer to sow my earliest spring broccoli outdoors in the garden late in April and overwinter small plants. Works much better.

Brussels Sprouts Don't go for an early start or you'll fight aphids—and lose the battle. Better the crop is direct seeded mid-December so that harvesting begins in autumn. Brussels sprout makes larger more vigorous seeds than most other brassicas so it is one of the easiest coles to directly seed.

Cabbage For earliest heads, grow like broccoli. Use a quick-maturing early variety. Varieties bred for autumn/winter harvest often make pointed, poorly formed heads when started in spring.

Cauliflower started in spring is more sensitive to chilling than cabbage or broccoli. Grow seedlings like broccoli but do not start seeds before the end of August. After mid-September cauliflower is better directly seeded. Many otherwise excellent varieties make low quality heads when spring sown. I recommend Snow Crown Hybrid, commonly used in North America and Europe. Farmers can access varieties like Snow Crown but unfortunately, no Australian garden seed supplier currently offers this one or anything nearly as useful. Good luck!

Celery/Celeriac In early August, shallowly sow a pinch of ten to twenty celery seeds in a 50 to 75 mm pot or cell. Seeds take two weeks to sprout, best at 15°C to 18°C. Don't rush thinning. Take at least one month after germination to arrive at one plant per cell/pot. Grow at 18°C to 24°C during the day, 10°C to 15°C at night. Celery requires more than two months of bright light in a loose growing medium to attain transplanting size. Move to a cold frame for the last weeks but not before night-time temperatures in the frame hold above 7°C. Too many hours exposure to temperatures below 7°C makes celery seedlings go to seed (bolt) prematurely. I prefer to direct-seed celery about when I set out tomato seedlings, while coolish weather makes germination possible outdoors but nights aren't so cold as to induce premature flowering.

Sweet Corn One corn seedling quickly fills a small container with roots. One week before the last usual frost date sow 3 seeds per 75 mm pot. Germinate at 21°C. Thin promptly to two plants per pot. Do not let them become pot bound. Transplant seedling pairs 450 mm apart in rows 750 mm apart. You might harvest one week sooner than had you direct seeded one week after the tomato seedlings went out. Might.

Cucumbers Start seeds one week after tomato seedlings are transplanted out. Given good growing conditions cucumber seedlings fill containers in short order. Sow two or three seeds 25 mm deep in a 75 mm pot. The ideal germination temperature is 24°C. Cucumber seed will sprout well at 21°C but take a few days longer. Be sure to remove the poly bag as soon as the first shoot appears; this lowers humidity and prevents disease. Grow under lights for at 21°C to 24°C in the daytime, over 13°C at night. Thin to the best plant per pot before the second true leaf fully develops. Transfer to a cold frame for a few days of slight hardening off; it is impossible to make cucumbers (or melons) very hard. Transplant very gently; cucurbit roots are easily damaged.

Eggplant grows like capsicum, but note that young seedlings are more sensitive to temperature under 10°.

Kale grows like super-broccoli, so vigorous that direct-seeding is preferable. Kale is much better tasting in autumn/winter than it is during the heat of summer. Raising transplants seems pointless to me.

Kohlrabi Don't raise transplants! I always direct-seed mid-September through October 1st and harvest them at full size well before hot weather hits. For autumn harvest, direct-seed during February. This vegie makes strong seedlings that cope outdoors.

Leeks If summertime harvest is desired, raise seedlings indoors using the same procedure for growing huge onions. Use a variety intended for late summer/autumn harvest. If autumn/winter harvest is desired, direct-seed in a nursery bed outdoors during October (see chapter 9/Alliums/Leek). For more on raising seedlings, see "Onions" below.

Lettuce Raise seedlings only to achieve the earliest possible spring harvest. Start them early August; otherwise grow like broccoli. I find it much easier and totally reliable to harvest as early as is possible in spring by overwintering lettuce outdoors. Sow seeds late April. See: Chapter 9/Greens/Lettuce.

Melons Grow like cucumbers but melons are more sensitive to low temperatures and damp conditions.

Onions Raise transplants only if your goal is to raise prize-winning lunkers or to have the earliest possible spring onions. Start seeds early in August. The best way is to carefully place four seeds per centimetre of furrows 75 mm apart on a 300 mm x 300 mm seedling tray filled to the brim with container medium. If using cell trays, sow four to six seeds per 50 mm cell. Sprout seeds at 21°C. Grow at 10°C to 18°C in the day, 4°C to 10°C at night. You'll be using long day varieties; keep them on 16 hours light/8 hours dark so as to not trigger seed making. Do not thin. After seedlings have grown about 100 mm tall, using sharp scissors take the top 25 mm off the leaves—a 25 percent haircut. This promotes sturdy leaves and better-developed roots. After the next set of leaves grows 50 mm taller than the previous haircut, cut 15 to 25 mm off of them. Etc, repeat. Transplant when stems are over 3 mm in diameter, or at the latest, early in October no matter their size (as long as they're large enough to survive transplanting). Onions transplant bare-root so separate the seedlings by shaking them apart or washing the soil away in gently running water. Please believe me, you'll get bigger onions by direct seeding early September into very airy fertile soil.

Parsley seeds are slow to germinate so parsley is often transplanted by most gardeners. Grow parsley transplants like broccoli, but note that germination can take 14 to 17 days, best at 15°C.

Peppers Many gardeners set peppers out at the same time as tomatoes, thereby subjecting the seedlings to overnight lows they can't handle easily. It is far better to first put pepper seedlings through a few more weeks of hardening off. Start seedlings six weeks before the last expected frost. In each 75 mm pots or 50 mm cell, sow four seeds. Sprout this heat-demanding seed at over 21°C (best at 24°C). To achieve very strong seedlings grow them at 18°C daytime, 12°C to 15°C in the dark period. Thin progressively to one plant per pot or cell. Immediately after tomato seedlings have been planted out, pepper seedlings should be potted up a size and hardened off in a cold frame for a few weeks before setting them out.

Tomatoes. Best results come if you grow seedlings under lights, at least for their first few weeks. Start August 1 if you use fluoros or the window ledge; start August 15 if its an cmH lamp or LEDs. Sow four seeds in each 50 mm to 75 mm pot or cell. Sprout at 21°C to 24°C. Make temperature 18°C to 21°C in the day, 10°C to 15°C at night. Thin gradually to one plant per pot. Pot up as necessary. And then harden off. While hardening off protect against night-time lows below 7°C. If possible, hold the seedlings in 250 mm pots in the cold frame until you've got 450 mm-inch-tall plants already bearing fruit. That way you *might* start enjoying ripe tomatoes before Christmas.

Zucchini and pumpkin (squash). Squash of all kinds are hardier than cucumbers but are equally difficult to transplant and require bigger pots than cucumbers because the seedlings start out larger and grow faster. I suggest germinating squash seeds at 21°C to 24°C. One week before the last anticipated frost, sow three seeds in a 100 mm pot. Once germinated, thin each container to two plants and move them immediately to a cold frame if available. Grow the pair of seedlings until their roots have developed enough to hold the soil ball together—four to seven days. Then transplant. In these days of hybrid variety dominance open-pollinated summer squash varieties often throw off-type plants. Start out with two plants per position. Best to delay thinning a single plant per position until the pair of plants have formed their first few fruit.

Chapter 8
Pests

Soil microorganisms interact with higher plants. Given identical soil conditions the composition of the microflora changes sharply with the type of plants growing on that soil. Plants are a very strong ecological factor, favouring certain species of bacteria, fungi, actinomycetes and other inhabitants of the soil while discouraging others. As a result of wrong agricultural practice the soil becomes infested with harmful microbial forms. By use of suitable plants in the crop rotation, one may change the microflora of soil in the desired direction, and eliminate harmful organisms, in other words—restore the health of soil.

– N. S. Krasil'nikov, ***Soil Microorganisms and Higher Plants****

Sir Albert Howard, founder of the organic farming and gardening movement, asserted that before a plant visibly suffers from insect or disease it already was malnourished. Today's organic gardeners still believe if their soil contains enough worms their garden would have few to no disease or insect problems. Most often this is correct. When a problem does appear the organic crowd opines that their long term solution is even more compost, resulting in even more worms. I have already made the point that this belief is incorrect. Plants can have problems for many reasons. Here are some examples:

First, the usual thing—poor nutrition. One spring early in my gardening career I had three excess cabbage seedlings from a purchased punnet of six. Rather than bin them I planted them in a never-before-used never-fertilized never-limed spot on the garden's fringe, fed them only cheap chemical lawn fertilizer that provided too much N and no trace elements. I spread no lime nor did I dig dug in compost. These seedlings were promptly attacked by flea beetles, which I sprayed. Then one plant was killed by cabbage fly larvae—this pest does not live in Tasmania. The two small heads I eventually harvested tasted foul. The same batch of cabbage seedlings growing in my garden beds had no problems of any kind and tasted delicious.

I grew a brussels sprout variety trial involving 96 plants—8 plants from each of 12 varieties. Aphids can be counted upon to infest any variety that starts forming sprouts before autumn. Well before any of those 12 varieties had begun forming any sprouts, all eight plants of one variety were destroyed by aphids while the other 88 plants of the other seven varieties were untouched. I concluded at the time that particular variety was poorly adapted to my type of soil.

In another variety trial an undiagnosed disease picked off a single tomato plant while adjoining plants of the same variety that were touching the diseased plant remained healthy. Did something damage that plant when it was a seedling. Or maybe it was a genetic mutation. Or maybe that spot got too little COF. Or maybe that spot got too much COF. Or maybe . . .

Rather than exercising your mind about minor losses like these, use that energy to enlarge the garden. I think it is far better to produce a big surplus; then you can afford to lose a few plants. Make space to grow several varieties of important crops instead of just one variety. If a crop doesn't start out right then immediately start it again in another bed and *do not worry, do not fight.* Insects frequently nibble a bit of this and that, make a few holes in leaves, suck a dead spot in one tomato out of 10—but rarely is the crop ruined. For minor issues the best thing is to do nothing. Or give the garden a foliar feed on general principles.

When early summer weather has been poor, tomato will handle that stress and grow okay until fruit starts ripening. The straw that breaks the camel's back can be the added burden of forming seeds. There was an unusually cold wet summer in Cascadia in the 1980s; all tomato plants were weather stressed and then they started ripening fruit. And then a totally destructive disease called late blight raced through Washington and Oregon states, scything down every tomato plant except for a few in greenhouses or that were positioned against a sun-facing wall with a roof overhang.

In Tassie the summer of 2014-15 was cool, often overcast and rainy; fortunately we didn't see tomato late blight although there were a lot more green tomatoes than usual at summers end and many of these had black disease spots on them. That year we also met several kinds of annoying insects that never before had made themselves known. When this sort of thing happens the most important thing a gardener can do is to not blame their method. Stuff happens.

Pesticide?

Give it a patient think before spraying pesticide. When leaf eating insects do slight damage why bother to spray; loss of less than ten percent of a plant's photosynthetic capacity reduces the outcome by the same minor percentage. Leaf eaters of all sorts are usually a small ignorable annoyance in my garden. When young seedlings in spring are being chewed down as fast or faster than they are growing the real problem may be that crop was started too early. Sowing again a few weeks later when the soil is warmer and the sun stronger allows seedlings to outgrow those losses without you even noticing.

With extra seedlings in the row or position that'll need thinning out anyway, a gardener can allow biology to thin out the weaker individuals. Snail baits may be a valuable short-term springtime solution while waiting for growth rates to accelerate. Try a foliar feed; then plants may outgrow insect damage or become so healthy nothing wants to eat them. On the other hand spraying pesticide may fend off the problem until weather conditions improve or the pest pressure lessens by itself. Or maybe sowing again is a better fix.

Globe artichoke, celery, celeriac, melon, salad radish and cauliflower all demand loose open soil; in clayey ground these vegetables are often attacked. There is little or nothing that can be done short of importing a deep bed of light soil. On the other hand, brussels sprout prefers heavy loams; many brussels sprout varieties cope poorly with sand. It may be that your garden simply can't grow brussel sprout well but will excellently grow radish and cucumber.

Chilly nights and weakening light at summer's end trigger diseases in heat-loving fruit-bearing crops *because* these plants are exhausted after heavy bearing; these plants are hardly worth fighting for. If you want to harvest top quality French beans or a great many zucchini in March then start a few more plants around Christmas that come into bearing mid- to late February. This strategy is a form of gardening aikido.

Aikido is a soft defensive martial art (as opposed to "hard" styles that focus on attack). It uses avoidance techniques while simultaneously redirecting the opponent's movement so that they injure themselves with their own force. I admire that form of natural justice. So I prefer to think of pests as helping me in the same way ethical gardeners help seed merchants perform to a higher standard by returning empty non-germinating packets and politely requesting a refund. An important step along this gentler path is to grow enough excess to be untroubled by minor losses. Some lousy summers the sun just doesn't shine often enough, some tomato varieties will get diseased, cucumbers will succumb to powdery mildew, eggplants won't set fruit, peppers are few, small and not as juicy or as sweet as usual, corn matures very late, French beans have aphids. But take comfort—at least you can eat a lot of greens and root crops.

I avoid much fighting by rejecting the Australian Sanitary System, which to me resembles its acronym. The opinion asserts that food should never show that a bug ever touched it. I say accept insects! Remove them when the vegies are washed and then, if you must, take your glasses off at table. To me a few holes in the leaves don't matter if the plant is still growing fast. And what's the worry about an occasional scar on a cucumber's skin! What's the worry if stink bugs blemish 15 percent of the tomatoes; you'll still have plenty.

Pest Control

Some circumstances demand a pesticide. Usually there is an effective naturally occurring poison that has been approved for use in certified organics. The newest organic pest controls are biological, including cultured bacteria, viruses, predatory fungi, living parasitic nematodes and beneficial insects as well as microbially manufactured poisons like spinosad, which is extracted from cultured bacteria. Antibiotics are produced the same way. Bacillus thuringiensis (Bt) is probably the most familiar biological; it is a virulent disease that only targets leaf- and fruit eating caterpillars.

All but a few organic pesticides require that the victim directly contacts a spray droplet. Once the droplet dries the spray becomes ineffective. So spray thoroughly; especially cover the undersides of leaves, leaf notches and inner recesses where eggs and juveniles are hiding.

Insects develop resistance to naturally-occurring poisons the same as they do with synthetics, which is why it is wise to alternate products if you must spray the same pest more than one time. Many pesticides that are approved for use in certified organics kill bees *if they contact a spray droplet before it has dried out* so the best times to spray are early mornings before the bees get active or shortly before dark.

Recommended pesticides described

Pyrethrins instantly kill almost any kind of insect on contact but become ineffective when the spray droplets dry out. Pyrethrins control aphids, flea beetles, asparagus beetles, cucumber beetles, leafhoppers and cabbage worms. If I were uncertain of which pesticide to use I'd try this one first. Certified organic producers are no longer allowed to use pyrethrin products with added piperonyl butoxide which is an organic synergist extracted from cherry pips that makes pyrethrins more effective. I have no concerns about using piperonyl butoxide. A high concentration pyrethrin product, say five percent, works better on adult hard shelled insects. Pyrethrins may require respraying every few days. I suggest if that happens, try using spinosad instead.

Bt (Bacillus thuringiensis) is not a contact insecticide; it is a bacteria that must be eaten in order to kill. Bt lethally infects one entire family of moth larvae. The grubs become too sick to eat within a few hours of ingesting even a tiny amount. Susceptible pests include all three species of cabbage worm we contend with as well as corn ear worms, tomato fruit worms and horn worms as well as apple worms. Be sure to add no more than three drops of mild dishwashing liquid to each litre of spray or else spray droplets roll off leaves.

The most readily findable Bt product is called Dipel, which is distributed to gardeners by Yeats. Bunnings price for Yeats Dipel in 2024 amounted to about one dollar per litre of spray. I am thrifty. I also want the best possible result so I purchase 500 grams of *industrial strength* Dipel powder from ServAg, a Tasmanian farm supply and advisory business. A 500 gram jar is the smallest quantity ServAg sells; the last jar I bought cost $80. Industrial strength instructions recommend dilutions ranging from 1 gram per litre down to one-quarter gram per litre. So I can make either 500 full-strength litres at 16 cents per litre, or 2,000 minimum-strength litres at 4 cents per litre. I can't help but wonder which strength the Yeats product provides. Bt powder remains active for at least two years if it is stored at normal household temperatures. My supply is kept under refrigeration; it has remained effective for a great many more years than two. I spray Dipel once a week when cabbage grubs are active. I include apple trees when I spray Bt, which means we have very few apple grubs. Dipel mixes nicely with NTS 10-10-10 but if you're going to spray NTS 10-10-10 that often use it at 5 ml/litre.

Spinosad is a poison extracted from a culture of *Saccharopolyspora spinosa,* a bacteria. Yeats calls it "Success." Spinosad kills cabbage worms, leaf miners, apple codling moth larvae, thrips, mites, aphids, flea beetles and whiteflies. Spinosad kills honeybees too so spray when they are not present. It is more than a contact poison. After spinosad dries it remains effective for a week or more when a sprayed leaf is eaten.

Mavrik. Yeats distributes this synthetic pyrethroid. I thoroughly researched Mavrik; I believe that it is entirely harmless to humans. I find it effective against cabbage worms, coddling moth larvae and probably a long list of others. The effect persists for about a week. For diamondback moths I mix both Mavrik and Bt in the same spray tank and get better control than I get from Bt alone.

Neem oil is pressed from the seeds of the neem tree (*Azadirachta indica).* Neem oil is safe for mammals. It has been used medicinally for centuries in India. Its extremely bitter highly persistent flavour doesn't wash off and is so horrible nothing will eat anything sprayed with it—you included. Neem can work well on seedlings or half grown vegetable plants as long as no edible parts have formed yet. Neem oil is not considered a threat to birds, earthworms or beneficial insects if it is not applied directly to their primary food source. After spraying you should clean the sprayer with hot soapy water because even a trace of neem oil leaves a very unpleasant taste that just won't go away.

Insecticidal soaps. When dishes were washed with soap instead of with detergents, when municipal water did not reach rural- and small town kitchen sinks, people noticed that dirty dishwater poured over vegetable plants killed bugs. The insecticidal power of soaps varies greatly according to the kind of fat used to make the soap. Soap spray must contact the insect directly; make sure it heavily covers the entire plant. Soaps are useful against aphids, thrips, mites and leafhoppers, and less so with larger insects. Soap can cause sunburn on leaves, especially on seedling-sized cole crops and spinach, so test before dosing the whole crop. Do not spray insecticidal soap when the sun shines intensely.

Horticultural oils kill insect eggs, larvae and adults of soft bodied species like spidermites. The product may be a single type of oil or combination formula involving paraffinic, canola, fish or sesame oil, possibly in combination with rosemary, eucalyptus, garlic, clove, etc. Oils disrupt feeding and/or smother pests. To be effective the oil must thoroughly coat the foliage but leaves must breathe in order to function normally and the oil inhibits this to some degree, more so with some species. Do not use horticultural oil when temperatures are over 30°C. Be sure to water the bed the day before spraying. Young plants, plants with thin delicate leaves, plants under moisture stress are likely to be more susceptible to injury so test first.

Bromakil Super Rat Drink. Farmers put this stuff into drinking stations in barns troubled by rats because unlike mice, rats must drink water. It is not sold at garden centres or big box shops. I was informed that Bromakil also kills English sparrows. The person who told me about Bromokil also told me how they use it. Of course I would never do what I am about to describe because this particular application is not an approved use on the label but in case you would do what I say I wouldn't do, read the label carefully and *honour the handling instructions.* The label says it is dangerous stuff! In a large glass jar add 25 ml Bromakil to 175 ml water, then add enough feed wheat to reach the top of the liquid. Soak for 36-48 hours. If a small part of the liquid hasn't been absorbed at this point, stir in enough pollard or chicken feed pellets or stale bread to soak it up. Do not touch the stuff! Put tea mug sized mounds of bait where sparrows are active. Try to have another batch ready when the previous lot has been consumed, usually in one day. Continue feeding until they stop gorging on it and you won't see very many sparrows the rest of the summer. I'm told that native birds do not feed with the sparrows.

Pests A to Z

Aphids (plant lice) cluster on leaves and stems. They suck sap; their feeding curls leaves. Sometimes there are only a few aphids that cause no *apparent* problem. However, aphids transfer potato and strawberry virus diseases; infection can't be prevented by spraying because disease transmission needs only one aphid. Aphids stunt plants. They multiply rapidly.

Aphids can overwhelm stressed plants; they usually ignore healthy fast growing plants. When something has more than a few aphids on it the most likely causes are crowding (root zone stress), moisture stress, weather stress and/or out of balance nutrients. Your initial questions should be: Have the plants run out of uncontested space to grow into? Is the entire root zone moist? Is there adequate soil fertility? If the crop has been bearing fruit for awhile has it become exhausted?

I have read that some kinds of ants raise aphids in order to milk a sweet secretion from them. I've never yet met any aphid-farming ants. However, I have had occasion to eliminate ants invading my kitchen benches and cabinets. The ant baits you can buy these days are based upon borax, which happens to be an essential plant nutrient. Inexpensively make your own bait by mixing 1 gram or ¼ teaspoon of borax into a tablespoon of honey. If you haven't included so much boron that the ants refuse the bait an intense feeding frenzy soon develops. Then the ants fade away.

Aphids can be temporarily blasted off the plant with hose and nozzle. Pyrethrum is instantly effective—very temporarily. So are insecticidal soaps. But either way, if the underlying stress remains then the cure may have to be repeated daily until you give up. To eliminate aphids on newly forming brussels sprouts during the month of March, grow later maturing varieties that don't start to form sprouts until mid April. See Chapter 9/Brassicas/Brussels sprout. Aphids sometimes appear on fruit-bearing plants at the end of summer; remember that for every crop there is a season. Ignore the aphids and start eating the cool season vegetables. Besides, the fruit coming from those exhausted plants won't taste nearly as interesting as it did three weeks previously. I would interpret the arrival of aphids at this season as a prompt for me to clear and remineralize those beds right away whilst there remains time to sow them to winter lettuce or other leafy crops.

Beneficial Insects. Gardens near diverse unsprayed vegetation usually have plenty of helpful bugs. It is possible to buy large populations of some beneficials but this possibility is more relevant to commercial greenhouse operations than to gardeners. Pest-eating predators travel in search of prey. If the immediate surroundings naturally feeds predators they should arrive right along with their next meal. To help beneficials prosper use the surrounds to grow plants that support them. Sweet alyssum will self sow although not invasively. It has the type of flat shallow flowers that small insects feed on for nectar and pollen; beneficials eat them and hang around. Amaranth, asters, thyme, dill, cosmos, calendula, sunflowers and borage also help. Cover crops provide habitat for beneficials. The best spot to release beneficials is in a permanent patch of perennial and annual ornamentals.

Cabbage grubs are moth larvae. Most years, they and their close relative, the apple codling moth, are the only pests I directly fight. Tasmania has three species of cabbage moth. The big green caterpillar that gardeners notice is present from January through April. It quickly grows over 25 mm long. They hatch from clusters of small yellowish eggs laid on the undersides of leaves by white-winged day-flying moths. Every gardener sees them flitting about. In the same months a similar larvae comes from a night-flying brown moth. In my garden almost unstoppable severe damage comes from diamondback moth larvae. Their parents appear in October; they're mostly gone by Christmas. These moths are so small I often fail to notice them until the damage their tiny larvae cause can not be ignored. I avoid stress by starting most kinds of brassicas after mid-December.

Painstakingly hand-picking the larger larvae and tossing them away from the plant can be sufficient control in a small garden—but only after the tiny diamondback larvae have gone. I use Bt (plus Mavrik for diamondbacks). The spray is effective for about one week.

From whenever the diamondback moths begin fluttering about like mossies (mid-October) and continuing well into March (and some years until mid-April) I spray all brassicas except kale, turnip and swede, one or two days after each irrigation or rain. Starting in March I spray every two weeks until the white moths are no longer around. Spray into the growing point; these tender new leaves are especially damaged by larvae. If your intensive layouts or sandy soil require frequent sprinkler irrigation then I suggest spraying once a week in the morning on a day you do not water.

Cabbage family vegetables often make water-repellent leaves. To make Bt stick better mix a few drops of low sudsing dishwashing liquid into each litre of spray. The right amount of detergent makes water droplets spread out on the leaves instead of beading up and running off. More detergent than may harm the bacteria. Do not use anti-bacterial dishwashing liquid.

For many years I confidently asserted that in order to grow fancy brassicas to a high standard required multiple sprays against cabbage grubs. But lately I've seen how regularly foliar feeding Nutri-Tech 10-10-10 makes the waxy coating become thicker and very shiny. I now opine that if brassicas are foliar fed a mixture of NTS 10-10-10 at 5 ml/litre and Dipel every 10 days from the time they have formed two or three leaves they can become immune to the *large* cabbage grubs after a few sprays. The moths still lay eggs and I suppose the larvae hatch but the larvae must starve soon after hatching because I find almost no grubs. I do not believe that any degree of improved plant nutrition can defeat diamondback moth larvae.

Slugs and snails are fewer in a clean garden. They shelter under debris during the day so promptly move garden waste to the composting area and eliminate daytime hiding places such as tall weeds around the garden's fringes, boards, sacks or buckets resting on the soil. If snails or slugs are eating too many seedlings in spring try sowing again a few weeks later when seedlings can grow faster. Sowing more than the minimum number of seeds and then thinning progressively provides some for them and enough for you. Side dressing COF along seedling rows or around transplanted seedlings might increase growth rates enough that minor nibbling can be ignored.

Gastropod populations can be reduced. A traditional trapping method uses wooden planks laid on garden paths. Gastropods shelter under them as the sun comes up. The gardener turns the boards over, hand picks and drops them into a jar of detergent solution or salt water. Or feed them to the chooks. This works on medium- and larger sized gastropods; getting tiny slugs seems too painstaking. That's why I don't do this.

Slug and snail baits made with metaldehyde are acceptable to me because I don't allow our dog into the food garden. Metaldehyde is chemically similar to methyl alcohol and is equally poisonous. It quickly breaks down into harmless substances. Gastropods love to intoxicate themselves to death with metaldehyde in the same way they'll happily drown themselves in a dish of stale beer (ethanol also attracts and poisons gastropods). Bait need not be scattered amongst the vegetables; it may be put on paths and surrounds. I suspect that slugs travel at random; snails seem to know where they are because they to return to the same shelters every morning (or are these different snails, same hideouts?). A bait barrier will kill those entering the area while ones already in the garden will feed on the baits when crossing a path.

Serious gardeners can save considerable money by investing in a 10 kg bag of Meterex purchased from a farm supply shop. It contains the same poison at the same concentration as the stuff in the garden centre, but ends up costing much less because Meterex pellets are miniscule and hard so they persist much longer and cover far more area with less weight. Don't use methaldehyde baits if dogs may get at them—metaldehyde attracts some dogs and is fatal to canines even in smallish amounts. Meterex pellets are so small they don't interest pets.

To get gastropods out of your food submerge vegetables in cold water for ten minutes and then rinse well; slugs suffocate and sink to the bottom; snails climb the sides of the sink.

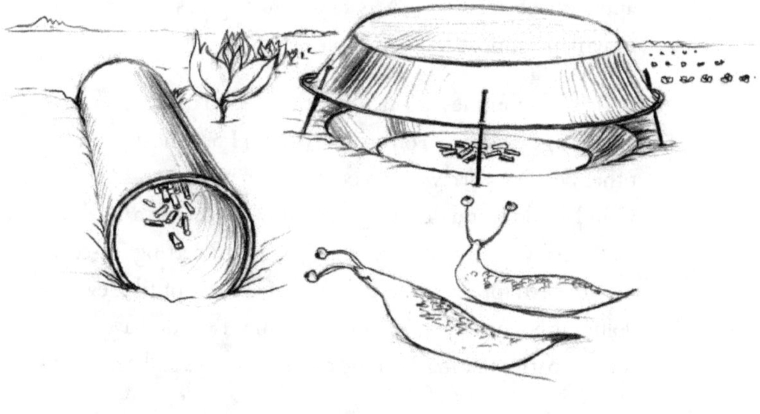

Leaf miners are fly maggots that tunnel through beetroot, silverbeet and English spinach leaves; they'll also mine bean, blackberry, onion and lettuce. Spinosad works on miners even though they are inside the leaf. The DPI says we have leaf miners but I have never noticed any. I once gifted a section of spun-fibre row cover to a gardener who complained of leaf miners ruining every beetroot crop he planted. The gardener carefully covered most of a beetroot bed after the seedlings had gotten large enough to thin and weed and kept the cover in place until harvest. His unprotected plants were thoroughly ruined. Under the row cover there was a fine harvest, though the fabric did reduce light levels so the plants made smaller bottoms. This minor light reduction could be compensated for with increased interplant spacing.

Flea beetles are tiny, black, fast-moving insects that make pinholes in leaves. They primarily feed on members of the cabbage family, beetroot and tomato seedlings. They like thick juicy brassica cotyledons (the first leaves that emerge after germination). They especially go for weak plants or ones in shock. Rarely are fast-growing healthy plants seriously damaged.

Overwintering adults come from surrounding fields in spring, feed on leaves and soon lay eggs in the soil. During the summer their larvae feed on various roots including potatoes, usually without doing much more than slight skin damage. After maturing into adults, the beetles feed until they hibernate in autumn.

I knew this insect all too well in Oregon. In Tasmania I've only seen a few but this pest is worth mentioning, just in case. Management can reduce flea beetle damage to a tolerable level. If you transplant brassica seedlings harden them off before setting them out so they don't go into shock. If you direct seed don't do it too early, sow twice as much seed and thin progressively. When seedlings are heavily damaged they're probably not growing fast enough. In that case, try a drench of liquid fertilizer. If the slow growth was due to harsh weather resow. A bed thickly sown to cheap radish seed, raab, rocket or turnips may attract flea beetles and take the pressure off. As a last resort spray pyrethrins, Mavrik or spinosad.

Wildlife. Some gardeners feel the need to net their entire garden against birds. Fortunately (so far) I only hear about other peoples' currawongs, cockies and feral turkeys. At Grindelwald wood ducks grazed on my pea shoots for a few weeks every spring but very lightweight bird netting tossed over the bed for a few weeks discouraged them until they voluntarily started feeding on something else. I do have fearless parrots eating ripening apples—but we still get plenty for ourselves. Some years English sparrows are at plague levels (see page 114).

Wildlife that walks can be fenced out. Except, that is, for mice, young bandicoots, rats, bluetongues and well-established wombats with unchangeable habits. Mice and rats cause me only minor annoyance because their numbers are greatly reduced around the garden by only one bait station. Bluetongues have gotten stuck in my strawberry net (against blackbirds). They get gently unsnarled and relocated. Bandicoots do no harm and receive admiration if I spot one. I'm told a fence will work against a wandering young wombat looking for a territory but not when a wombat already walks a traditional path through a proposed garden site.

For keeping out roos, wallabies and their smaller relatives, bunnies and possums, if you can make a proper braced corner with treated pine posts and pound star pickets then you can keep them out. I don't recommend blocking walking wildlife with an expensive colorbond fence 1,200 mm high; it works so long as no tree on the wildlife's side overhangs the garden, no vine, shrub or tree growing on the garden side makes a tangle on top of the fence or forms an overhanging branch where it could be marked by a possum leaping 1,500 mm above the ground. I actually witnessed a mortally stabbed brushtail leap over a fence more than 1,500 mm high but unless that distressed they won't leap over a 1,200 mm high colorbond wall or wildlife mesh fence when they have nothing at the top to grab on to. Colorbond works because it can't be climbed. The colorbond's bottom must be close to the soil line with footing wire extending 300 mm into the wildlife's side. But solid fences do not make the best windbreaks. And colorbond creates shade.

You can't entirely keep out possums with a dog. Dog's sleep at night; possums do not. Someone gardening in or near the bush using a fence that keeps out roos and bunnies but that isn't possum proof—and can calmly accept some losses—can keep a dog or three really healthy by shooting them a possum nearly every night. Dogs thrive on uncooked small animals because they get the bones, the brains, heart, liver and all the other organs. I've never seen anyone reliably stop possums with a floppy overhang. Something always goes wrong with these complex structures; a weak spot inevitably develops. And let me tell you possums are smart! This isn't something I only read about. I once nurtured an orphaned possum; I was its mother (baby brushtails know nothing of fathers). I was a good mother; I helped mine survive initiation by the possum clan that owned my bush property. I had long been friends with that mob; I fed them on the deck almost every night. I was especially good friends with Possie, a male that would sit on my lap and accept a few pets. So I can tell you from close experience that possums are smarter than dogs. They also are natural burglars, totally persistent, intensely curious and when one of one of them learns how to get into something the entire clan knows how to the next day.

To stop wallabies I make a farm-field-like fence of hexagonal wildlife mesh which is like heavy gauge chicken wire with a smaller grid pattern. Unless there are large roos about, I suggest using the less costly 900 mm mesh instead of 1,050 mm because it perfectly fits ordinary star pickets. One hundred metres of perimeter encloses a space containing about 500 square metres, which is plenty for a food garden and a few fruit trees. You've paid for the corner posts anyway; a few additional star pickets don't cost all that much more so if possible erect the whole 100 metre roll because you'll probably find use for protected garden space. Make ordinary field-fence braced corners with treated pine posts. I like using gripples and a proper grippling tool to tighten brace wires. Make absolutely sure the top of *every corner post and gate post stands exactly 1,000 mm proud of the soil line plus or minus not very much.* Drive an ordinary star picket every two metres along the fence line. Stop pounding when the picket's bottom hole is 25 mm above the soil line. If the picket is the ordinary sort and has been set the correct depth then its top hole now stands 1,025 mm above the soil line, plus or minus not very much. Then three high tensile wires are stretched from corner post to corner post. I tension them with gripples too. The bottom wire is 25 mm above ground; the top one is located one hole down from the top hole in the star pickets (these two wires should be 900 mm apart). One more wire in the middle stiffens the mesh. First the mesh is hung from the top wire with ringstaples; it is stretched minimally tight and then it is attached to all three wires with a ring staple every 450 mm. There is no need to strongly tension the mesh because wildlife do not press against a fence to get in; not the way livestock do when trying to get out. That fence stops roos, wallabies, potteroos and any escaped livestock except goats.

In order to stop bunnies unroll 300-mm wide footing wire outside the entire perimeter. It extends into the wildlife's territory. Attach it to the bottom of the wildlife mesh with ringstaples 300 mm apart. The footing wire lies (more or less) flat on the earth. Soon grass and weeds will make it disappear. In spots where it doesn't lay flat snip a few wires so you can flatten it or temporarily put a big rock on it until the grass grabs it. When a bunny comes along and tries to dig under the fence they are stopped. The bunny may back up a little and try again, but again hits the mesh—and gives up. And goes away. If a wallaby tries to put its nose under the fence it too is stopped. And what about possums?

To keep them out it only takes one hotwire supported on insulators placed in the top hole of the star pickets. Where there is a wooden post an insulator is nailed into the top. Touching a hot wire doesn't traumatize if the animal is not in good electrical contact with the soil. Clinging to the wildlife mesh definitely earths the possum. A possum could avoid the hotwire by leaping from the ground to a wooden post that extends more than a few inches above the hotwire. Do not attach insulators to the side of a post that extends above 1,000 mm; make sure the posts do not extend above 1,000 mm.

The gate must also be impossible to climb over without contacting a hotwire. My garden gate is wide enough to comfortably pass a wheelbarrow. To possum proof the gate I stretch a wire-impregnated bunge cord across it just below the top, not quite touching the gate when it is closed. Gate kits like this come with insulated handles. No way a possum could climb the gate without touching the bunge cord. I allow nothing above the bunge for the possum to leap up and grasp from ground level. To allow me to pass, the handle is detached from the fitting it is hooked on when stretched across the gate, moved to the other side and temporarily hung on something.

Chapter 9

How to Grow It

The gardener is the servant of the plant.

Louise Howard, ***The Earth's Green Carpet****

This chapter provides the details to help you to grow vegies that are equally attractive as anything from the supermarket—and taste better. Much better.

This chapter is divided into two parts. Use the larger part of this chapter like consulting an encyclopaedia; it is not intended to be read from beginning to end.

The introductory part of this chapter is only a few pages long. It points out essential aspects of my method. The first few pages should be carefully considered and fully assimilate to make the best use of the how-to-grow-it encyclopaedia.

Family groups

Vegetables in this chapter are grouped either by botanical classification, such as "alliums" (onion family) and "brassicas," (cabbage family) or else by similarities in how they're grown, such as "root crops." This organization creates an effective crop rotation if, after harvesting something belonging to one group, you grow something on that spot belonging to a different group.

The vegetables in each group are managed similarly. If you're new to food gardening after you succeed at producing one vegetable in a group then the others in that group should seem easy to grow.

These are the groups:

Solanums

eggplant, pepper, tomato

Legumes

bean, pea, lentil, chickpea, green manures

Greens

celery (and celeriac), endive and escarole, corn salad (mache), lettuce, mustard, English spinach, silverbeet, rocket (arugula), coriander

Brassicas

broccoli, brussels sprout, cabbage, Chinese cabbage, cauliflower, collard, kale, kohlrabi, swede, turnip

Roots

beetroot, carrot, parsley (both leaf and root types), parsnip, potato, radish

Cucurbits

cucumber, melon, pumpkin, zucchini, marrow

Alliums

garlic, shallot, leek, onion

Miscellaneous

asparagus, sweet corn, horseradish, globe artichoke, okra. I consider each vegetable in this section to be unique and ungroupable.

Planting dates

Sowing as early possible in spring rarely brings much benefit and often brings disappointment. Seeds for some frost hardy crops may germinate after mid-August but they take a long time to come up and grow very slowly until mid-September because light intensity is low, days are short and the soil is still chilly. I suggest delaying spring planting until seeds can germinate rapidly and seedlings can grow fast from the start. Exercising patience in spring results in healthier plants and a larger harvest that usually begins days later than had you sown a month sooner. The dates in my sowing calendar are the product of many many years of experience. Please try them.

The exercise of patience also applies to heat loving crops. Except in a poly tunnel these species grow slowly during October. In my experience setting out heat lovers two weeks later than your neighbours do means *your* plants do not get killed by frost and if there is no more frost that year then your first harvest still happens only a few days later than theirs. Some years October weather is extremely unsettled, the early sowings get shocked so often and stressed so severely that they do poorly for the rest of the summer. Starting the same vegetable early in November can result in harvesting a few days sooner than a mid-October sowing, and harvesting a lot more. Please exercise patience in spring.

Depending on your location the best planting dates for your garden may differ by a few weeks from what this book suggests. I think you'll be better able to modify my dates by knowing where I was living at the time of writing this chapter. I have already mentioned that Annie and I moved house in 2020 and now live near Chudleigh, which is not as warm as Grindelwald.

Grindelwald is located 20 km northeast of Launceston on a hill overlooking the Tamar Valley. My garden was exactly 100 metres above sea level and close enough to the Tamar that the estuary slightly moderates night-time low temperatures. The entire Tamar estuary is a banana belt. People living in nearby Exeter at about my elevation but one kilometre further from the Tamar than I was got spring frosts that my garden escaped. I nurtured a thriving lemon tree in a protected position but I failed with lime. People at the bottom of Grindelwald hill are closer to the Tamar; they enjoy lime and grapefruit. I reckon my garden's climate was close to average for northern Tasmania.

South of Launceston, in the Midlands and positions more than a few kilometres inland from the Bass Strait are always a few degrees colder in winter than where I lived and are far more likely to have frosts. Autumn and winter crops grow more slowly inland than they do near the Tamar or the coast, so they must be started a week or two sooner than my planting calendar suggests. Cold season crops in harsher districts don't grow as large as they do near the Tamar so they may not need as much growing room as I suggest. Where elevation exceeds 300 metres cool season varieties sourced from Mainland suppliers may not survive winter. Still, winter gardens may pass unharmed through repeated frosts and even occasional snow if you're using proper seeds.

Positions in sight of the Tamar, within a few kilometres of the Bass Strait and especially near the east coast, are all milder than where I lived. Spring in these areas starts earlier; frost danger ends sooner and returns later. Coastal gardeners can start spring and summer crops a week or three earlier than my planting calendar suggests. North Coast and East Coast gardeners enjoy gentler winters. They often see significant growth from mid-May through August. So coastal gardeners may take their time about sowing winter and overwintering crops and will have a bigger result from winter crops. All their winter crops may benefit from more growing room than I specify.

I lack experience to provide as much detail regarding Hobart and other southern Tasmanian communities. I notice they are cooler most of the year than where I am, so heat lovers will take longer to ripen and autumn/winter vegetables should be started sooner than I did. However, Hobart and vicinity occasionally get quite a bit hotter than the North.

A new gardener or an experienced one that is new to Tasmania will need a few years to work out their best planting schedule. I suggest that you start with mine, it won't be off by more than a week or two.

How much to grow?

Yield depends upon soil conditions, plant spacing, that year's weather, on the variety—and your skill. I can't know how many sit at your table or what foods they prefer. I feel inadequate to say how much area to devote to most vegetables. So in what's to come I share what I do. I always try to produce at least half again more food than Annie and I use. We are a two person vegetableatarian household. I like inspire others by giving away the best tasting vegetables our friends and neighbours have ever had. We believe in making nutrient-dense vegetables be at least half our total food intake. We believe that is the most healthful lifestyle for us—and for you and yours as well. I supply our table with a broad abundance of fresh vegies, twelve months a year. I'd like to see your family similarly blessed.

Planting Calendar*

March

All month: overwintering cabbage, broccoli and cauliflower, corn salad, arugula (rocket), small salad radishes, lettuce, English spinach for winter

First half of month: coriander, endive/escarole, large winter radish, mustard greens, turnip

April

First half of month: winter-hardy lettuce for spring harvest, corn salad, garlic, English spinach

Last half of month: garlic, green manures like broad bean, tic bean, Shaftal (Persian) clover, cereal rye

May

All month: garlic, shallot, overwintering bulbing onion, green manures like tic bean, broad bean, Shaftal clover, blue lupin, cereal rye

June

21st: Traditional Tasmanian day to plant garlic.

August

First half of month: earliest peas, especially slower-to-mature climbing peas, broad bean

Last half of month: radish, lettuce, English spinach, broad bean, peas, mustard greens, bulbing onion, spring onion

20-25th: I start tomato seedlings indoors; people in cooler areas may do this a few weeks later

September

All month: pea, lettuce, beetroot, kohlrabi, broccoli, English spinach, small salad radish, spring onion

First day of the month: pepper and eggplant seedlings indoors

First half of month: turnip, mustard greens, last chance to sow broad bean.

Second half of month: early cabbage, early cauliflower, lettuce, leek nursery, early potatoes under frost cloth

October

All month: early cabbage, broccoli, celery (direct seed), parsley, parsley root, carrot, silverbeet, beetroot, spring onion, leek nursery, lettuce, summer varieties of English spinach, radish

Second half of month: runner bean, sweet corn, tomato seedlings go outside, French bean, zucchini and pumpkin

November

All month: lettuce, cabbage, broccoli, parsley and parsley root, silverbeet, beetroot, spring onion, English spinach, French- and runner bean, carrot, cucumber, zucchini

First half of month: zucchini, pumpkin, pepper and eggplant seedlings go out, cucumber, melon

December

All month: lettuce, cabbage, broccoli, English spinach, carrot, zucchini, cucumber

Second half of month: brussels sprout, kale, end of summer cauliflower

January

All month: cauliflower, kale, Brussels sprout, English spinach, lettuce, broccoli, carrot, cabbage, swede, endive/escarole, fennel

February

All month: endive/escarole, cauliflower, winter radish, lettuce, English spinach, beetroot, silverbeet, broccoli, purple sprouting broccoli, kale, Chinese cabbage

First half of month: cauliflower for autumn and winter, swede, carrot for autumn/winter harvest

Second half of month: overwintering (spring) cabbage, turnip

** Everything is directly seeded unless transplanted seedlings are specified. Direct seeding includes cucumber, pumpkin, zucchini, melon, celery, the entire cabbage family and other things many gardeners usually transplant. How to avoid transplanting will be explained in detail through the encyclopaedic section to come. Not transplanting makes gardening much easier and far more certain of success. Dates are for warmer districts like the Tamar Valley. Adjust them to suit your location.*

Varieties

This chapter recommends excellent varieties for Tasmanian conditions. I urge you to try them. Take it from an ex-seedsman—choice of variety often makes a huge difference. Heat-loving varieties that are productive and delicious on the mainland often fail to perform as well when they experience cool Tasmanian summer nights. Mainland cool season varieties too often fail to survive Tasmanian winter. Onion varieties that work fine around Sydney or Brisbane don't do so well when attempted in our latitude. Sometimes seeds for varieties that are extremely useful in Tasmania are not available in Australia. In that case I point out what could be purchased by someone willing to import and cope with Quarantine. I hope increasing gardener demand will prompt a Tasmanian seed seller to offer these varieties.

Plant spacings and cultivation methods

Most of the suggested layouts in this chapter refer to slightly raised beds that are 1,200 mm wide. These are discussed in Chapter 4, "Planning." My suggested plant spacings allow the crop to completely fill the bed if the soil provides the level of fertility COF produces and if the soil is kept moist. My suggested spacings produce a very large yield. When I compare my result with other gardens I've seen, I conclude my method produces the most food for the least work.

Providing highly fertile soil is essential. I suggest using Complete Organic Fertilizer on all crops. COF is not the only way to grow a successful garden but it is a certain to give you a great result. The amount of COF a crop needs is distinguished as either "low-," "medium-" or "high-demand." All this is discussed at length in Chapter 2, "Soil."

Low-Demand Crops

grow great on the basic amount of COF—6 to 8 litres evenly distributed over 10 square metres.

Medium-Demand Crops

need more soil fertility. Start them off like low demand crops but be prepared to side-dress another half-dose COF once the crop has started growing fast.

High-Demand Crops

need even more nutrients but rarely more than eight additional litres of COF side-dressed on 10 square metres.

Buying seeds

This chapter recommends specific varieties and their suppliers. Contact details are in Chapter 6, "Seeds." In order to save space, these abbreviations will be used:

ADA	Adaptive Seeds, Oregon USA
BIRD	Birdland Seeds, VIC
FOT	Mr. Fothergill's
JSS	Johnny's Selected Seeds, Maine USA
SH	Southern Harvest Seeds, Kingston
TSC	Territorial Seed Co, Oregon USA
MOLES	Moles Seeds, UK

Fertigation and dry gardening

This chapter suggests ways to make the garden require less water, less often. I have much more to say about this in Chapter 5, "Water." Any household depending on rainwater capture tanks, a very limited bore or a less-than-abundant dam to irrigate their food garden should pay close attention to Chapter 5 and put these methods into practice.

Root system drawings

This chapter provides drawings of actual root systems that developed on deep open fertile prairie (aka krasnozem) soil in Kansas, USA. Krasnozem is a soil type that does not form a distinct clay subsoil. Deep sand soils allow vegetables to make similar root systems. Where there is a clay subsoil, called "duplex soil" by agronomists, the root system will not go as deep but will be every bit as broad, if not broader. In short—if you give them space, they will fill it up.

Solanums

Tomato, pepper and eggplant are members of a botanical family named solanum. All three vegetables are heat-loving frost-intolerant perennials that behave like summer annuals when they are grown in temperate climates. Solanum varieties that are productive in Victoria often don't get enough heat in Tasmania to perform as well. Many mainland solanum varieties only set fruit during our warmest nights. Cool conditions retard fruit ripening, make the fruit smaller and have less flavour. Varieties demanding the most heat will survive summer on Tassie but never set any fruit. We need to use solanum varieties that are adapted to Tasmania's climate. But mainland seed suppliers have little or no motivation to seek out varieties that thrive when midsummer night-time lows occasionally drop to 6°C and often are barely over 10°. Taswegians, *including our seedling nurseries,* have long made the best of varieties we can get conveniently.

Trying to compensate for lack of heat, Tasmanian gardeners set out solanum seedlings as early as possible. But often, instead of a bountiful harvest the seedlings either get killed by a late frost or else they become stunted or diseased. Things go much better when we don't rush to set them outside.

Most people gardening around the Tamar put out tomatoes on Launceston Show Day. Mid-October is safer; November 1st is better for planting out pepper and eggplant seedlings. Patience pays off with more fruit of higher quality from healthier unstressed plants whilst getting the first ripe fruit only a few days later than those who danced with frost and cold nights.

Near the Tamar tomato plants grow slowly in October; eggplant and pepper can't grow fast until at least mid-November. Some folks err by transplanting solanums into heavily fertilized soil. This practice may work against the gardener's hopes. The plant *must* uptake nutrients held in the soil moisture. But a non-growing plant can't build new tissue with these nutrients, nor can it eliminate them. So nutrients in the plant sap can reach toxic concentrations, stunting it, maybe weakening it to the point that it becomes diseased. It is far better practice to transplant into soil of moderate balanced fertility. And then side-dress solanum seedlings *after* they've started growing fast.

When tender greenhouse-grown tomato seedlings experience a chilly spring night (5°C to 6°C) within a few days of being put outdoors, they cease growing for a few days. Nights below 5°C, especially nights that approach but do not quite reach frost, can stun a nursery-raised seedling and may prevent growth for more than one week. Pepper seedlings are even more sensitive. They can be mildly shocked at about 8°C and may be stunned at 5°C. Eggplant is even moreso. Putting a greenhouse-grown seedling straight into cold soil creates a shock all by itself. Seedlings that grew to transplanting size under cooler conditions would not be bothered nearly as much. Chapter 7, "Seedlings," tells how to grow your own strong chill-resistant solanum seedlings and also how to gently strengthen purchased ones before transplanting them.

Most garden books say tomatoes prefer acidic soil. Actually, garden solanums can grow well with soil pH anywhere between 5.5 and 7.5. What they can't handle is a shortage of calcium. The aglime in COF slowly lifts soil pH and provides calcium. Because COF also contains (slowly soluble) gypsum it provides plenty of available calcium even when soil pH is still low.

Solanums can make use of a lot of nutrients *when environmental conditions allow rapid growth.* Start them as low-demand crops and then side-dress mid-November and again after Christmas. The rate of growth inevitably slows after mid-February so do not side-dress solanums after mid-January. COF provides roughly equal quantities of N and P and K. This balance is excellent for making strong healthy vegetative growth. But when solanums start setting fruit they will make stronger bushes that carry more- and larger fruit if they get half as much N compared to the amounts of P and K provided. Tomato vines won't run rampantly. Peppers will make stronger branches that won't break so easily. So I reduce the amount of canolaseedmeal by half in COF when I mix it for side-dressing fruiting solanums. The same thing holds true when using NTS 10-10-10 to fertigate solanums that are making fruit. The NPK ratio is similar to COF and by itself it provokes too much leaf and stem and reduces fruit set. What I do to remedy that is to add enough monopotassium phosphate to Triple Ten to make the NPK ratio 1-2-2. MKP is compatible with Triple Ten. MKP is a frequently used greenhouse fertilizer that is available from ServAg in 25 kg bags; that much will be a lifetime supply for most people. I suggest this recipe for fertigating solanums that are ripening fruit: saturate the entire rootzone with 10-10-10 at 5 ml/lt plus MKP at 2.5 ml/lt (measured by volume). Please don't make it any stronger than that. Repeat every ten days. Stop fertigation in March.

Follow solanums with tic beans, lupines or cereal rye. The next major section, "Legumes," provides information about growing these green manures.

Solanum flowers are self-fertile. Small insects (not bees) may cause occasional crossing in pepper; less frequently in eggplant; never in tomato except with a few heirloom tomatoes that no one grows any longer. Separating pepper and eggplant varieties by 10 metres insures enough seed purity for home garden use.

Tasmanians should make smart choices about solanum varieties so as to obtain a long abundant harvest period. This especially applies to eggplant. Most "early" hybrid eggplant varieties failed in my trials because they are only early in warm climates. Hybrid vigour can treble eggplant yield. A few open pollinated pepper varieties are productive here. Fortunately, we now have Tasmanian seed suppliers that offer superior varieties. Saving seeds from open pollinated solanums is easy.

Eggplant

(Solanum melongena)

Yes, most varieties will form an attractive broad-leaved bush with large (usually) purplish potato-like flowers but . . . seeing those flowers become little eggplants is another matter because cool nights stop most eggplant varieties from setting fruit. What constitutes "too cool" depends on variety; my observations suggest it can be anywhere from 10°C to 18°C. Spreading a sheet of black plastic over the eggplant bed can raise nighttime temperature a degree or two; that small difference can make all the difference.

Culture: At Grindelwald I planted out eggplant seedlings November 1. To grow them at Chudleigh a polytunnel is a must have. Eggplant is a medium-demand crop but prepare their bed with only enough COF for a low-demand crop. Then spread a sheet of black plastic over the entire bed surface. Make the plastic wide enough that it extends over the edges of the bed. Anchor the edges with soil, planks or rocks. When doing this keep soil off the plastic to have as much heat-adsorbing black exposed to the sun as possible. Make the planting positions 75 cm x 60 cm apart. Cut an "X" with lines about 150 mm long over the centre of each planting spot.

Black plastic soaks up more solar energy than lighter-coloured soil does and then insulates that heat, which creates slightly warmer nighttime air temperatures immediately above the bed—a difference that allows an early eggplant variety to set fruit. Black plastic also serves as a weed stopper. And warmer soil accelerates growth. Plastic also makes a safe habitat for slugs and snails; they can destroy new seedlings. So through the "X" insert a few snail pellets between plastic and soil. Do this the day before you transplant.

Side dressing is impossible when black plastic covers the bed. Irrigation can't be done quite as usual either. Immediately after the first sprinkler irrigation or rain, poke holes in the plastic with a fat nail. Make one at every low spot in the bed to let the water through (little puddles will form at those places). If growth slows, fertigate every few weeks. Keep them growing fast until mid-February in order to produce the largest possible harvest.

Gardeners east of Wynyard and close to the coast, near the east coast or close to the Tamar where nights are warmer might forego the plastic and still have good results, especially if they have dark coloured soil.

Garden planning: Eggplants do best in a sheltered position; their thin leaves are susceptible to wind damage. One excellently grown plant of a well-adapted variety may produce six to ten large fruit during summer and be carrying another half dozen or more tasty half-developed fruit at the end of March. Well-adapted small-fruited varieties can produce 20 or more fruit per plant in a good summer.

Insects and disease: Well nourished eggplants are rarely bothered by anything except strong wind and low temperatures. Late season insects should be ignored; the plants are exhausted at summer's end in any case. If you got *any* fruit, give thanks.

Harvest: Eggplant tastes best if it is harvested just before the fruit reaches full size, before any seed has developed, whilst the skin is still shiny and thin. Half-developed eggplants taste as good as full-sized ones. The plants stop setting fruit when high-summer ends, certainly before mid-March. At this point harvest all large and mostly-developed fruit; that unburdening encourages smaller fruit to enlarge and also helps the plant cope with chilly nights and weaker light.

Saving Seed: Seeds mature after the skin has toughened and lost its shine. Allow one of the first fruits to hang on the bush until the skin wrinkles and develops a brownish tint. Then the seeds are ripe. One good fruit provides a home gardener with enough seeds for many years. Crush the pulp in a large bowl of water with your hands. As you free the seeds they settle to the bottom. Skim off and remove the pulp. Catch the seeds by pouring through a tea strainer. Finally, dry them on a sheet of newspaper at room temperature.

Hybrid vigour in large-fruited varieties makes all the difference in our marginal conditions. As far as I know Australians can access only one productive open pollinated variety. It has made lots of seeds for me.

Varieties: Our seedling nurseries seem addicted to easily-sourced mainland varieties. I hope after enough Tasmanian gardeners have read this book that they will motivate our seedling growers to do the right thing.

I'll start this review with those big blocky supermarket types. Any variety with the name "Beauty" in it, such as U-Beaut, probably derives from the heirloom Black Beauty, a heat-lover if there ever was one. Beauties make fruitless bushes in Tasmania.

Bonica Hybrid works here. Black Italia certainly works! Asian varieties make fruits shaped like cucumbers; a few of them, like Orient Express (SH) and Millionaire, are earliest of all in Tassie. It is not possible to import solanum seeds at present without biosecurity procedures. Diamond (SH) is OP. It produces a good yield of medium-sized fruit in my garden and also makes lots of strong seeds. None of the many other open pollinated eggplant varieties I've trialled at Grindelwald generously yielded or produced ripe seeds.

Dry gardening: Increase interplant spacing to 900 mm x 900 mm. Use black plastic. Fertigate. Give each plant 3 to 4 litres every few weeks during December and 10 litres every few weeks during January and February.

Pepper: capsicum and chilli

(Capsicum annum)

Culture: Peppers are a medium-demand crop. Gardeners in the midlands and at higher elevation almost have to use black plastic to warm the pepper bed, the same as for eggplant. Gardeners in warmer microclimates will harvest more-, larger- and sweeter fruit if they cover the bed with black plastic.

In average microclimates set out peppers October 20 to 30. The middle of November is better around Chudleigh. Peppers should be positioned 60 cm x 60 cm up to 75 cm x 75 cm. Use the wider spacing when growing naturally larger varieties, or if irrigation is limited, and/or if you enjoy a warmer microclimate. Sidedress peppers as soon as the plants start growing fast (usually late November at Grindelwald) and sidedress again early in January. Use COF but with half as much canolaseedmeal because when peppers are overfed on nitrogen they make weak branches and set fewer fruit.

Branches that are weighed down with nearly mature fruit may break when wet, especially this is so if the wind also blows. With some varieties place short wooden stakes or strong bamboo canes where branches fork so they take some weight off the branch or else tie branches to them.

Garden planning: Well-adapted open-pollinated large-fruited capsicums (bell pepper types) may produce ten or more fruit per well-grown plant. Smaller-fruited varieties are usually better adapted to Tasmanian conditions. They will make dozens of capsicums or hundreds of small chilli. Capsicums ripen in February and March. I like hot sauce; some years I grow four chilli varieties even though one good plant yields enough for us.

Harvest: Most varieties, hot or sweet, start out with green (or pale yellow) fruit and ripen to deep red or intense yellow, orange, purple, even "chocolate," acquiring thicker juicier flesh and a sweeter taste in the process. Fruit that ripens when the sun is stronger will be sweeter (or hotter). Chilli plants always carry a great quantity of unripe fruit at summer's end. Just before the first autumn frost, or if there has been no frost, then before too many cold rainy days ruin the fruit, pull the plants roots and all, shake off all soil and hang them upside-down under the veranda or in a shed or garage. Most of the chillis will ripen as the bush dries out.

Here's how to make an easily prepared, unfired hot sauce that can be stored for more than one year in the fridge. The richest tasting sauce is made from red-ripe chillies but green ones also make delicious sauce but with a different flavour. Every variety makes its own unique flavour. Using a meat grinder, mince a few kilograms of destemmed chillies, seeds and all. I put a few garlic cloves through the mincer at the same time. Into the bowl containing minced chilli (and garlic) rapidly pour (and stir a bit) enough household white vinegar to barely submerge the minced fruit. Allow the vinegar to soak into the chilli *for no more than one minute* because you do not want your hot sauce tasting strongly of vinegar. However, that brief soak lets an opened jar keep much longer in the fridge. Promptly drain the vinegar by pouring the chillies into a big strainer. Extract as much vinegar as possible. Then put the drained chilli into another bowl and stir in enough (relatively tasteless and less costly) light olive oil to generously coat every piece. Then fill small glass jars with oily chilli. Press the solids down with the back of a spoon; make sure there are no air bubbles. Add more oil if needed to eliminate all bubbles. Leave a one centimetre of air space at the top and then add more oil such that four or five millimetres of pure oil covers the solids and that there is at least a five mm air space on top (so oil won't leak out if there's a bit of fermentation during storage). Unopened jars last at least 12 months in our fridge; opened jars go off in a month or two so best to use small jars that'll be consumed quickly. Oh! Remember that vinegar. By itself it makes an interesting and very long keeping piquant vinegar.

Saving seed: Tasmania is too cool to grow commercial pepper seed; the yield here would be way too low and seed vigour would not be great. Still, the home gardener can produce useful seed. Allow a few fruits to get beyond ripe—let their skins shrivel a bit if possible before picking them. Be aware that the first fruits to set (on chilly nights) may be seedless, or nearly so. Usually, these seedless fruit are also half-sized. Better to take seed from fruits that set early in January; these will ripen in February whilst the sun is still intense enough that the seed will be vigorous. Before extracting the seed, let the ripe fruits cure indoors for a week allowing the seeds to fatten more. Spread the seeds on a sheet of paper to dry at room temperature.

Small crawling insects make occasional crosses. If you can't allow 10 metres of isolation, then at very least separate chilli from capsicum by that distance.

Quarantine restricts importation of capsicum seed. Because of that, I'm sure SH would be delighted to hear from a serious Tasmanian home gardener or market gardener who can produce genetically pure, vigorous pepper seed by the one hundred grams. I'm sure SH would happily pay a high price for strong pepper seed.

Varieties: Antohi (SH, BIRD), is a highly productive OP; it is early, heart-shaped fruit, thick-walled, intensely red and intensely sweet. I cheerfully substitute Antohi for supermarket-type capsicums.

Open pollinated capsicum varieties like California Wonder produce well enough on the mainland and in polytunnels but set only a few fruit that ripen rather late when grown outdoors in Tasmania. Hybrid varieties are far more likely to be productive here. *Small-fruited peppers, be they hot or sweet, are earlier and more prolific.*

I've had good results with Chilli Inferno This small-fruited variety is commonly found on garden centre seedling benches. It has a pleasant flavour in addition to sufficient piquancy and is early enough to ripen more than half of its heavy fruit load by the end of March in a decent summer. However, making a large quantity of hot sauce with such small chilli requires painstaking harvesting and destemming.

I avoid "Diablo," from my local garden centre. It produces a fair yield of large chillies but usually they are not very hot (an occasional plant throws overwhelmingly hot chillies) and is quite late to achieve red-ripe; I can well imagine some might prefer this one for its (usual) lack of potency. However, now there is a better medium-hot OP called Hot Portugal which is reliable, prolific and early enough to produce strong seeds here.

There are many Jalapeño strains, most of them are hybrids; most are quite late and fail to make red-ripe fruit. The Jalapeño seedlings I've purchased from the garden centre yielded little. However, open pollinated Early Jalapeño does excellently here, at least in respect to forming a lot of full-sized sufficiently potent green fruit on a strong, tidy bush that forms unbreakable, wind-tolerant branches. Early Jalapeño usually is the last pepper plant still alive in my garden in autumn. It would be a great service if someone on the east coast or someone with a polytunnel large enough for 20 plants (10 square metres) would provide Southern Harvest with seeds for it.

Thai Chilli, found in most garden centres, is too hot for my pleasure and has too little flavour to savour once you get past the fire. The same is even more so of the heat-loving tropical variety Habanero, a chilli so hot that many Mexicans are afraid to eat it, fearing a ring of fire the next day.

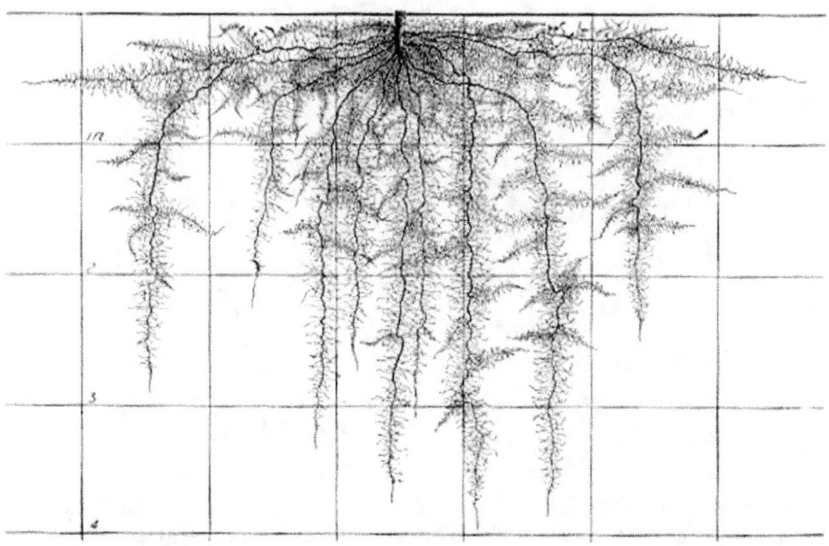

Root system of a mature pepper plant. Each square is thirty centimetres on a side. This plant is capable of extracting all the soil moisture from a circle over 1 metre in diameter.

Hungarian Hot Wax produces abundantly but is not very potent. When used for my raw chilli recipe, Hot Wax makes a delicious mildly piquant sauce that can be use in abundance without burning out the tastebuds. This hot sauce can be mixed 50/50 with tomato sauce/catsup and then used generously without making the portion too hot for the uninitiated.

Dry gardening: With limited irrigation grow small-fruited types. These make a larger root system. Space plants 900 mm x 900 mm. On deep soil, fertigate every two weeks. Start with about four litres on the first fertigation; increase the amount as they grow into big plants.

Tomato

(Lycopersicon esculentum)

Culture: Harvesting buckets of green tomatoes at summer's end is not the point. Our game is won by getting the plant to set fruit as soon as possible so that it'll provide vine ripened tomatoes for more weeks than it otherwise might have. The difficulty is that tomato flowers fail to pollinate on chilly nights—then the flower aborts, no fruit forms. The critical minimum pollination temperature differs by variety; it ranges from 10°C to 15°C and maybe even higher than 15°C for tropical varieties. So the key to achieving the first ripe tomato by Christmas is to encourage a variety that is genetically well-suited to setting fruit during Tasmania's chilly nights.

Tomatoes are a medium-demand crop that benefits from side-dressing *after* they begin making rapid growth. The last side dressing should happen early- to mid-January. Best to side dress with the aforementioned modified version of COF that provides less nitrogen.

Tomato varieties are either determinate or indeterminate. Determinate varieties make compact bushes that ripen fruit sooner than indeterminates. Attempts to trellis, prune, stake, or cage determinate varieties don't work very well so cheerfully accept that some fruit will be lost to slugs, some rots where it contacts the soil; some fruit will be overlooked; but these losses are more than offset by earlier ripening and ease of growing. Some early determinates may be crowded into 90 cm x 90 cm centres. Lustily growing determinates like Legend or Rouge de Marmande could use 120 cm x 120 cm centres. Determinate varieties can fill up even more space in a polytunnel.

To get ripe fruit sooner transplant a few already flowering early determinate seedlings into a 1,200 mm wide tunnel cloche two- to three weeks before the last usual frost date. Allow them to grow under plastic until the plants are pushing against the sides. Then, with chilly nights safely behind, remove the cloche—ripe tomatoes start appearing almost immediately.

Set out unprotected tomatoes after there is no danger of frost. And safer, wait ten to fourteen days after all your neighbours put theirs out even if you must pot them up a size in order to hold them back without making them potbound. You can grow these big seedlings in a protected position and bring them indoors on very cold nights. Despite being held back for a few weeks the first ripe tomato may happen sooner than had those plants struggled in the field.

Indeterminate varieties take a few weeks longer to ripen their first fruit than determinates do. They also make ever-expanding vines that should be supported so they don't rest on the soil. Indeterminates should be spaced *at least* 1,500 mm x 1,500 mm apart; most indeterminates benefit by owning all the space inside a circle extending *at least* 1 metre from their stem (positioned 2 metres x 1.5 metres). Indeterminates will make a hard to harvest tangle that conceals a lot of spoiling fruit if they are allowed to sprawl without training or staking. So indeterminates are propped up in cages, tied to trellises or to wooden stakes. And they should be pruned or else they make smaller fruit with less flavour.

The pruning method is simple. Indeterminates form a side branch at every leaf notch, usually in a pattern of two weak side branches and then a strong one, repeat. Every weak side branch should be pinched off as soon as it is seen. Only strong side branches are allowed to develop. This action produces larger, earlier ripening, tastier fruits that can be seen before they rot.

I've have used several tomato training systems that are frequently recommended in garden literature. I'll briefly and fairly describe one method. Seedlings are pruned so as to make only one or occasionally two vines (I've done it both ways) which are then trained to grow up strings and entirely prevented from making *any* side branches by pinching them all off as fast as they form. Please look at the illustration on page 70. A 3 square metre tomato patch grown this way will hold 18 plants. There will be an impressive yield—in the beginning. But by the end of January the crowded plants will be stressed for lack of rootzone. Then the yield drops a lot; disease/insect pests may appear.

Garden books suggest wire cages to keep the fruit off the ground. Vines can be trained up a trellis. Etc. All those worked for me. But I always seek out what takes less effort and gives more result. So these days I tie the vines to 1,200 mm hardwood stakes that are pounded in where needed as the vine expands as it pleases. While transplanting out indeterminate seedlings I set a wooden stake close to each one and loosely (because it'll grow very fat) tie the main leader to it. From that point every weak side branch is immediately pinched off; every strong side branch is allowed to grow. When a strong branch has grown over 750 mm long it is tied 300 mm to 450 mm above the soil to another stake. The stakes are put in where the vine naturally goes and eventually form roughly concentric rings. By the end of February each plant will have ten to twelve stakes around it. The last stakes to go in could be 1,500 mm from the plant's centre; many of those stakes will have several main leaders tied to them at different heights. If you envisioned what I said then you're imagining a plant that is well over two metres across with a root system just as extensive. I grew them that big outdoors and unprotected in Grindelwald. In chilly Chudleigh we can only achieve a high yielding plant like that in a polytunnel.

Garden planning: These days for two oldies I grow only one Siletz, a very

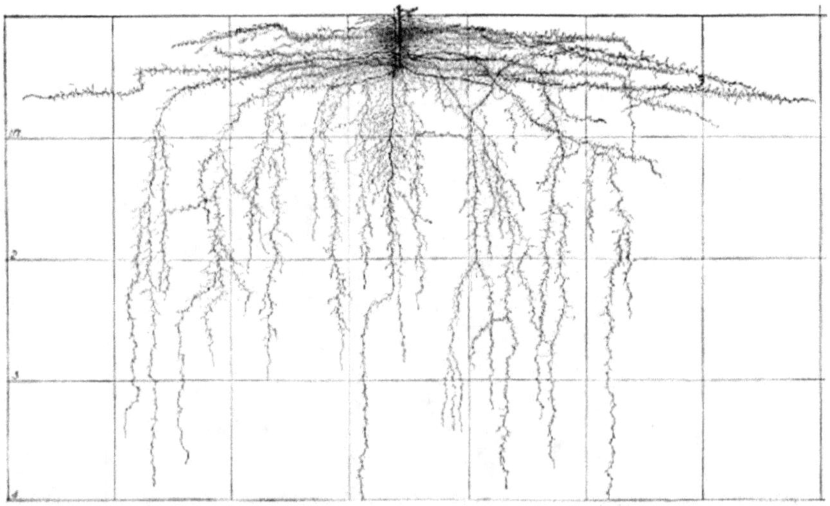

Indeterminate tomato plant only eight weeks after transplanting; note the roots fully occupy a circle about 120 cm in diameter. As the vines continue to spread the roots will spread too, as well as penetrating deeper. Even if the plant is trained up a trellis or constrained within a cage, if the roots find unoccupied growing room they will still expand into unoccupied soil, mirror imaging untrained vines.

early determinate, to fill the gap until the best-tasting varieties start ripening. I also grow three indeterminate varieties, one plant of each. I provide a 1,500 mm wide bed for them. Because I give them barely enough growing room these four plants produce plenty of tomatoes for our needs and as much again to give away.

Insects and diseases: I have never seen a catastrophic insect problem although we expect to lose a few fruit to insects and blackbirds. Tomato fruitworms are a close relative of the cabbage grub but they aren't present every summer. When fruitworms are around, losses can be minimized with Dipel (Bt). Spray every two weeks. In the (non) summer of 2014-15 those strong triangular "stinkbugs" that wreck raspberries (and taste foul if you accidentally bite into one) damaged around 20 percent of our tomatoes. Nothing like that ever happened before. I could have sprayed the stinkbugs every few days but did not bother; we still had plenty of undamaged fruit.

Most of the diseases that tomatoes have been bred to resist concern commercial producers using soil has lost a lot of organic matter and is remineralized with little more than chemical NPK. Garden tomatoes sometimes do show a bit of disease in very poor weather but now that my soil has been properly remineralized even Golden Jubilee, the most heat loving variety I grow, has no problems.

Two phenomena appear to be diseases but aren't. When large amounts of water are added to dry soil, tomatoes may respond by temporarily curling their leaves; the gardener can prevent leaf curl by maintaining higher minimum soil moisture. The blossom ends of fruits may blacken and rot. This often happens to the first few fruits that ripen, then end rot stops happening all by itself. A shortage of calcium can cause blossom-end rot on fruit that ripens later. Fertilizing with COF and a generous dose of good compost before planting time *was* the cure. COF prevents calcium shortage; compost dug in through the entire potential root zone increases calcium uptake. If you are trying to cure blossom-end rot in already growing plants, keeping a steady moisture supply may reduce the problem but the best cure can only be effected by fertilizing better next year. Top dressing 1.5 litres of gypsum per 10 square metres of root zone should help a lot.

I don't believe the oft-repeated warning that overhead watering gives tomatoes diseases although this might be the case where summer is hot and humid or when the soil is badly out of balance.

Harvest: Most determinate varieties overbear—like apple trees do. Even if the determinate you're growing doesn't seem to be doing that I suggest reducing its fruit load. When the first fruit shows signs of ripening start removing at least two-thirds of all new flower clusters. This makes bigger, better-tasting tomatoes.

If tomato fruit worms or other insect pests are troublesome or the cunning blackbirds are too cheeky, pick the fruit when it first starts turning orange and let it ripen indoors. It'll taste almost as good as had it completely vine ripened. Gently harvest all full sized green or half ripe tomatoes just before the first frost or else before deteriorating weather conditions cause skin damage. We bring in buckets full of green fruit early in April that ripen during April and May. These won't have quite the vine ripe flavour but still are far tastier than what is on offer at the supermarket. You may read about time-consuming methods promising more success with indoor ripening of green fruit and about a very late ripening variety called Longkeeper that produces green tomatoes especially for ripening indoors. Longkeeper is an excellent variety but we find that when large clean unblemished green tomatoes of any variety are stored in a single layer in a cool part of the house, are checked every few days for colouring up and those that do start to ripen are put on the kitchen bench, most of the tomatoes ripen and very few rot.

Saving seed: Tomatoes self-pollinate; naturally occurring crosses are nearly impossible except with a few very old heirlooms. Tomato seed lacks vigour if it is extracted from fruit that did not get fully vine ripe. Remove the seedy gel from a few *fully vine ripened* tomatoes (overlooked or damaged fruit are ideal for this purpose), put this in a small glass jar on the kitchen counter to ferment. Loosely cover. Within two days the pulp will start bubbling, mould may form on top. Stir or swirl once daily. Conduct the fermentation speedily which means at a temperature around 20°C. Cold, slow-going fermentations lasting more than one week result in dead seed. At normal summertime room temperatures most of the seeds from most varieties will settle to the bottom after fermenting for three days. Then, slowly add water until the jar is nearly full. After the seeds have resettled on the bottom, carefully pour off most of the pulp. Repeat this wash several times until the seeds look fairly clean. Have no concern about light-weight seeds that float away with the pulp; these are not ripe and would fail to germinate well. Then pour the seeds into a tea strainer and wash them thoroughly in cold water. Then spread them out to dry on a sheet of paper.

Fermentation does more than conveniently separate seeds from pulp, the procedure also removes naturally produced sprouting inhibitor chemicals. This accomplished, the seed germinates much faster. Fermentation is a far better seed-extraction method than the traditional home-gardener's technique of drying pulp and seed together.

Varieties: I dug my first Tasmanian garden the first week of November, 1998. We had just moved in. It was too late to start my own tomato seedlings. So I purchased an assortment at the local garden centre. The disappointing result reminded me my first year growing tomatoes in Oregon when I also bought seedlings from the garden centre. I soon discovered that these seedlings were not well adapted to Oregon. The varieties on offer were what every Oregonian used *before* Dr. James Baggett's varieties were released.

Most American garden seed sellers are located in the heavily-populated East where summer resembles eastern NSW. But when varieties that work in most of the northern United States are used in Oregon they are far slower to ripen than advertised; the supposedly delicious flavour doesn't happen; there are heaps of unripe green tomatoes at the end of it all. This was just like my result the first year in Tasmania.

So I surveyed all the garden seed sources in Australia, I talked to local gardeners and to Quarantine. I drew out the owner of a large Tasmanian seedling nursery. And this is what I discovered: The tomato varieties that our garden centres provide are on offer because Tasmanian seedling nurseries conveniently obtain their seeds from mainland sources. I reckon the results we get from mainland varieties are accepted because Tasmanian home gardeners know of nothing better.

Mainland varieties do produce a moderate (but late to start ripening) yield—except when we cop a cloudy cool humid half-summer that better suits brassicas. During a cabbage year the fruit ripens very late; we end up with more black-spotted green tomatoes in April than all the ripe ones harvested during summer.

So, after a disappointing tomato result in the summer of 1998-99, no matter what barriers Quarantine had erected and no matter how much Q was going to charge me, I imported seeds for a dozen early open pollinated tomato varieties that work well in Oregon, including six of Dr. Baggett's varieties (plus a dozen packets of the earliest open-pollinated pepper and eggplant varieties still available in the States, which is why Antohi, Early Jalapeño and Hot Portugal are now available. Because I explained why I was importing so many small packets of these restricted species Tas Quarantine generously allowed them to enter without the usual fees. Next summer I trialled them. The year after that I began producing seed for the best of them and encouraged Tasmanians to try them. Baggett's tomato varieties proved to be the best by far.

Dr. James Baggett was Oregon State University's highly-respected plant breeder at the same time I was in the vegetable garden seed business. He was a kind and generous man who taught me a great deal. Dr. Baggett developed a family of tomato varieties by crossing delicious American home garden varieties with a unique strain he received from Russia. The Russian tomato had very little to recommend it except for one valuable and rare (in tomatoes) genetic trait—it was parthenocarpic, meaning it had the ability to set seedless fruit on cold spring nights instead of aborting its flowers—which is what the usual varieties do. Those first fruits ripen weeks ahead of anything else—and are entirely seedless because the flower was not pollinated.

Four of Baggett's varieties proved well suited to Tasmania and especially delicious: Gold Nugget, Siletz, Oregon Spring and Legend. Gold Nugget is covered with rich-flavoured deep yellow cherries (at least the first thirty to fifty cherries are rich-flavoured; after that the variety's overbearing tendency dilutes the flavour but by that time there are better and bigger tomatoes getting ripe). If you really fancied Gold Nugget you could remove most of the flower clusters, thus greatly improving taste and increasing fruit size. Gold Nugget is guaranteed (by me) to ripen ten days earlier than anything else you can find. The tidy bush is under one metre in diameter.

Siletz makes large, thin-skinned, soft (but firm, not watery) fruits with an interesting complex enjoyable flavour. It makes few seeds even when the fruit does pollinate. The early fruits entirely lack seedy gel-filled cavities. Siletz makes a compact determinate vine rarely exceeding 1.2 metres in diameter.

Legend is a vigorous determinate that spreads to a diameter of 1.5 metres and sometimes 2 metres. It sets heaps of big red tomatoes that taste so much better than Siletz that we stop eating Siletz when Legend starts ripening, which usually is about two weeks after Siletz starts. Legend's harvest continues to the end of summer. When Annie and I supplied Daniel Alp's gourmet kitchen he opined that Legend tastes better than Brandywine—which is our favourite large red variety.

Tasmanians are slow to change. As far as I know, seedlings for Dr. Baggett's varieties are still not sold at garden centres. However, these varieties are so early that you can direct seed them and still get ripe fruit as soon and as abundantly as you'll get from planting seedlings for mainland varieties.

I once had enough youthful enthusiasm to supply SH with seed for Baggett's tomato varieties. In order to simplify the process and increase the seed yield significantly I direct seeded the crop. I proceeded exactly as I would to grow a broccoli plant. At Grindelwald, around 5 October, I sowed pinches of seeds about 1 cm deep. This is about the same date that tomato seeds left by last years rotting tomatoes naturally start coming up. I progressively thinned each position to a single plant. Direct seeded plants end up a few weeks of vegetative growth smaller than transplanted seedlings at summer's end. So Legend was positioned on stations one-metre apart; Siletz got 600 x 750. Directly seeded plants make their first flowers five or six weeks after they germinate but by late-November when this starts happening the nights have become warmer. So the first fruits on direct-seeded parthenocarpic tomato varieties usually have seeds in them . . . and the very first ripe tomatoes happen about three weeks later than the first ripe from the same variety set out as a ten week old seedling in a 250 mm pot.

Please, if you have space for an experiment, direct seed one Legend tomato plant. If you haven't yet grown one of Dr. Baggett's varieties you may be delighted. If you have been raising and transplanting your own seedlings in the usual way, then direct seeding one plant will give you an illuminating experience. I predict you'll get higher quality fruit in March from direct-seeded plants than you've ever had from seedlings grown in the usual manner.

Southern Harvest offers a broad choice of well adapted varieties. Sam Bayley asked me to specifically mention that he considers the apricot-sized fruit on Kotlas to be the earliest ripening variety that has really great flavour.

Because Tasmanians are slow to change I suppose I should review a few of the locally popular mainland varieties. Rouge (de Marmande) makes a larger plant than most determinates do and has long been one of the earliest varieties on the garden centre seedling bench. It tastes pretty good but seems watery and seedy to me compared to Legend. Many gardeners around here sing the praises of Grosse Lisse which is, no doubt, as the German translates, big and smooth (and hard, and thick-skinned and to me, rather tasteless). Apollo ripens many fruit of acceptable table quality.

Every spring mainland seed sellers and TV presenters rave about one or two newly released varieties. My gardening friends are surprised that I am disinterested. Introducing new tomato varieties every year is a standard garden seed business practice because it encourages hope for a better result than the disappointments of last summer. Trouble is: new mainland varieties rarely please in Tasmania.

Gardeners who make sauce or paste from table varieties are wasting energy—both hydro and their own. Salad or slicing tomatoes have a high water content: a full pot cooks down to only a little seedy sauce. Processing varieties are bred to have a high percentage of solids and fewer seeds. They cook down more rapidly into a thick sauce; some processing varieties will hold a firm round shape for whole-pack canning. My favourite for sauce is the pink-skinned rather late ripening indeterminate Mama Mia. What a flavour! Such thin skins; they disappear without having to be removed. And so abundant (in a hot summer). Mama Mia is supposed to be a hybrid but I've grown my own seed for it through many generations and in my opinion it actually is an OP. I've also had good results with Roma, a well known determinate that is better adapted to cooler microclimates than Mama Mia.

I reconsidered the previous paragraph in preparation to reprint this book in 2019. I wondered if Mama Mia was still available anywhere or was I wasting space praising a variety no one could obtain. I found one garden centre in Saskatchewan, Canada had it. The only Australian source I could find is United Nurseries in VIC. They do not sell seeds; they sell seedlings to garden centres.

In the same way that small-fruited capsicums outdo the big ones in marginal conditions, most cherry tomatoes ripen their first fruit earlier than large-fruited varieties and almost all cherry varieties are wildly aggressive indeterminates. Mainland cherry varieties usually do fine on Tasmania. I prefer Tommy Toe. Annie fancies Sweet Bite. Yellow Pear and Yellow Plum are heirlooms, both are incredibly aggressive, both taste great but ripen rather late here.

Heirloom varieties are always indeterminate. Most heirlooms do not develop full flavour in Tasmania's cool nights; many prove too late to ripen much at all. So try heirlooms cautiously. My favourite variety of all, Golden Jubilee, isn't quite an heirloom unless I am one too. It was a brand-new variety in 1943 (one year after I was born); it was released with much fanfare by a major US seed company. Jubilee produces absolutely the most delicious, firm, huge yellow-orange slicing tomatoes. Golden Jubilee usually leaves a lot of green fruit at summer's end; in a poor summer this one is the variety most likely to get diseased. However, when full-sized (but still green) Golden Jubilee tomatoes ripen indoors through April and May, they'll taste nearly as good as they did in midsummer. Longkeeper, the variety that ripens over many months of indoor storage, was probably bred out of Jubilee.

Lately we've been favouring Brandywine. Comparing the ease of growing Legend to the time spend staking and training Brandywine—I choose Brandywine.

Dry gardening: Indeterminate varieties make root systems that will, if they can, extend far beyond what most people expect is possible. Indeterminates are the best choice for water-short circumstances. Legend is determinate, but is so vigorous it does nearly as well. The maximum useful outdoor spacing for indeterminates in this climate seems about 1,800 mm x 2,000 mm. Grown this way on deep moisture-retentive soil, a vine may yield modestly through an entire summer without rain or irrigation. But fertigate each vine every two to three weeks during summer and you'll harvest several fold more. Small-fruited varieties dry garden best of all.

Legumes

There is much incorrect information circulating about legumes that has been re-repeated by several generations of copycat garden writers and by vegans writing about healthful eating. To me this situation demonstrates the propagandist's maxim that the oft told lie becomes the truth. I hope what is on this page will disabuse your belief that major health benefits come from eating legume seeds for protein.

Garden books and magazine articles often assert that legumes supply nitrogen to non-legumes sharing their root zone and that garden beans and peas leave useful amounts of nitrogen in the soil for the next crop. The truth is: very little nitrogen leaks into the soil from living legume roots and very little remains in legume roots after harvest. It is true that legumes can manufacture at least part and sometimes all of their own nitrogen requirement. This is done in collaboration with a family of soil-dwelling bacteria called rhizobia, whose colonies form pinkish nodules on legume roots. Legumes without rhizobia have to obtain all their nitrogen from the soil just like non-legume species do. However, virtually all rhizobially manufactured nitrogen becomes part of chlorophyll, the dark green protein in the leaves.

Many legume species that farmers grow have the ability to self-generate their entire nitrogen requirement. But some farm soils have been so totally mined out that no rhizobia are present. Without them already in the soil a legume crop must be inoculated with rhizobia before sowing. Seed inoculation is a common farming practice. Garden soils that are fed compost already have rhizobia; garden peas and garden beans shouldn't need inoculation. Besides, the large amount of nitrogen in garden soils from decomposing organic matter, from chook poo pellets, bloodandbone and other nitrogen fertilizers inhibit rhizobial fixation of nitrogen. Don't be concerned if beans and peas in your garden fail to develop well nodulated roots. Be concerned instead about soil fertility in general and about the amount of soil organic matter.

During winter, instead of mud, weeds and rotting crop waste you could be viewing vibrant green patches of small-seeded broad beans, clover or lupins. Turning under an actively growing legume green manure does effectively increase both soil organic matter and soil nitrogen. Overwintering green manures, be they legumes or another species, also preserve soil fertility by capturing nutrients that might otherwise be leached. A dense stand of vegetation transpires so much moisture during spring that it allows tillage of heavy soil weeks earlier than otherwise might be possible. All these benefits accrue in exchange for establishing a green manure crop in autumn.

Clovers are excellent nitrogen fixers; tic beans are better yet. A strong stand of clover that is turned under *when flowers first start to form* can supply more than enough N from its own rapid decomposition for a low-demand crop such as carrot or beetroot. Digging in a strong stand of tic beans may quickly release enough nitrogen to supply a medium-demand crop.

There is much misinformation about eating legume seeds. They do contain a lot of protein but I don't think it's best dietary practice to satisfy the body's protein requirement with them. Besides, there should be no concerns about protein. An Australian would have to *almost entirely* eat potato crisps and sugar drinks in order to develop a protein deficiency (but would develop many other nutrient deficiencies). The best way to intake vegetable protein is by eating large servings of dark green leafy salad and cooked greens like spinach, mustards or silverbeet. The green colour is chlorophyll which is a complete protein with an amino acid balance that is perfect for humans.

Yes, legume seeds are high in protein but they are equally rich in carbohydrates. Most human stomachs don't properly digest cooked proteins and carbos at the same time. That's why pea soup, baked beans, hummus, lentil soup, etc, cause intestinal gas in almost everyone. Wind is my least concern. Attempting to digest this difficult combination generates toxic waste products that degrade health and cause disease. Vegans often fret about getting enough protein; they often eat a great many cooked legume seeds. These folks develop the same deadly diseases that people eating too much overcooked red meat and potatoes get. If you want a high protein vegan meal I suggest filling the belly with leafy green salad and steamed French beans.

It isn't lack of protein that is causing our steadily increasing amount of degenerative illness. Our collective poor health isn't caused by pesticide residues in our foods either. These toxins would only be minor irritations to well nourished bodies. Actually almost all Australians are suffering from a lack of nutrient density in almost everything they eat. Had farmers put the full range of plant nutrients into cropping soils—lime and sulfur, trace elements and micronutrients *and* NPK—there would be much more nutrition in our foods.

Very early sowings of pea may fail to germinate if the soil is too cold. Broad bean seeds will usually come up eventually but can get badly set back by too much struggle.

Similarly, garden beans are often started before the soil has warmed up enough to really suit them. Germination is more certain if these large seeds are first chitted, presprouted. (see Chapter 6, "Seeds")

The key to getting the strongest planting seed from beans and peas is growing the mother plants in fully remineralized soil and then allowing the pods to dry down completely on the plant without exposing them to rain or irrigation. In a garden this last requirement may prove to be impossible. If end of summer weather turns rainy or if you must irrigate the area where bean seeds are drying down, then first pick any bean or pea pods that are at least half dry and bring them inside to finish. However, do not pick any pod before its vascular connection to the plant has ended. This is revealed when the stem end of the pod gets thin and floppy (wilts). From that point the pods are not receiving any more food from the plant so they may as well dry indoors as hanging on the bush. Do not remove half dry seeds from the pod because they are still soft; the delicate embryo within may be bruised. It is not well protected until the seed gets hard.

French Bean, Bush

(Phaseolus vulgaris)

The wild ancestor of *P. vulgaris* is a rampantly growing semi-tropical vine. Domesticated climbing varieties will cover a two metre tall structure and then some. Bush varieties were bred from climbers to lower production costs. Some bush varieties mature in such a concentrated fashion that they can be mechanically harvested. Unfortunately, the flavour (and probably the nutritional content) of the very best bush varieties can't quite equal that of the climbers because their crowded leaves shade each other whilst the well-separated leaves of climbing beans can gather more direct, unfiltered light. Similarly, a climber's root systems is more aggressive than bush (dwarfed) varieties. In this respect, bush beans resemble early determinate tomatoes that set a huge quantity of less tasty fruit because it is supported by less leaf area per fruit and a diminished root system. Some bush varieties are flavoursome, but when climbing types are available I rarely eat bush beans.

Culture: *P. vulgaris* beans grow best in warm soil. *Vulgaris* seeds rot in the ground instead of sprouting when soil is wet and chilly. Because of this sensitivity I make my first sowing about the same time I set out tomato seedlings. Sowing a week earlier than that usually results in hitting a patch of chilly wet weather; if I do get some germination I still end up with stunted, low-production plants. So why create stress! My garden abundantly provides a broad choice of vegetables in all seasons. We can wait another week to eat the first French beans.

Garden beans are a low-demand crop. Sow 2 to 3 cm deep, each seed 5 cm to 8 cm from the next in the row, 60 cm between rows. Seedlings start growing fast about a week after they emerge unless the weather is poor. Progressively thin to 25–30 cm apart in the row. If a few days of chilly or rainy weather happens between sowing and emergence then any seedlings that do come up may be exhausted. Even if the sun returns they won't grow fast for awhile. The best thing to do when bean seeds go through several consecutive days of bad weather before emerging is to sow again (between the original rows if that works); do this as soon as the weather improves. And if that sowing also hits a bad patch, resow yet again. Whichever sowing gets going the best will soon dominate the space even if other seedlings had come up sooner.

Garden planning: Bush beans produce the most in the first weeks of harvest. To harvest plenty all summer, make another sowing every three weeks. The last crop should be sown late in December; it will yield in March. The harvest from three square metres of bed provides more than twice as many beans as we two oldies can eat fresh. To achieve the earliest-possible harvest, bush bean seeds may be sown in tunnel cloche about two weeks before the last usual frost date; keep the plants under plastic until the harvest starts.

Insects and Diseases: There should be no worries. Problems will arise if the patch was sown too early, if soil fertility was inadequate or when the patch is overcrowded. Focus on those concerns as well as the pest or disease.

Harvest: Bush bean plants are easily damaged; handle them gently when harvesting. *P. vulgaris* doesn't thrive in windy locations for the same reason; ground-hugging bush varieties handle wind better than climbers. Thorough picking done every other day extends the harvest period because if seeds develop in more than one or two pods, the set of new pods declines.

Saving seed: Naturally occurring crosses between *P. vulgaris* varieties are extremely rare; isolation is unnecessary. Mutations are not so rare. If the plants show variations save seeds from one ideal plant—tender, earlier, slower to develop strings and seeds, etc. Allow all subsequent pods on the ideal plant to form and mature seeds. Bean seeds that dry down late in March won't be as vigorous as seeds drying down when

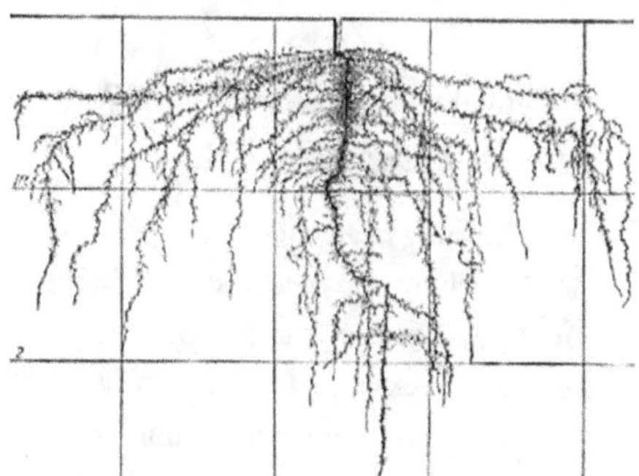

Roots of a two-month-old bush bean

light is more intense. In my opinion any gardener buying bean seed for any other reason than to try a new variety wastes money. The vulgaris seed I grow retains good germination for five-plus years.

Varieties: Green, "blue," yellow, filet, flageolet, haricot vert, Dutch, English, Guatemalan, purple-mottled, longpod—just about every one of the dozens of dwarf *vulgaris* varieties I've trialled has yielded well enough although some varieties form their first pods a week earlier or a week later. The pods of traditional varieties *quickly* form strings and seeds (and stop being tender). These include Tendergreen, Brown Beauty, Pioneer and Provider. Modern varieties are much slower to form seeds and strings so they do not have to be picked as promptly. My favourite at the moment is Bountiful Baby (FOT); it is nearly as tasty as the best climbing varieties I know. Purple podded varieties like Royal Burgundy or Purple Queen usually yield sooner under cool conditions. Purple-coloured pods turn green when cooked.

Dry gardening: If in-the-row spacing increases to 450 mm apart and there is 1 metre between rows, then bush beans may grow steadily in some soils without being irrigated at all, especially this is so of the older varieties. Experiment—there's considerable varietal difference in root-system vigour. Where water is really short I suggest growing climbing varieties, especially Kentucky Wonder Brown Seeded. I harvested an abundance of seeds from that one at the end of an entirely rainless hot Oregon summer without any irrigation.

French Bean, Climbing

(Phaseolus vulgaris)

Climbing beans need a few more weeks than bush types to start yielding but most climbing varieties produce for eight weeks *if picked thoroughly and frequently*, ultimately providing a great deal more from the space. I've trialled climbing varieties that yielded from Christmas until mid-March.

Culture: This is a low demand crop that might benefit from light side-dressing if yield falls off. Climbing vines naturally wrap around rough poles, a trellis, a fence or strings. Early settlers grew them up tall tripods made of skinny rough poles. In this case sow clusters of three seeds at the base of each pole, placed 3 cm deep and thin to one or two plants per pole. If the vines are to climb netting then place each seed 50 mm to 75 mm apart in the row. Once they have become established and are growing well, thin to 150 mm apart in the row. If superoverenthusiasm causes more than one row to be grown make the between row space at least 1.5 metres because if climbers don't run out of below-ground growing space they'll produce longer.

Garden planning: Three row metres of climbers produce over two times more than our family can use fresh. To have a stable supply through the entire summer I suggest making two sowings; the first sowing when the tomatoes go out; the second six weeks later. Bean fanciers might also sow a bush bean variety under poly; it will cover the plate until the climbers yield.

Insects and diseases: Same as dwarf beans. Some climbing varieties are intensely touchy about windy sites. And the rest are only fairly fragile.

Harvest: Like bush varieties; the pods of climbers are better-eating if they are picked at three quarters of full size. Should the position be so well protected that the plants experience no winds strong enough to rip off old blistered worn out leaves, then you might remove them yourself, exposing potential growing points to more light, which will then respond by developing bearing side branches. But if the old leaves are allowed to choke the plant then its yield will taper off.

Saving seed: Like bush beans. You're a spendthrift if you don't save your own seeds. I let one or two plants go entirely unharvested; they supply more than enough seed for me and all my neighbours.

Varieties: Blue Lake Pole has especially slow seed- and string development and makes longer, better-flavoured pods than bush Blue Lake varieties. Either variant of Kentucky Wonder, brown- or white-seeded has a richer beanier flavour than Blue Lake. Brown-seeded Kentucky Wonder is the finest all-purpose variety, nicknamed"old homestead" for good reason; it's the best one I know of for dry-gardening. Its pods have great flavour, it is pretty good for shelling beans and/or dry beans, too. Purple King starts yielding earlier and does better in chilly microclimates.

Dry gardening: Most climbing varieties do quite well without irrigation if they are given sufficient growing room and deep open soil. Each plant stands 300 mm to 450 mm apart; if more than one row make them 1,800 mm apart. Fertigate every three weeks.

(Scarlet) Runner Bean

(P. multifloris)

English people usually opine that *P. vulgaris* beans do not have as much flavour as *P. multifloris*. I agree. Runner bean forms delicious fuzzy pods that settle as satisfyingly in my stomach like beefsteak. Runner beans start bearing a few weeks later than *P. vulgaris*. Their vines may run longer distances than *P. vulgaris* climbers—over the top and hanging half way down the trellis. No matter how much growing room they have they seem to fill it up. But once they fill their allotted root zone the yield declines to very little.

Culture: Grow this low demand crop like pole beans—with differences. Provide each plant with *at least* one square metre of root growing room. If you hope to harvest a lot for a long time I can't stress how important it is to give them as-yet unoccupied root zone. The vines must climb something. I suggest a pair of 2.5 metre tall tripods that are two metres apart centre to centre, one tripod for each plant. Strongly anchor the legs! The vines fill gaps between the tripods by twining around strings tied from tripod to tripod.

Sow when you transplant tomato seedlings. I put three seeds in the centre of each tripod and thin to a single plant. Each plant soon forms many vines. Runner bean seeds take longer to germinate than vulgaris beans so chitting brings the first harvest forward about one week.

P. multifloris can be perennial, regenerating each spring from a clump of dahlia-like bulbs. For this reason runner beans are sometimes termed "seven year beans." However, I suggest digging up the root-bulbs in autumn (my friend Mary's pigs relish them). Start afresh from seed every spring because pod quality will be higher and the first harvest will be sooner.

Insects and Diseases: At first the vines bloom prolifically but no pods are set. Then pods start appearing. More pods will be set if you mist the vines with hose and nozzle just before sunset so that the vines are wet at dark.

Harvest: Take pods before any seed development starts. Pod set decreases when even a very few pods are forming seeds so harvest thoroughly. You can cook immature (still soft) seeds.

Saving seed: Runner beans are *mostly* self-fertile but bumblebees make crosses so seed savers should grow only one variety. Some varieties have white flowers, some have red. I inevitably overlook a few pods every year; these form seeds for next year's patch. Discovering an occasional runner bean seed in the soup makes an interesting experience. If grown entirely as a seed crop a very high seed yield would be a half-kilogram per square metre of root zone.

Varieties: Improved varieties feature much slower seed- and string development and longer more refined better-tasting pods. The Scarlet Runner seeds you are offered by many garden seed sellers probably are (more or less) the First Nations variety adopted by the English when they started settling North America. It produces short irregular pods with extremely rapid seed development which means the pods get tough and stringy just as fast as the seeds form. Birdland has a much better Scarlet Runner strain. Southern Harvest offers better varieties. A neighbour may grow a superior local variety.

Dry gardening: Very suitable. Give each seedling at least two square metres of uncontested root zone. Fertigate each plant every two weeks.

Broad Bean, large seed

(Vicia faba)

Large-seeded varieties have long been eaten by Europeans. Their small-seeded relatives are called tic beans if used for spring-sowing in the UK; they are called winter beans if the variety is hardy enough to overwinter. In Tasmania small seeded broad bean plants are fed to livestock or used as green manure. These seeds do not taste good. However culinary-quality small-seeded broad bean seeds are a delicious dietary staple in western Asia.

Culture: Broad beans are a very low demand crop. Their bed usually doesn't need COF if it received some compost within the last year. Many large seeded varieties survive frosts of minus 7°C. Territorial Seed Company once produced seed for an extra hardy large-seeded variety that started from a few Aquadulce Claudia plants that survived three continuously below-freezing days, the coldest morning of those three days was minus 10°C. Some small seeded varieties are even hardier.

Start overwintering broad beans between mid-April and mid-May. Position each seed 20 cm apart in rows 75 cm apart. Thin the row to 40 cm apart when the seedlings are well established. The later in May that they are sown the less likely the plants will grow excessively tall and then fall over (lodge) from the weight of developing seeds. You can insure germination of a late sowing by chitting the seeds. However, most years they will shoot anyway, chitted or not, and it is advantageous when it takes several weeks for a late May sowing to finally emerge because the plants won't grow as tall by spring. Around mid-August I suggest pruning back the stalks of overwintered plants to about 20 cm tall so that each plant puts up many shorter stalks.

Spring sowings don't grow as tall; the plants usually form only one stalk. At Grindelwald I spring-sowed broad beans mid-August although those further inland might wait until September. You'll want spring sown plants up and growing as soon as possible so chit the seeds. Sow 25 mm deep, 30 cm apart in a pair of parallel rows about 60 cm apart running lengthwise down a raised bed that is about 120 cm wide. Every already-sprouting seed will emerge.

If you are new to gardening be not dismayed when broad beans flower and flower and flower without setting pods. Eventually pods *will* appear—after conditions warm up enough.

Garden planning: Overwintered plants start bearing two or more weeks sooner than spring-sown plants. I no longer grow broad beans from a spring sowing because the pea harvest starts about when the overwintered bean harvest ends—and by then I've eaten more than enough broad beans for the year. Three row metres fills a big pail several times a week for several weeks.

Insects and diseases: Black spots on leaves and pods are usually related to poor winter drainage. Perhaps another part of the garden is less soggy? Disease also comes from too many days of poor weather. Increased interplant spacing increases light penetration to the lower leaves, increases air circulation and reduces or prevents disease. *Do not crowd broad beans.*

Harvest: Pods fatten first nearer the bottom of the stalk. Harvest progresses upward. Pick pods before the seeds reach full size because mature seeds lose sweetness and toughen.

Saving seed: Dry pods of large-seeded varieties securely retain ripe seeds so harvesting them need not be rushed.

On the other hand, tic bean seeds readily shatter from thin brittle pods. This type should be harvested promptly or else many seeds will be lost. My suggestions for cleaning dry bean seeds (soon to come) also apply to tic beans.

Broad beans cross pollinate more than occasionally. Different varieties should be separated by 30 metres or more. The large-seeded "variety" I started with in 1998 came from Waratah Distribution. Their half-kilo bag proved to be a blend of different varieties (and their crosses). From this diversity I saved seeds from two especially pleasing plants—one tall with very large seeds; the other shorter with medium-sized seeds. Then I had two varieties; both suited my soil and situation.

Varieties: U.K. seedsmen offer many excellent varieties. Unfortunately the home gardener can not comply with AQIS import restrictions on beans although importers of food-grade broad beans seem to have no barriers because I have seen many types being sold in ethnic food shops; these will sprout and grow. You go figure! Southern Harvest offers several. Red Epicure (BIRD) makes intense red seeds with excellent flavour.

Dry gardening: Broad beans grow in a season when the soil is reliably kept moist by rainfall and their seeds mature when Tasmanian conditions naturally dry out. Taswegians trying to create maximum self-sufficiency could cook dry seed from large-seeded varieties instead of eating vulgaris beans, which require irrigation and richer soil than broad beans need to yield big.

Dry / Shelling Beans

(P. vulgaris)

P. Vulgaris matures seed from February through March depending upon variety and also upon how early your microclimate allows you to sow them. March can present heavy dews that slow or prevent drying. And rain is more likely then. This makes early finishing varieties desirable.

Culture: Like dwarf French beans.

With irrigation: sow seeds 10 cm apart in rows 45 cm apart. Thin when established to 20 cm in the row. Moisture stress will accelerate ripening and stop the formation of new pods. So greatly reduce (light soil) or entirely stop watering (heavy soil) when the first pods start drying down.

Without irrigation: sow seeds 15 cm apart in rows 100 cm apart. Thin when established to 30-45 cm in the row; in-the-row spacing depends on your previous experience with that variety. First timers should err on the side of more interplant spacing. *Keep the patch extremely well-weeded; a hoe applied shallowly and frequently maintains a loose-soil mulch that reduces moisture loss.* Moisture-stressed beans yield less but dry down sooner.

Garden planning: Irrigated yields depend upon the variety being grown and will be from 25 kg to 50 kg per 100 square metres. Unirrigated yields are lower; the amount depends upon summer rainfall and the moisture supplying ability of the soil as well as on the variety's ability to handle moisture stress.

Harvest: Ideally, pull the plants when 90 percent of the leaves have yellowed and all the pods have dried completely but before many seeds shatter. Only a few varieties can reach this stage of maturity in Tassie. Most years the almost done plants have to be pulled from the earth, roots and all, and then hung in bunches under cover, such as under a veranda roof. When drying plants are thinly spread on a tarp turn them over every day at first. Thresh the seeds when the plants have become crisp. Threshing can be done with a flail or by scuffle-dancing on a foot-thick layer of plants spread on a tarp, or by banging the plants (held by the stems at the root-end) against the inner wall of a metal petrol drum; they may be threshed by crushing the pods between the palms (consider wearing gloves). Then clean (winnow) the seeds by slowly pouring them from one large plastic bucket into another in a moderate breeze.

Saving seed: Vulgaris beans very rarely cross. Some varieties are naturally stable; others are more likely to mutate and throw off-types. Uniform seed stocks are maintained by choosing a few perfect plants each year, harvesting them separately and planting this selected seed next year. For the highest possible uniformity, start with one perfect plant, then grow out the seeds from each pod on that plant in its own line. Then increase perfect lines.

Varieties: Dry beans sold at the supermarket will come up if you sow them but the varieties will almost certainly require more heat than Tassie can provide; likely they're produced in Queensland's cool-season. But if you fancy a particular kind of bean you'll never know how it'll grow here until you try. With beans, one or two plants per variety is enough for a trial. Most garden seed companies offer a few dry bean varieties. For over 30 years Black Coco has been my head and shoulders above all others favourite.

When I taste-test a new-to-me dry bean variety I soak one heaping tablespoonful of dry seed in water overnight and next day simmer these seeds for exactly two hours without benefit of salt or seasoning. A desirable variety will become quite tender in that much time and have flavour good enough to enjoyably eat just like that. However, a bean that remains tough after two hours of cooking may not be an undesirable variety. It may just be old seed. Bean seeds develop an impervious skin when in storage for a year or more. In the seed trade this phenomena is called "hard seed." This is undesirable because hard seeds are slow to take up moisture when sown. Latin Americans depend on beans; they avoid old bean seed. Asians similarly dislike old rice.

Peas

(Pisum sativum)

Most people have never tasted barely cooked freshly harvested garden peas. Or never experienced the pleasure of eating some raw as the patch is being harvested. Raw absolutely fresh peas are more delicious than the fanciest frozen and light years ahead of supermarket "fresh" peas.

The shelling pea harvest usually ends around Christmas when the first hot days of summer trigger diseases. The harvest can be made to start much earlier in spring by sowing mid-April and keeping the patch weeded during winter. It also is possible to grow at least one variety of snow pea *(mangé tout)* during summer. Shelling and snow pea may also be grown in a polytunnel for winter harvest but I don't bother because the peas or snow pea pods forming without intense sunlight are not very sweet.

Culture: Pea seed should be sown early enough that the harvest finishes before hot weather arrives. Vigorous pea seeds germinate well in cool soil; weak pea seeds may shoot okay after the soil warms up. But germination, even of strong seed, usually fails when the soil is cold *and* soggy *and* stays that way for many days. Gardeners coping with clay soil may not be able to sow the earliest peas unless they pre-prepared the bed the previous autumn. To do this, in April remove weeds and crop residues from the intended pea patch. Then hoe in 15 mm of compost and establish a green manure. I suggest using tic beans or rocket. In August, the green crop can either be pulled out (and composted) or else just the tops are cut off close to the soil and removed (and composted). Either way, the crop has formed a dense network of fine, rapidly decomposing roots that eliminate the need to deeply loosen the soil. Then spread the basic amount of COF, chop the surface with a strong hoe, thus making a very rough seedbed. Then cut furrows with the corner of a hoe and sow. Carefully place chitted pea seeds in furrows about 2 cm deep, one seed every cm in short rows arranged 45 cm to 60 cm apart across the bed.

As soon as my earliest patch emerges I sow another patch. This time I do not bother with chitting. As soon as the second patch shoots, I sow a third one, and so forth, proceeding this way until it is too late to sow peas—which is mid-October at Grindelwald and probably early November at Chudleigh, but I am not yet sure about Chudleigh, I need a few more years gardening here before I know for sure.

I do not thin a row of pea seedlings unless clusters emerge.

Some years at Grindelwald the mid-October sowing was harvested before hot weather diseases took it out. Some years this one failed. Either way, we enjoyed an abundance of fresh shelling peas before the first French beans were forming.

Keep the isles between rows weed-free until the pea vines cover them. If there is one pea plant every one or two centimetres in the row, and there are several rows across the bed then the vines will soon form a self-supporting tangle. Old garden books say peas need supports to climb. Few modern dwarf varieties will climb. You may read about providing support for peas in relatively new garden books too, or on a TV gardening show, but that's because many garden writers and TV show presenters learn more from earlier erring copycat garden writers than from their own experience. There may be heirloom pea varieties still in use that need something to climb.

For a tall heirloom climber like Telephone (Alderman), sow seeds along a two metre tall trellis and thin to 4 cm apart; tall varieties take longer to begin yielding than dwarves but yield over a longer period. Start climbers as early as possible if you hope to harvest much before the heat of summer arrives.

Garden planning: Four rows of dwarf shelling peas across a 1,200 wide raised bed yield more than enough for two oldies for about two weeks. That's why I sow a succession of patches. To freeze enough peas to provide two generous serves twice each week through autumn and winter requires harvesting 10 to 20 square metres.

Any bed that grew winter vegetables makes a good candidate for shelling peas. If the bed space is needed before harvesting the peas pull the vines before any seeds form. Pea's rapidly decomposing *dense* root system lets the bed be planted with shallow hoeing.

Insects and diseases: Peas get diseased when days turn hot no matter what a gardener does or doesn't. Young pea vines do not become diseased because of hot days until they start forming seeds. If you want to grow peas in summer, use the highly disease resistant snow pea variety bred by Dr. Jim Baggett and make sure to harvest every pod before the seeds in it start to form. Don't miss picking any.

Harvest: Pick peas every day or two. Best to take shelling peas when the seeds within are only two-thirds developed; just one day older and the peas in that pod will be getting tough and starchy. Pods that are at the correct degree of maturity to harvest are easily recognizable once a variety has been learned (by munching raw peas as you harvest). Removing overmature overlooked pods may encourage slightly longer production; leaving them in place to fully mature yields planting seed for next year. Commercial freezing varieties fill almost all their pods at once; this trait suits machine harvesting. Home garden varieties fill their pods over a longer period.

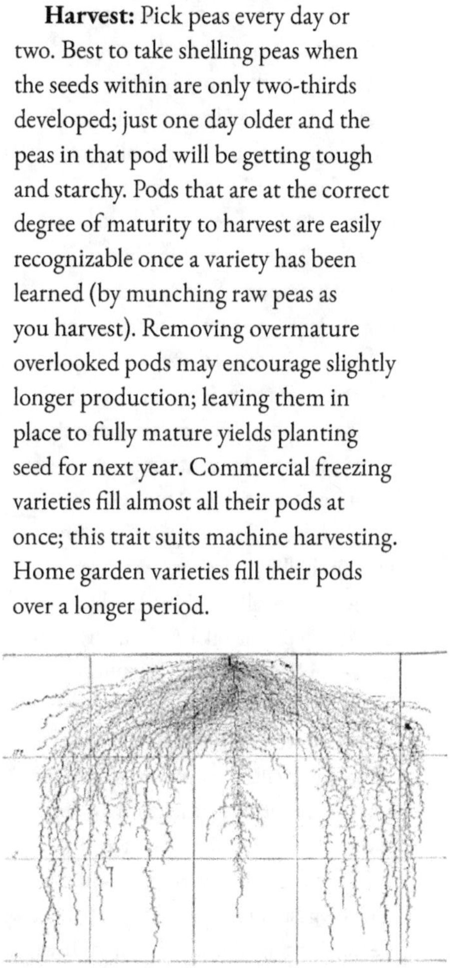

Pea vine at maturity

Heirloom snow pea varieties should be picked when pods reach 2/3 full size, well before string and seeds form. The Oregon snow pea varieties from Dr. Baggett don't toughen their pods rapidly. If these are allowed to develop a string and half-sized seeds they'll be sweeter. Most varieties of snap pea become tastier if they're harvested when the pad has begun to fatten seeds and form strings. The strings can easily be stripped from the pods before cooking.

Saving seed: When harvesting for the table I inevitably miss a few pods but usually spot them a few days later because they're turning pale yellow. I leave them on the vine to mature because they'll provide enough seeds to plant for the table but not enough to use to grow as green manure. Pea seeds will germinate better if the partly dry pods aren't remoistened by rain or irrigation so I harvest them partly dried. I handle them gently because the seeds within are still soft. Spread out half-dry pods indoors. Remove seeds after the pods have become thoroughly crisp.

Peas occasionally cross pollinate. They'll more than occasionally cross in gardens that are not sprayed with insecticides. Crosses aren't made by bees but by small crawling insects. Each generation of seed saved with insufficient isolation introduces an ever higher percentage of undesirable plants. A precious rare variety can be purified by growing out lines, as is done with vulgaris beans. Prevention is a lot easier; separate varieties by 10 metres.

Varieties: *Shelling peas:* The finest tasting shelling peas I've ever eaten come from a tall climbing heirloom called Telephone (aka Alderman). Most seed suppliers offer Tall Telephone. Telephone comes with downsides. It is slow to start yielding and climbs a two metre tall trellis. Telephone is only very slightly tastier than quicker maturing modern varieties that don't require support so I have given up growing it. The biggest culinary difference between pea varieties is seed size. I prefer Onward for its large seeds and hefty yields. But you should make your own choices; do a variety trial.

Snow peas: Yukomo Giant (SH) is a tall climber with exceptionally broad pods that must be picked before any seed development starts. It handles summer's heat and features purple-pink flowers. Southern Harvest is deeply interested in pea varieties. They sell Dr. James Baggett's Oregon Sugar Pod and his newer one, Cascade Giant; both are non-climbing varieties, both are highly disease-resistant. They can produce in hot weather. They are very slow to form string and seed. In cool weather the pods can be allowed to fatten with half-developed seeds and get much sweeter without getting tough and fibrous.

Snap peas make thick fleshy pods that are eaten like French beans. Snap peas can be allowed to form almost fully developed seeds before picking, which makes them sweeter. As seeds fatten strings also form. We prefer snap peas with seeds inside and find stripping out strings to be no bother. The original Sugar Snap resulted from a chance mutation. It was the first variety of its type and still is the best tasting snap pea variety. It makes a tall-growing vine requiring a two metre trellis. The original Sugar Snap is slightly slower to start yielding than the dwarf snap varieties that came after it; dwarves are slightly less tasty than the original but trellising does not fit into industrial agriculture. Recently a new half-tall climber was released, Sugar Snap Cascadia (SH). It tastes 90 percent as good as the original Sugar Snap; it only climbs about 1,500 high; it clings to the trellis more strongly than the original—all plus points—and like all of Dr. Baggett's varieties, it is highly disease resistant. Cascadia has a down side—it was bred to be very very slow to form seeds and strings because the supermarket wants snap pea pods that are flat and seedless. When I trialled it I waited until seeds did develop, then its pods became fibrous and they didn't get any sweeter as they fattened, not the way the original Sugar Snap does.

Soup peas: Southern Harvest provides "Purple Podded;" actually this is an old Dutch variety called Capucijner. The seeds may be cooked when green and fresh or else allowed to dry, to later be rehydrated for soup making.

Dry gardening: As with broad beans. They will not require irrigation. Sow 1 seed per centimetre. Use 45 cm interrow spacing.

Garbanzos and Lentils

(Cicer arietinum and Lens culinaris)

These two legume species grow small frost-tolerant bushes with leaves resembling those on a pea vine. The seeds dry down early in summer, which suits our climate. Best to position them where irrigation may be withheld when harvest approaches

Culture: Prepare the soil for a low-demand crop. Sow around mid-September when the soil has become warm enough to sprout the seed. Place garbanzo seeds 2 cm deep, 5 cm apart, in rows 60 cm apart if you can irrigate them; make the rows 75 cm apart if you can't or don't wish to irrigate. Plant lentils on the same spacing but the smaller seeds should be positioned about 1 cm deep. Thin seedlings after they are well established: garbanzos to 20 cm apart; lentils to 10 cm apart; if you don't irrigate thin garbanzos to 30 cm apart; lentils to 15 cm apart. Keep well-weeded; without irrigation yield will be less if spring is unusually dry

Harvest: Like dry beans, but harvest occurs early in summer. Self-sufficiency-minded Taswegians wishing to depend on legume protein should try growing their own.

Saving seed: When you grow them to eat, you've also saved seed to replant.

Varieties: I find the small black garbanzos from Afghanistan particularly tasty and tender—300 percent better than the familiar big yellow seeds. This is an occasion when I'd buy my initial planting stock from Greenpatch or Eden. Any lentil or garbanzo variety from a food shop will probably sprout and grow. When I was still living in Oregon Carol Deppe gifted me with seeds for a dozen garbanzo varieties. There were black, brown and yellow seeded varieties; large seeds and small ones. Some of them didn't seem very tasty but those varieties probably had other uses such as grinding into flour. One unusual variety made popping seeds that were dry-roasted and became a crunchy nut.

Dry gardening: Much easier than *P. vulgaris* beans. Keep the patch thoroughly hoed; then the soil probably won't become stressfully dry.

Green Manures

Some farm suppliers sell green manure seeds by the kilogram. Some garden centres provide lupin and tic bean seeds as well as green manure mixtures and shelling peas in half kilo packs. The home gardener should choose green manures according to the *difficulty involved in removing the vegetation.* In a fertile garden all green manure crops grow great without COF.

Shaftal (Persian) Clover

(Trifolium resupinatum)

Biennial clovers like Shaftal are easily terminated, which for green manuring purposes makes them far more suitable than perennial clovers, which are the usual thing found in paddocks. Shaftal doesn't grow well on poorly drained, highly acidic or infertile soils. Any soil that grows winter vegetables well should be more than good enough.

Start Shaftal April to early May as ground becomes available. After that the soil gets too cold to germinate the seed. One kilogram of strong seed broadcast over 100 to 150 square metres and then mixed into the surface inch should thickly carpet the bed with seedlings. Persian clover grows slowly over the winter, accelerates in spring, hopefully it gets to be hip high before it starts flowering. If the vegetation is spaded in before it opens any flowers it will decompose within two weeks, leaving a fine seedbed. Let it flower and the stems rapidly become lignified (woody,) harder to dig in and take a lot longer to break down. If the crop has gotten too forward because the heavy ground it is growing in hadn't yet dried out enough to dig, then instead of digging it in and robbing the soil of nitrogen whilst it decomposes all that fibre, better to scythe the clover down with a weedwacker or else yank out the vegetation, which is not hard to do with Persian clover in my soil, and compost it. Then shallowly hoe the bed. Stubble and roots quickly decompose, putting the bed in fine-enough condition for spring sowing. When Persian clover is only knee-high it may be hoed in, tops and all. The succulent young material rots rapidly, making easy sowings of mustard, spinach and peas.

WARNING: Persian clover makes delicate pinkish flowers with separate petals that do not look at all like the flowers paddock clovers. Persian is biennial and therefore, easily eliminated. Beware of *perennial* clovers. These form strong spreading clumps that eagerly re-establish even after a thorough mauling with spade and hoe.

There are several Persian clover varieties that suit different soils. Ask. And if you ever encounter seed for crimson clover (almost certainly in a bag marked "Halsey, Oregon") I suggest that you give it a try. Crimson is also biennial. I got some old weak crimson clover seed from Roberts many years ago so I say this from experience—in Tasmania crimson grows way better than Persian.

Tic Bean

(Vicia faba)

Small-seeded broad beans make excellent green manure. They grow taller than large seeded varieties, produce more organic matter. Dense stands effectively shade out weeds. Tic beans frugally provide many more seeds in each low-priced kg.

Sow tic beans as space becomes vacant during April and the first half of May. Position each seed about 10 cm apart, 2 cm deep, in rows 30 cm apart, which barely allows hoeing between the rows until the plants shade the isles. Or else broadcast about one kg per 10 sq. metres and shallowly hoe them in. That much seed makes a superdense stand that soon suppresses almost all the weeds.

The brittle stalks can be cut off close to the soil, gathered up and composted. The stubble is easily turned under. Before seeds start forming I can spade in a waist-high stand of tic beans. I use my feet to flatten the plants immediately behind where I'm digging. That way, as I dig my way backward, the spade cuts these long stalks into manageable lengths that easily get turned under. Before seed formation begins tic bean plants are so brittle they may be tilled under with a garden-sized rear-end rotary cultivator (without tangling the tines). But once seed formation begins the stalks wrap around the tines instead of breaking, creating tangles that stop the machine from digging.

Blue Lupin

(Lupinus angustifolius)

Resembles a short tic bean plant with much prettier flowers. In April/ May, sow one seed every 5 cm, 2 cm deep, in rows 30 cm apart—far enough apart that you can hoe between the rows until the plants grow tall enough to form a canopy. Or else, broadcast about 500 gm of seed per 10 square metres and chop it in with a hoe. The plants may reach 600 mm tall. Dig in the vegetation in before flowers do any more than start to form or else pull out the plants soon after they start blooming and make compost with them. Lupin rots rapidly if turned under before seeds start forming.

Corn Salad, Mache

(Valerianella locusta olitoria)

This vegetable may be used as a green manure/cover crop that also supplies winter salads. The plants overwinter and bloom in September. When in bloom the vegetation still remains so tender that it may be easily chopped into the bed with a hoe. Then it rots rapidly and forms a fine seedbed.

In early April clear vegetation left from a summer crop and then *shallowly* hoe the surface until the soil is loose to the depth of about 1 cm. Then *uniformly* broadcast and *shallowly* hoe in 30 gm to 50 gm of the fluffy light seed per 10 square metres of bed. Thin the bed for salad greens all winter. You may have to produce your own seed to afford using this much. Seed saving info is given in the next major section, "Greens."

Rocket

(Eruca sativa)

Rocket is fully discussed in the next section, "Greens. " Rocket can be used as a quick green manure crop during spring or summer. Broadcast and rake in or shallowly hoe in 25- to 50 grams of seed per 10 square metres. If sown in autumn it grows for several months before flowering. Sown spring or summer it quickly puts up seed stalks. If spaded in when seedstalks first appear the still tender plants will decompose quickly. If they grow another few weeks the now-woody plant are easy to pull out. April/May sowings overwinter; in spring they will be waist high and forming seeds—and be way too woody to be dug in. Instead, pull them out, which is easy to do, and use the vegetation for making compost. Or else allow one square metre to ripen around 500 gm of seed.

Grains

(Grammineae spp.)

Grass grains like wheat or oats may be used as green manures. Sow April to early May. Scatter from 250 to 500 grams of seed over 10 square metres. Till-, rake- or hoe in the seed 25 mm deep. Let it grow. In spring, turn it under. Seems simple, eh! It might prove not to be so simple.

The first potential glitch comes from sowing too much seed; overcompetition makes the plants grow too tall. Then if there's strong wind or heavy rain it all falls over and makes a tangle that isn't easy to mow or remove. When this catastrophe happens to farm crops it is termed "lodging."

Any winter-hardy cereal works—wheat, barley, oats, corn rye—but before you try this, understand that leaves and stalks become decomposition resistant when seed formation initiates. On clayey soil a rainy spring can delay turning under cereals. Before seed formation starts the leaves contain a lot of protein so they break down rapidly when turned into the soil. But as seed making progresses the seedstalk (and leaves) become increasingly woody, "lignified" is the proper term. Tender young cereal leaves decompose after two weeks. But once seed stalks start reaching upward if you turn the plants under they will rot so slowly that another crop can't be started for a month or more, resulting in a very late garden—or a very poor result if the gardener ignores all that decomposing straw and sows anyway.

Farmers say winter wheat yields to the disc most easily of all the grass grains. Tasmanian-grown wheat seeds suitable for green manuring can be purchased at farm suppliers who sell it as livestock and chook feed. However, there's a downside with wheat. Newer varieties are very very short and don't make much biomass. I would not use wheat unless I got the seed from a farmer who raised a taller variety. I also would not sow wheat berries from the bulk bin of a health food shop because most likely you'll get a mainland variety which responds to that daylength pattern, not Tasmania's. Oats create much more biomass than wheat.

If you have use for very long, unusually strong straw that is especially good for insulating compost heaps or for summertime mulching, then grow cereal rye, often called corn rye. Cereal rye makes the most biomass of all the grass grains and is my choice to prepare ground for large sized hot weather loving plants like zucchini, pumpkins, cucumbers, tomato, pepper and eggplant. By "rye" I do not mean ryegrass as found in pastures. Use seeds from a whole foods/health food shop for grinding rye flour to make bread.

Cereal rye grows tall. The seedheads top out at two metres. *Please,* never ever never never consider turning cereal rye under unless you have sandy soil (that for absolutely sure allows early tillage) *and* have a strong tractor powering a heavy duty rotary cultivator to chop it up and put it under *and* are absolutely certain you can do this job before there is any sign of seed heads forming at the base of the plant. At this stage the leaves may be waist high and it'll be early spring.

I never consider digging rye under. There's a better way for gardeners. I let it grow on awhile because I plan to use that ground for sowing summer crops. I scythe down the rye with a weedwacker a few days after fully formed seed heads have released pollen and have set seeds. At Grindelwald this occurred between the last days of September and mid-October. The exact date will be strongly influenced by microclimate—in warmer districts like Grindelwald rye goes to seed sooner, which is helpful because mild locations allow an earlier start to hot weather crops. If I were to mow the rye before its seed heads have pollinated the plants will resprout and try to make new seed stalks. After pollination the plants die when they are cut off at the base. I have to warn you: If bad weather or other commitments were to cause me to delay mowing for more than a few days after pollination then the seeds might ripen as the straw dries out. And that would make a terrible mess of rye-weeds when I used the straw for mulching. After mowing I let the straw dry in the sun for a few days and then gather it up.

Decomposing rye roots put my ground in fine condition to plant the summer garden: tomatoes, peppers, eggplant, cucumber, pumpkin and zucchini. Cereal rye saves me a lot of work because digging the entire bed before planting is not required when starting these vegetables. Rye roots are so dense and so quick to rot that the soil loosens by itself. Tilling or digging the whole area would make sure all the stubble died-for-sure. However, rather than dig the whole area in a big rush during the period when I have many garden hours to put in and because I'm going to use this area for growing what will become very large plants, I only dig hills at planting positions.

A month later there'll be much less garden work. That's when I shallowly dig/hoe between the hills to kill the odd bit of rye stubble that tries to regrow as well as blend in COF.

Rye, being so tall, should make you especially wary of overseeding. Broadcasting 250 grams of seed per 10 square metres is plenty. A too-crowded stand competes for light by stretching, and falls over.

The Grass Ley

I strongly recommend periodically rejuvenating a vegie garden by resting it in unirrigated paddock grasses and legumes for periods of three to five years. Or even longer. The best result comes from using a wisely chosen mixture of grasses, legumes and herbs. The two best books I know of on this subject happen to be a lot older than the regenerative agriculture everyone in the know is talking about these days, but these two old books tell much the same story as the current buzz. They are Newman Turner's *Fertility Pastures and Cover Crops* (published around 1950, currently in print by Acres, USA) and Robert Elliot's classic *Clifton Park System of Farming** (around 1900). Both books recommend complex seed mixes and explain their benefits.

Tasmanians trying to purchase seeds for many of the species recommended by Elliot and Turner would almost certainly fail to find them. Trying to import some of them would raise your understanding of Biosecurity. Instead I recommend using this inexpensive mixture: a nurse crop of 250 grams perennial rye grass seed (any variety the nearest farm supply shop supplies), 1 kg cocksfoot, also called orchard grass, (a coarse, deeply rooting grass that is slower to establish than perennial rye), 100 gm red clover. Blend seeds together uniformly; sows 200 square metres.

Sow mid-April, certainly sow before mid-May; you also could sow very early in September. An autumn start eliminates the risk of the grass dying out during an unusually hot dry summer in its first year. First clear the area of vegetation and loosen the surface two centimetres, then broadcast the seeds and very shallowly mix them in with a hoe. If it's early autumn and rain doesn't happen, be prepared to water a few times until the seeds sprout.

Next summer, mow the area soon after the grasses start putting up seed stalks. Mow before grass seeds develop, which is something you don't want because forming seeds uses up the plants energy. You want the plants to be growing vegetatively, building more biomass. Mow high, about 100 mm above the soil line so that the grass regrows more rapidly. I mow with a weedwacker because grass that is making seeds grows tall and strong in what was vegetable ground and because cockskfoot is very coarse stuff. Allow what's cut to remain where it falls. If it rains much in November/December I may have to mow three times before the grass gives up on making seeds.

Leave the plot in grass for at least three years. Remove nothing. Because this minipaddock started out as fertile vegetable ground it'll develop an enormous quantity of biomass. After a few years of this when the sod is terminated the area will produce vegetables far better than before. Most likely you'll enjoy three to five trouble-free years of growing vegetables and will not need compost for the first two years. COF will be enough.

I sent a soil sample from a grassy reserve for lab analysis. The report said this land had built itself up to 8.5 percent organic matter. My going garden beds get compost once/year; they have 7 percent SOM.

The latest holistic farming approach is called regenerative agriculture. I urge you to do an internet search for it and spend some time reading or watching videos. There's been a lot of people jumping on the regen-ag bandwagon in recent years. The basic idea is that by growing complex mixtures involving at least five quite different species, the plants will make much more biomass and build far more soil organic matter than by just growing only two species such as grass and clover. Local farmers and Tasmanian forage seed producers are getting interested in regenerative agriculture. Our farm supply stores may start carrying seed mixtures for this.

Greens

The faster that leafy green vegetables grow the better they can taste. However, if greens are pushed hard by nitrogen fertilizer without providing the other essential plant nutrients in balance, especially the trace elements, they still grow big and fast but will be relatively tasteless, will appeal to insects and be subject to diseases. They will taste like what is found at the supermarket. Balanced, strong and complete nutrient support gives far better results. In soils that haven't yet come into balance it is smart to foliar feed greens with something that abundantly provides trace elements.

Modern varieties have been bred to grow tops faster at the expense of root development. But coping with moisture stress makes most leafy vegetables lose sweetness, they often become bitter. That's why it is essential to provide greens with plenty of soil moisture during summer. As an eager young seedsman I trialled every type of vegetable in every season it was barely possible to produce it. But now that I am just gardening for our own table I avoid making unnecessary difficulties. So I do not try to harvest a great diversity of salad greens during January and February. Instead, we eat more fruit in summer, and by fruit I mean the botanical definition of fruit that includes tomato, cucumber, zucchini and French bean.

Greens that suffer strong competition grow less quickly, which lowers eating quality. The longer that lettuce grows on past it's prime the more bitter it becomes. For both reasons I do not use cut and come again greens mixtures. I much prefer lettuce hearts taken at the peak of perfection. I like mild (very young) rocket and mizuna. So I start a patch of salad greens about once a month from early September through February. Most of it will be lettuce. That way there's always young plants to eat; overblown heads get fed to chickens. Early in March and again late in March I sow big lettuce patches. These supply raw salads through autumn and winter. I continue to sow lettuce in April and early May to overwinter for harvest next spring. If we don't use it all in salads these last lettuce sowings are considered green manure or else produce seeds next summer. In March I start minor greens that make our wintertime salads more interesting—such as rocket and mild mustards—and plant even more in April and May.

Gardeners waste money purchasing lettuce seedlings. Yes, true, lettuce is transplantable. But it is far less costly to direct seed it. And, there are interesting and extra tasty varieties available only as seed. And, sometimes starting from seed works a lot better. That makes three reasons to grow your own lettuce seed.

Celery *(Apium dulce)*
Celeriac *(A. rapaceum)*

Celery is frost-hardy; the seed germinates well in cool soil. Celery grows fairly fast (for celery) in September if it is transplanted or directly seeded. But chilly nights will trigger these seedlings into flowering prematurely. They'll continue growing for awhile after being triggered but about the point they've sized up enough to provide a few stalks these plants go into bloom—ending the harvest before it really began. What gets you celery to eat is to start it when you set out tomato seedlings. This way celery will act like the biennial it is, will grow on through summer, autumn and winter, and not go to seed until next spring.

Celery seeds are miniscule and slow-to-shoot; the thought of making these minute specks come up daunts most gardeners but it isn't too difficult to keep the seeds moist if sowing is done when tomato seedlings are safe to put outside. After the tiny seedlings emerge there will be mysterious disappearances, especially if the garden contains many slugs or other gnawers of the sort that breed up to large numbers under permanent mulch. That's why I sow a cluster of 20 or more seeds on each position and thin gradually.

Celery prefers mild temperatures and deep sand soil. Tasmanian gardens with deep sandy soil can grow celery to near-supermarket standards.

Culture: Celery makes a tap root, like carrot. Raising seedlings in punnets can take 10 to 12 weeks of patient nursing and after all that you end up with plants lacking taproots. *Direct seeded celery grows better and starting the crop that way uses far less of your precious time.*

Prepare the bed for a low-demand vegetable. Mix twice the usual quantity of compost into the surface inch; make it especially moisture-retentive. Tease all clods and lumps out of the sowing positions; you must have a finely textured seedbed. Sow or transplant on positions about 60 cm x 60 cm. Make a fist and gently press it into the seedbed, not deeply. Sprinkle a pinch of the minute seeds into a few knuckle dents in this shallow depression and cover them 4 mm to 5 mm deep.

Sow celery seeds soon after frost danger ends because it is extremely difficult to make miniscule celery seeds sprout in hot weather. Being so tiny they must be placed close to the surface where the soil dries out quickly. Celery seeds take 10-14 days to emerge; before shooting they require frequent watering, usually once every morning; sometimes again mid- to late afternoon if the sun has been intense, especially so if the breeze has been strong. Progressively thin each position to a single seedling by the time the plants are 10 cm tall. Be reluctant to thin celery. Anticipate that some seedlings will disappear for assorted unknown reasons.

Generously water celery during summer's heat. I locate the celery patch near the water tap. Every time I use the hose I give the celery some.

The plants must grow steadily or else the stalks become pithy and stringy. So I side dress celery for the first time when the seedlings are only 1 cm tall. I uniformly spread one tablespoonful of COF over a circle 75 mm in diameter with seedlings in the centre of it, avoiding getting it on leaves or if that happens, promptly spraying it off of them. When that circle has been covered by celery leaves I cover a ring around the plant's dripline with COF that is 75 mm across. I make the last side dressing about March 1st.

Celeriac is grown almost like celery. Sow at the same time on the same spacing. The difference is, if you crowd celery and/or don't fertilize it enough or fail to give it enough water you get smaller plants yielding shorter, somewhat fibrous stalks but the stalks will still be useful. If you crowd celeriac or don't give it enough water or nutrients you'll get nothing useful. Celeriac bulbs *have to exceed 125 mm in diameter* or else you end up peeling away most of the root and end up with almost nothing edible.

Garden planning: Two or three well-grown celery plants will provide more than enough to enliven the family's salads, juices and soups. Harvest starts sometime in January and continues until seed making starts which will be mid- to late September. If you intend to make seeds then celery occupies the bed from October through February of the year after next. Celery should have no problem surviving Tasmanian winter except perhaps in harshest interior positions.

When an enthusiastic younger Steve grew celeriac we ate about six over the winter and relished every bite of slow-butter-fried-browned celeriac chips.

Insects and diseases: The worst problems come about from attempting celery in unsuitable soils. Clays do not produce good results except perhaps with primitive varieties that resemble parsley. It is prudent to protect small celery seedlings with snail bait. Once the seedlings are 50 mm tall the usual population of slugs and snails (in an unmulched, tidy garden) no longer pose a threat. If mulch seems essential for celery then please apply it when summer arrives and remove it in April.

Harvest: Directly-seeded celery yields the first few snips in January. Or you can transplant seedlings and maybe harvest sooner. With ordinary celery we only eat half of the large stalks, leaving the rest to feed the plant. I suggest cutting off all the large stalks after the plant has formed secondary leaf clusters around the base. At the same time remove all but 2 or 3 of these secondaries. These will develop during winter—being smaller and younger and given more air circulation they'll resist humidity-induced diseases better. Celery can be harvested throughout winter. The unopened flowers and stalks below them (the tough stringy skin peeled off first) are good in salads.

Use celeriac like a swede after pealing off the thick rough skin. If you peal them before they exceed 125 mm in diameter you won't end up with much to eat.

Saving seed: Celery is biennial. Cold nights in the seedling stage makes it flower prematurely, a trait that plant breeders select against. Any plant that flowers before overwintering should be culled. Seed saved from a plant like that will have an even greater tendency to make seed the first year.

Celery is bee pollinated. It freely crosses with other celery varieties and with celeriac. Isolate similar celery varieties by at least 100 metres; isolate celery from celeriac by at least 1 km. Celery seed lives seven to ten years with decent storage. Celery flowers resemble those of its relatives, carrot and parsley but are much smaller. The nearly-dry seed is easily lost so take care when harvesting. Gently cut off branches when many of the flowers on that branch have formed light brown seeds. Spread the seed-laden branches on newspapers or a tarp under cover to finish ripening and drying.

Varieties: Celery is such a demanding crop that using cheap or amateur-grown seed that throws a large percentage of non-productive plants makes no sense to me. Tall Utah is a productive and good tasting. So too are any of the hybrid varieties.

Celeriac forms a rough-skinned, bulbous bottom that can be steamed, fried as chips, grated raw into salads or used in soups. Celeriac has little starch; it doesn't absorb fat. Quality celeriac varieties keep trimming waste low because they make fewer big side roots and are smoother. Never buy seeds of a variety named "celeriac" or "Prague," another name commonly used for cheap seed, much as "Vienna" always tells you that you're being offered bargain-basement kohlrabi.

Chinese, or leaf celery resembles parsley. It is much easier to grow than the fancy stuff. Although these wilder relatives don't make large stalks, they do provide fresh celery flavour in cooked dishes, soups and juices, and being nearly wild, are probably more nutrient-dense. ParCel is a superior variety of this sort.

Dry gardening: No way! Well, maybe using mulched ParCel with fertigation.

Coriander

(Coriandrum sativum)

Coriander leaf is used as an aromatic seasoning. It also forms whitish mini-carrot-like roots that are used in Thai cooking. It is a low-demand crop. Place seeds 1 cm apart in a furrow 12 mm deep. Thin the row to 3 cm apart. Harvest promptly because it bolts to seed quickly.

When experiencing long days (and moreso lengthening long days before the solstice) coriander goes to seed soon after it is barely tall enough to use. If not sooner. When experiencing shortening summer days it grows an additional week before going to seed. As the nights get longer coriander also grows longer before going to seed. The April sowing may last until winter before starting to flower. I suggest sowing a short row about once a month from September through April, maybe even early May. Half formed flower stalks may be chopped finely.

If you want to produce seeds for planting or for culinary use simply allow either an April sowing to overwinter or sow early in spring and let it grow on after it blooms. After most of the seeds are close to being ripe and about 10 percent of them have detached by themselves pull the plants, root and all. Spread the plants out on a tarp under cover. Provide plenty of air circulation while the seeds finish. Then strip seeds from the branches.

There are named varieties that are *supposed* to stand a few days longer before going to seed. I would buy planting seed at the health food shop.

Corn Salad / Mache

(Valerianella locusta olitoria)

In England, wheat, barley, rye and oats are collectively termed "corn." Corn salad was a low-growing biennial weed that came up in the stubble of harvested grain fields. In recent centuries the weed has been selected for increased leaf-size and better flavour but it still is pretty wild stuff. Allow a few plants to make seed each spring and it may naturalize into an edible weed that comes up by itself at summer's end.

Culture: There is no need to especially fertilize garden soil ahead of this crop. Naturalized or intentionally sown, the low-germination seeds rarely sprout until soil temperature has dropped well below the summer peak. I sow late March to early April. Space the seeds two per cm in a furrow about one cm deep, rows 30 cm apart. Thin any seedling clusters. (See the section on Green Manures for another approach.)

Garden planning: Corn salad may follow any crop that finishes before mid April. One row across a 1,200 wide raised bed yields a gracious plenty for me because I only use small quantities of the tender, mild-flavoured leaves. Corn salad leaves plus paper thin slices of mild onion or leek, shaved parmesan cheese and heavily slathered with olive oil is outright delicious. Corn salad goes to seed late August/early September; then the leaves become too bitter to eat.

Insects and diseases: None known.

Harvest: Take entire plants and thin the row as you do. Lift the base leaves with your fingertips so that you can cut the stem at ground level with a sharp knife. Lower leaves often conceal slugs so wash thoroughly.

Saving seed: The lightweight, irregularly shaped seeds fatten quickly, detach when they turn light brown and travel many metres in strong breezes. Slide a sheet of cardboard under the plant to catch falling seeds. Collect the seeds daily, dry them indoors. Corn salad seed lives two years.

Varieties: Many varieties are available in European seed catalogues but the differences are mostly in size of leaves—ranging from small to not quite so small. In Australia we're lucky to find even one variety.

Endive & other chicories

(Cichorium endivia)

To stay healthy in winter I've trained my body to enjoy large greens salads almost every day. Anything that breaks the winter's monotony of lettuce, then cabbage, then back to lettuce, repeat, strongly interests me. When I was in the garden seed business I carefully recorded overnight low temperatures and observed which varieties and species better handled frost and frequent rain. That's how I know the freeze-out temperature from a single frost for most lettuce varieties is about minus 6°C; a few varieties survive minus 8°C. *Protected* by a very drafty cold frame, I witnessed endive handily survive minus 14°C. measured inside the frame. In winter after some frost endive and escarole make delicious salad.

Culture: Endive/escarole seeds will germinate in cool soil but sowings made before mid-October go to seed prematurely. When harvested in hot weather it is far too bitter for me to enjoy. Best to sow from mid-January until mid-February. Sowings made later than that (except in polytunnels or cloches) may not get large enough. All chicories are low demand subsoil feeders. Sow seeds one cm deep, one cm between seeds in rows 45 cm to 60 cm apart. Don't make the isles narrower; good air circulation fends off leaf rot in chilly, humid conditions. Thin the rows progressively: to 30 cm to 40 cm apart in the row. Endive tolerates crowding in cloches because there is less humidity.

Garden planning: Unprotected plants may remain in decent condition throughout an entire sunny dryish winter with lots of hard frost. During rainy overcast mild winters the beautiful rosette may rot back to a stump. Plants from mid-February sowings will be smaller over winter, they'll have less trouble with leaf disease. I have eaten one dozen large heads of frisée from May through August.

Insects and diseases: Leaf rot can be vanquished but victory may take years to achieve because chicories are subsoil feeders. As my subsoil gradually loosened from applications of aglime and gypsum, as it remineralized with trace elements, diseases issues lessened, then ended. After I learned I should remineralize molybdenum the endive got sweeter.

Harvest: Winter's cold reduces bitterness. Even if there are rot spots on the larger leaves the smaller core leaves are often quite okay. There *will* be gastropods residing within. Soak the heads in water for ten minutes and slugs will soon be lying dead on the bottom; snails will be crawling up the sides of the sink. Our chooks cluck and flap wings for the trim and snails.

Saving seed: Chicories are self-pollinated biennials. Seed may be saved from only one plant. I've grown strong seed without any irrigation. The gnarled seed stalks appear after overwintering, soon reach one metre high, are covered with small blue flowers that become hard little knobs holding seeds. When (almost) no more flower petals are present, harvest the plant, roots and all, and finish drying it under cover. Then put it out in the sun on a few warm, low-humidity afternoons and *dry until it is brittle.* Some varieties readily release their seed after dancing on their brittle stalks. With some varieties I've had to pulverize the stalks with a flat-bottomed 6 to 8 cm diameter wooden staff (or a similar pounder) until the seeds separated. Then sieve to remove the big stuff. Then winnow away the dust and chaff by pouring it from bucket to bucket in a mild breeze. Endive seed is dense and easy to winnow. One healthy plant can produce up to 50 grams of long-lived seeds.

Varieties: Two general types are better known. One sort is called endive. It forms deeply-cut frilly leaves resembling Salad Bowl lettuce; extra finely cut varieties of this type are called frisée. Rhodos (SH) is an excellent variety of this type. Escarole, sometimes called Batavian, has broad plain leaves. Large heads of either sort form semi-blanched hearts. The hearts make tasty slightly bitter salads. Pain de Sucre (SH) is this sort; the inner hearts of this variety are slightly sweet. If you have problems with winter survival, check out Adaptive Seeds in Oregon. They offer extraordinarily frost hardy humidity resistant varieties.

Lesser known types of chicory are getting much interest from foodies these days and for that reason uniform productive varieties are appearing for these sorts. Radicchio makes an intense red, ball-shaped head resembling a small cabbage. Slower growing than endive, it is best sown during January. Thin progressively and thoroughly. If a basal leaf or two remains attached to the stump after harvest there will be leafy (non-heading) winter regrowth. The regrowth will be less bitter. Headed up radicchio rots outdoors in winter but it does okay in cloches.

Sugar Loaf (aka Sugar Hat or Zuccerhut) forms an impressive green conical head somewhat like Chinese cabbage. After the head is cut (May/June) there'll be loose, leafy regrowth. I find uncooked Sugar Hat to be too bitter for raw salad and hard to chew.

Grumolo is absolutely too bitter for me to eat during autumn. When I grew grumolo in Oregon the tops died back in winter. Very early in spring the regrowth formed rapidly and was much milder. At that time of year in Oregon anything useful in salads was a treasure. Tassie winter is much less severe.

Catalognia forms dandilion-like flower stalks that are picked before blossoms open. Cooked or raw it seems impossibly bitter to me but then, so does the tropical bitter melon. SH says it's good when lightly steamed.

Dry gardening: Sow early in November; put seeds 1 cm deep on positions 60 cm x 90 cm and spot water until they germinate. Once they're up, no more irrigation will be needed if the soil is deep and moisture retentive. Thin each position progressively to one plant. The leaves will be coarse, tough and bitter during summer. In early April carefully cut off the tops (feed this to delighted chooks), leaving a few bottom leaves still attached to the stem. If you don't destroy the growing point you'll harvest tasty regrowth in winter.

Lettuce

(Lactuca sativa)

Lettuce grows best and tastes best when the weather is on the mild side, something we Tasmanians enjoy much of the year. At lower elevations lettuce can be harvested twelve months a year. Interior districts can still produce a year-round supply but may require a wintertime cloche. And maybe not. The keys to producing beautiful heads are: *early and careful thinning,* fertile balanced soil, ample growing room and no moisture stress. Most types get tip burn (thin blackened edges on interior leaves) when given too much nitrogen and not enough calcium. Balanced fertilization, such as with COF, prevents this.

Lettuce stores water in a fleshy taproot that goes deep when soil conditions allow. It can pass through periods of moisture stress without seeming to suffer—but lettuce that is enduring does not taste good. Nor does it grow fast.

Culture: Sow loose-leaf varieties from September through April. Iceberg types head up poorly when the plant is stressed. Iceberg types don't form good heads during winter. Sow them October through mid-February.

Lettuce is a low demand crop. But nitrogen is released too slowly in the cold soils of early spring when it only comes from organic matter decomposition. Best to kick start lettuce with COF. In soil that has not yet come into balance it's probably helpful to side-dress COF close to the seedlings one week after germination. Sprinkle the seeds 1 per centimeter 1 cm deep in furrows 45 cm apart. *Thin progressively.* Encourage the formation of beautiful heads by eliminating competition. Eat the thinnings after they get large enough.

Garden planning: I eat a large (belly-filling) fresh leafy green salad almost every day. To achieve that for two like-minded adults I start a two square metre patch of mixed lettuce varieties every four weeks from early spring through summer. Starting in March I sow even larger patches every two weeks, continuing until late April. The last sowings grow slowly over the winter; these require meticulous weeding and thinning. That's good because smaller overwintering plants are less likely to be frost damaged. When daffodils appear I side dress the overwintered patch, provoking rapid growth. This lot provides for us until the first spring sown crop is feeding us.

Most crops do well following lettuce because its dense rapidly decomposing root system makes crumbly soil and also because lettuce root exudates do not seem hostile to any vegetable species, including itself. I have sown rows of lettuce seeds between half-grown rows of lettuce; making one patch produce a continuous harvest from early summer through winter. In this case I increase the between-row space to 60 cm. When the plants in the first sowing are 7 cm to 10 cm in diameter, new rows are sown between the old. As big heads are cut the younger rows are gradually thinned. As soon as the first sowing has been finished I hoe out the stumps while working in a bit of COF and then sow another lettuce crop, and so forth all summer.

Lettuce may be frozen out in the coldest districts but maybe not. Polytunnels and cold frames make surviving winter far more certain; they also make the first spring-sown lettuce harvest happen one month sooner and increase the size and tenderness of the heads during winter. Winter is much colder where I've been gardening the last few years. I'm pleased that Chudleigh has allowed us to eat unprotected winter lettuce.

Insects and diseases: I've rarely had problems except for slugs (and sometimes a few aphids) to wash out. If you have worse problems take another look at soil conditions. In the extremely humid summer of 2014-15 a small red long-legged never-before-seen insect multiplied ferociously; it invaded some of my lettuce plants (they seem to have had varietal preferences) but did no actual damage. We rinsed them out. I did nothing about it; the problem went away a few weeks later. However, something like this would make a market gardener's crop unsellable.

Harvest: I make salads with half grown plants when I thin them out but we prefer eating the tender inner hearts of full-sized looseleaf varieties. Most varieties become bitter soon after hearting-up so I start a new patch every month in which I sow several varieties needing different growing times. That way I always harvest top quality lettuce. Many garden books recommend another method that only *seems* simpler— harvest by snipping individual leaves from what is hoped will be an almost permanent salad patch. These books don't tell you that lettuce inevitably becomes bitter about two months after it starts growing. Rocket and some of the other species usually blended in cut-and-come-again salad mixes also get bitter when older.

Saving seed: Lettuce flowers are self-fertile and rarely cross-pollinate. No isolation is needed. I always grow my own mixture that includes I don't remember how many varieties— at least seven. I sow this mix from spring through April. Everything in it does okay in summer and everything in it is winter hardy because I only make seed from overwintered plants. About one plant in 100 looks unusual; it will be a cross that I wouldn't make seed from.

Early lettuce sowings will try to make seed in their first year. But seed making shouldn't be attempted that way because spring sown lettuce rarely ripens its seed in Tassie. Seed ripening stops mid February when nights lengthen. If the plants have unfinished seed at that time the seed never matures. Here's another reason to not spring sow a lettuce seed crop—going to seed quickly is not a desirable trait in lettuce. A spring-sown variety that goes quickly to seed provides a shorter harvest period. But only varieties that soon go to seed soon after getting large have a chance to ripen their seed from a spring sowing. Do not select *for* this trait. Tasmanians should grow lettuce seed by starting the seed patch in April and overwintering small plants.

Direct seeded lettuce makes a strong taproot so plants can survive considerable moisture stress whilst forming seed if the patch is kept weeded and is not crowded. However, without irrigation you'll harvest less seed and it may be less vigorous seed.

Lettuce seeds disperse when they get ripe. The sprays of flowers mature irregularly. When almost all of the flowers are maturing their seeds and a about ten percent of the seed has already shattered or is about to, then cut this plant close to the base and place it on a tarp under cover. Make sure there

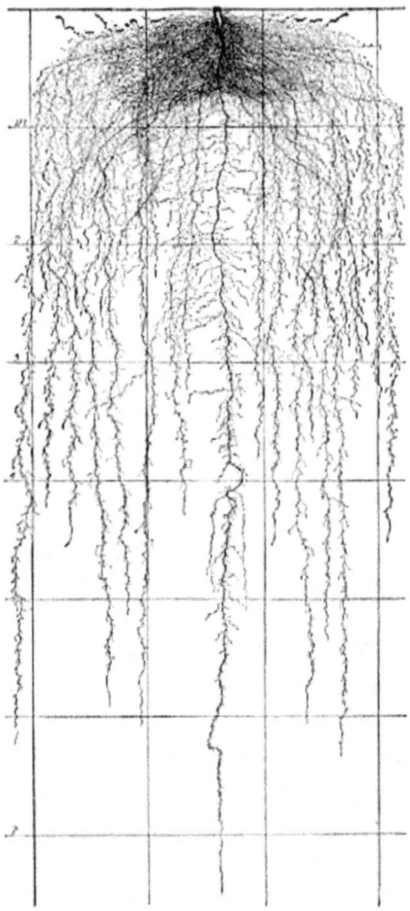

Lettuce root system at maturity. Note that if it could, this plant would use all the moisture in a circle one metre in diameter.

is plenty of air circulation; spread the stalks out. They finish ripening seeds as they dry.

Then thresh the seed. First, get the straw completely dry by dragging the tarp out in the sun from late morning until mid-afternoon. Do this late in February on warm sunny afternoons with light wind. It may take several days of drying before the stalks are crisp. Then rub the flower heads between your gloved palms or dance on them with much foot scuffing. Separate the seed from the resulting powdered dry leaves and other trash by first putting it all through a sieve to eliminate the big stuff and then pour the fine stuff (in a slow trickle) between two buckets in a *mild* breeze. *Beware:* if the wind is even moderate you'll lose many seeds. Sometimes I've had to hold the mix of seed and dry chaff in a large woven poly bag or bucket until the wind strength was just right. An electric pedestal fan in the shed might work better. If too much of the seed blows away in a gentle breeze, that suggests the soil that grew those seeds needs remineralization. As my subsoil got into better balance the lettuce seed it produced got much denser and germinated better. To better appreciate this please look again at the illustration on the previous page.

Varieties: Iceberg types demand near-perfect conditions to head properly. Southern Harvest offers Rein des Glace which provides much more flavour than the usual. Loose-leaf varieties are far more forgiving. Most loose-leafs can be sown from spring through autumn although thin leaved butterheads rarely make excellent heads during summer's heat. Mainland seed companies have no interest in discovering lettuce varieties that are winter-hardy in Tassie. Southern Harvest Seeds and Birdland offer many choices. My favourites are Winter Density, Little Gem, Buttercrunch and Red Cross. Marvel of 4 Seasons, aka Merveille des Quatre Saisons, aka Wonder of the Year Round, is a genuine heirloom and a possibly the most delicious butterhead of all. Sam Bayley especially favours Flashy Trout Back, a cos, and Maricella for its dark red leaves.

Dry gardening: A patch sown early in September with each plant given extra root zone may finish on soil moisture in a wet spring. I'd reserve as much water as I could through summer in order to start another patch (and other leafy greens too) in March for autumn and winter harvest.

Mustard

(Brassica alba, B. nigra, B. chinensis, B. juncea, B. rapa)

All types of mustard greens are easy to grow when they are started mid-February through March. All mustard species are extremely frost hardy; they can be harvested all winter. There is at least one type of pac choi that grows in all seasons. No insect in Tasmania much bothers this vegetable. Couldn't be easier!

Mustards comes in widely-differing leaf shapes, sizes, degrees of pungency, and colours. Cooked mustards are delicious. Young leaves of the milder sorts are a useful salad component.

Culture: Mustard greens are not so easy to grow in spring. Many gardeners, especially organic gardeners who mainly fertilize with compost, are disappointed when spring sown mustard goes to seed at a small size. More success in spring can be had by understanding the species and then helping it. Mustards entirely stop growing new leaves and only put up seed stalks when days are lengthening and have reached a critical duration. The initiation of seed making has little to do with how long the plant may have grown although it must have made at least a few pairs of leaves before it can bloom.

All mustard varieties I am familiar with are triggered into bloom by photoperiod except for one type of Pac Choi. Plants that started growing at summer's end will survive the winter and then go into bloom in spring. In order to get much to eat from a spring sowing it must germinate early in September—better, around mid-August. And then proceed to grow very fast. A spring sowing did well to reach useful size before going to seed.

Your success with spring sown mustards and with other spring crops as well may be improved by this brief science lesson. Every material has a measurable property called *specific heat.* Water has a higher specific heat than soil does. Water in fact has a higher specific heat than a chunk of iron has. "Specific heat" means the amount of temperature increase that occurs in a substance from adding to it a measured amount of heat energy. It takes more heat energy to raise the temperature of water than it takes to raise the temperature of the same weight of iron or of soil. Quite a bit more energy. In fact, water adsorbs more heat energy than any common substance. That's why solar home designers store heat in water tanks.

The high specific heat of water has big effects on gardening. Sandy soil has about one-third the water-holding capacity of clay. Thus, wet sand has a much lower specific heat than a wet clay does. Consequently, sandy soils warm-up sooner in spring. Wet clay soil must absorb much more solar energy to heat up to the same temperature as sand. Consequently clay soil will be several degrees colder than a sandy loam in September and October. Eventually the differences even out.

Soil temperature strongly influences the speed of plant growth. Mustard seeds will germinate in the chilly soils of early spring but if the plants are to achieve useful size before seed making starts they must find an abundance of nitrogen so they can grow very fast. The natural release of nitrogen from decomposing organic matter is insufficient to spur fast growth when soil temperatures are low. Only *strong* organic fertilizers release enough nitrogen in cold soil to spur mustard forward.

Raised beds help spring mustard grow slightly faster because the surface of a raised bed dries out (and warms up) sooner than flat ground does. Raking in organic matter instead of digging it in adds more air in the top 50 millimetres, and that also lowers specific heat, which raises soil temperature.

When I gardened at Lorane, Oregon on silty clay subsoil (all topsoil had been eroded away by extractive farming before I bought the property) I prepared the spring mustard seedbed the previous autumn. I shallowly chopped in a thicker-than-usual layer of compost and planted tic beans or crimson clover. The soil would be light and loose early next spring when I'd pull out the green crop, broadcast complete organic fertilizer and hoe the surface. Then I'd rake out a rough seedbed and plant mustard seeds in furrows about 1 cm deep, one seed per cm, the furrows about 45 cm apart.

To accelerate seedling growth in cold soil side-dress mustard seedlings with bloodandbone. Use very little! Place this powerful fertilizer close to the seedlings. Thin progressively. By the time the plants have grown to about 15 cm high they should stand 15 cm apart.

Mustards for autumn and winter harvest are so much easier! Consider them a low-demand crop. Sow mid-February through mid-March. Make the between-row space 60 cm because the plants will grow all winter. Gradually thin the rows to 30 cm apart.

Garden planning: A few rows across a raised bed provide a few serves during the short spring harvest period. On very heavy slow-to-warm-up soils it may be essential to sow spring mustard under a cloche.

Mustard grows steadily through winter; two rows 1,200 mm long provides more than we need.

Summer pac choi has a relatively brief harvest period because when it gets too large it loses quality and eventually (or quickly with some varieties) goes to seed. I treat this type like lettuce, intending to harvest each sowing for about three weeks. I start a few rows across the bed every month from October through February.

Insects and diseases: Some spring-sown seedlings will inevitably disappear soon after emerging. The best solution is sowing more seed and progressive thinning. In colder districts cloches and frames help spring crops outgrow nibbling. I also use snail/slug bait.

Harvest: Regarding spring crops and summer pac choi: Progressive thinning allows you to eat entire (small) plants until the in-the-row spacing is 30 cm. From that point if the spring crop is going exceptionally well (and showing no signs of bolting yet), pick off larger outer leaves as needed. Or continue to take whole plants. Garden food is scarce in spring; as yet unopened mustard flowers substitute for broccoli.

In autumn, thin progressively. In winter take individual leaves. A few small young leaves improve a salad; too many ruin a salad.

Saving seed: Mustards are bee pollinated. There are several closely related mustard species that sometimes make interspecies crosses with turnips and Chinese cabbage, producing interesting but often not-too-edible progeny. I manage that confusion by not letting more than one variety to form flowers in spring. Mustard seeds usually last at least seven years, sometimes a lot longer. The seed saver may produce seed for quite a few different varieties by alternating years.

Producing mustard seeds on a small scale is practical. Most mustards aren't highly refined; varieties may be maintained through many generations from a dozen plants in each production.

The small yellow flowers develop into brassica-like pods containing several seeds each. When half of the pods have browned off (some of the first-formed ones will have already shattered and dropped seed), cut the plants and let them finish drying on a tarp under cover. Then, one sunny morning, drag that tarp into the sun and let the straw bake until it is crisp. This should happen by mid-afternoon. Then gather the straw into a heap and thresh the seed by walking, jumping, dancing, scuffing feet or otherwise carrying on until everything has been crushed. Sieve out the big stuff and then winnow by gently pouring between two buckets in a mild breeze.

Not removing mustard flower stalks from the bed will almost certainly result in a self-perpetuating overcrowded mustard patch that needs only an annual dose of COF, a thin mulch of compost and a bit of by-hand weeding.

Varieties: I suspect that all mustards originated in the Orient because their deeply cut frilly leaves on long graceful stalks are beautiful works of art. There are a great many varieties. Some varieties are extremely pungent, others are quite bland. My preference is Miike (Red) Giant; it is an extremely hardy variety with reddish-purple leaves and broad thick stalks. It is peppery but also sweet and flavourful.

Tai Sai/Pac Choi makes celery-like stalks and broad spoon-shaped leaves essential to Oriental cookery. There are a few special strains like Canton White (SH) that can be sown later in spring and harvested in summer. I go to considerable trouble to keep Black Summer (JSS) in my seed box. It not only refuses to go to seed in summer, it also grows in all seasons and is the most delicious variety of its type. Market gardeners: when Black Summer is about 150 mm tall (half of full size), it makes the handsomest rubber-banded bundles you ever saw. It's especially tasty when small. I sow it about once a month, eat it small and give it to the chooks at full size.

Mizuna is only suitable for autumn/winter cropping. It bolts too quickly to be useful when sown in spring. Mizuna looks like friseé and has little pungency. Mibuna is a sort of mizuna forming a rosette of small spoon-shaped leaves on long, thin stems.

Writing this section brought to mind the extremely wide choices amongst Asian mustard greens so I searched the net for "asian seeds australia" and turned up several websites. Maybe my experience in the seed business can save you from losses. All but one of those vendors sell some unproductive varieties. I know that because I searched their catalogue for "brussels sprout" and Long Island turned up; so I assume I'm looking at a junk seed seller in Asian attire.

Spinach, English

(Spinacia oleracea)

Much like mustard, spring sowings of English spinach must be encouraged to grow very fast so they get large before being triggered into seed formation by increasing daylength. Fortunately there are bolting-resistant long-day summertime varieties that work in spring too. These do not need to be sown as early as possible nor pushed to grow as fast as possible. Sowings made at the end of summer for autumn/winter harvest survive winter's humidity better under plastic. Unprotected plants survive winter better when they are started mid- late March so they're smaller and don't trap as much moisture.

Culture: *For spring harvest* sow mid- to late August if possible instead of September. Spinach seed often shoots in chilly soil. *For summer harvest* sow in October/November and use varieties intended for long days. Summer varieties could produce if they are sown December and January but hot weather often wrecks germination; I sometimes can get a row to establish in summer by sowing thickly, moistening the bed daily and correctly anticipating a week of cooler weather. I suggest substituting silverbeet for spinach during high summer. *For autumn and winter harvest* sow mid-February through March. *For early spring harvest* (or to make spinach seed) sow in April and overwinter small plants because small plants better resist humidity-induced diseases.

Spring spinach is a medium-demand crop that responds to side-dressing. Sow seed in furrows 1 cm deep, 1 seed per cm, in rows 35 to 45 cm apart. In spring I side-dress blood-and-bone immediately after germination.

Thin progressively but delay the first thinning until the seedlings have one true leaf and are growing fast because mysterious disappearances of new spinach seedlings has been the usual thing ever since I started gardening. I prefer to thin spinach by separating top from root with a small kitchen knife; I use the thinnings in salad. Full sized plants should stand 30 cm apart. Given this much space the plants make leaves the size of book pages. I snip leaves this large off their stems with a fingernail and quickly fill a bucket. How delicious! Time saved washing greatly exceeds the time spent thinning.

Garden planning: I locate spring-sown spinach where a half-grown tic bean or blue lupin green manure was dug in two weeks previously. A few square metres sown in spring produces all the salad leaves and cooked greens our family can use. With ordinary varieties the spring harvest period is only a few weeks. To have a long stable supply sow few square metres every three to four weeks from September through November. Start a few patches between mid-February and the end of March. My final sowing is made late in April to overwinter for early spring harvest or to make seed. Areas assigned to autumn/winter crops are larger because winter growth is very slow. Hopefully it'll be a sunny dryish winter so they'll keep producing. At worst the winter will be more rainy than average and the plants will succumb to disease. *The key to success with unprotected winter survival is increased air circulation.* So thin thoroughly and keep spinach well-weeded during winter. It may seem unpleasant to weed in winter but if the plants survive then a side-dressing in early August results in abundant September harvests.

Insects and diseases: Spinach tolerates frosts that are far more severe than Tasmanian winters serve up. But high humidity, pounding rain and low light levels—all these insults combine to make the plants susceptible to disease. Fully remineralized soil helps fend off problems. For winter harvest thin the row such that air can move freely around leaves. Spinach overwinters reliably and makes more growth under a cloche or cold frame—it is like endive in this respect. Finally, removing deteriorating leaves in winter allows more air circulation.

Saving seed: Overwintered plants and early spring sowings go to seed soon enough to mature seed during summer. Later sowings in spring try make seed that probably will not mature. Best locate seed crops where general garden watering won't touch them. Seed producing plants finish irregularly over a few weeks. When most of the seeds on one plant have become light brown, give the stalk a gentle upward tug. If it lifts easily from the soil then that one was ready to harvest. If there's any resistance wait a day and check again. Repeat. Spread the plants on a tarp under cover and dry to a crisp. Strip the seeds by pulling the stalk through your (gloved) hands. Then rub the seed clusters between your palms to break (most of) them up. Then winnow to eliminate the dusty waste. Spinach is wind-pollinated and readily outcrosses; varieties must have at least 1.5 km of isolation to maintain purity.

Spinach seed may end up dead if it ripens in hot weather. That is why 90 percent of the world's spinach

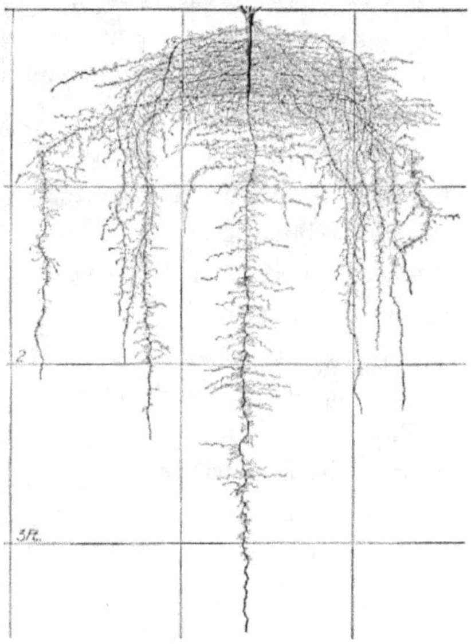

Ten-week-old English spinach

seed is produced in the Skagit Valley, Washington State, USA, where dry mild summer weather is the usual. However, most summers my Tasmanian spinach seed productions have succeeded.

The species makes two types of males as well as females. Male plants put up flower stalks before the females do. Males open small sacks that release dust-like windblown pollen. The very first few plants to go to seed may be "dwarf males" that should be pulled out before they can contribute pollen.

Varieties: Bloomsdale and its variants are traditional open-pollinated varieties for spring and autumn. Their thick savoyed (crinkly) leaves have extraordinary flavour. Bloomsdale strains vary as to disease-resistance, bolting date and cold-hardiness.

There are many spinach hybrids; most taste more or less the same. Some leaves are flat; some are crinkly (savoyed). Most hybrids are slower to go to seed than the Bloomsdales and survive winter better. Tyee F_1 (SH) is slower to bolt in spring than any other broad-leaved savoyed type. Southern Harvest offers many varieties.

Silverbeet

(Beta vulgaris cicla)

Silverbeet easily withstands Tasmanian winter. Silverbeet can *exist* in infertile soil; it will survive being moisture stressed all summer but it will produce a lot more and taste its best if it is fertilized and watered.

Culture: It is possible to start this low-demand vegetable from September until mid-February. I suggest sowing between October and mid-December because the seed germinates more reliably after the soil has warmed up; it also sprouts far better when the soil isn't too hot. When silverbeet is sown late in February the plants will be small during winter but still useful. Side dressing increases leaf production.

Place seeds 2 cm apart in furrows 1 cm deep, rows 60 cm apart. Thin progressively until each plant stands at least 30 cm apart in the row. Eat the thinnings once they become large enough to bother with. Having gaps between plants during winter lets in more light, which makes more new leaves appear.

Garden planning: Waiting until the soil warms up (October) makes establishment a lot less worrisome. Our spring sowing gets harvested in summer, autumn and through winter before going to seed next spring. Because younger plants make tastier leaves I could start patches mid-December and mid-February. But we prefer English spinach.

Insects and diseases: After the seedlings outgrow snails we have no problems except with nesting sparrows—their babies prefer bits of leaf torn from silverbeet.

Harvest: When thinning silverbeet we eat every other plant in the row. Once plants stand 45 cm apart in the row we take individual leaves as needed. If growth is too slow, side-dress. Increased interplant spacing and removal of large deteriorating leaves results in higher production. Half-sized young leaves taste better.

Saving seed: Silverbeet crosses with beetroot. See "Roots/Beetroot." Seed-production is just like beetroot although examining the roots is not necessary so transplanting is not required. Do not save seed from any plant that goes to seed a few months after being sown. Silverbeet is a biennial that should *not* go to seed the first year. Only poorly selected varieties do that.

Varieties: All varieties are winter hardy. Ruby, aka Rhubarb Chard ("chard" is what Americans call silverbeet), has one downpoint; it often bolts prematurely if sown before November. Rainbow is the latest sensation, providing a mix of stalk colours from one packet. I haven't bothered to grow it yet but I do produce my own seed for a variety with chrome-yellow stalks that we consider to have a superior flavour. Fordhook is the most commonly found type; it's an heirloom. Perpetual Spinach (SH) is but another kind of silverbeet.

Dry gardening: Silverbeet forms a taproot that goes very deep and stores heaps of water, making it useful where water is scarce. For dry gardening, sow silverbeet on the early side so it'll get a taproot far down before hot weather comes. Position plants 90 cm apart in

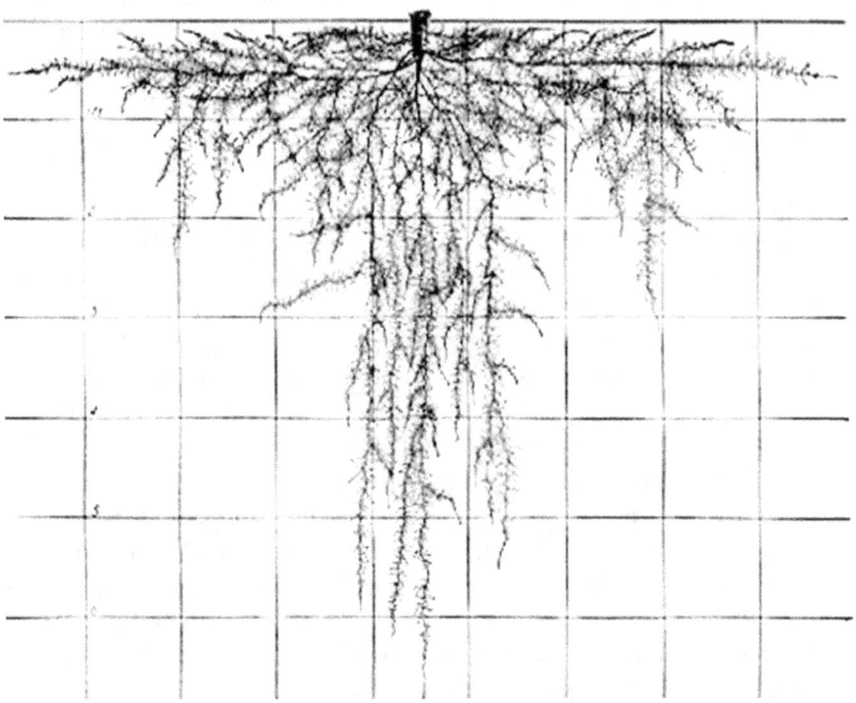

Silverbeet at mid-summer. One plant could use all the moisture and nutrients in a circle over 150 cm in diameter.

rows 120 cm apart. The patch might not produce much per square metre during summer but once the rains return it'll burst into new growth, especially this will be so after being sidedressed.

Miscellaneous cooking greens

Santoh is a non-heading Chinese cabbage that may be slower to go to seed in summer than heading types. I say "may be" because there are many varieties used in Japan but we're lucky to access any of them. Santoh survives winter better than heading sorts. It compares to Chinese cabbage much as collards relate to regular cabbage. (see Chinese Cabbage in the section on Brassicas)

Raab (rapa) is a type of turnip grown for edible greens. Raab provides cooking greens sooner than any other spring-sown crop. It goes to seed very quickly; fortunately the unopened flowers are as tasty as the leaves. Raab is not nearly as good to eat as mustard greens. I can't imagine why anyone would choose to grow raab other than to have something, anything, to eat as early in spring as possible. That strategy was sometimes necessary in Oregon because a severe freeze would completely wipe out the winter garden about once in five years. This hasn't happened since I settled in Tassie.

Edible chrysanthemum aka **Shungiku** is a dwarfed chrysanthemum used in Japanese cookery. It creates the unique flavour of sukiyaki. Shungiku may be started from October through mid-March. It should be harvested before the flavour becomes far too spicy, which happens when the flower bud appears. For a continuous supply start a few plants every three weeks.

New Zealand spinach *(Tetragonia)* is a hugely abundant producer during summer. It may barely tolerate slight frost. In fertile garden soil the fast growing ground-covering plants need constant cutting back (harvesting). If you eat the last 150 mm or so of every stalk the plant will regrow even more tips. If you don't harvest it regularly then the patch becomes a nasty tangle of decaying older leaves covered by younger branches that still produce useful tips. About two weeks after the tomatoes go out I suggest sowing 2 seeds per position 2 cm deep, positions 45 cm x 45 cm. Thin to a single plant per position and have no worries if an occasional spot comes out a blank; the entire area will still be lushly covered before the end of January. Lightly steam the tips, including the stems. The flavour is naturally salty. Intuition suggests this is due to an extraordinarily high concentration of minerals. You may find this plant growing wild on salt-sprayed sand next to the Bass Strait.

Malabar spinach is a heat loving climbing vine. In semi-tropical climates it grows aggressively but in Tasmania it is unlikely to need more than a metre-tall stick to wind itself around. The thick leaves remind my mouth of okra. There are two varieties, red and green. I prefer green. The first time that you grow Malabar spinach try positions 40 cm x 40 cm. Do not sow it before the soil has warmed up very well.

Miscellaneous salads

These leafy greens add interest to salads. Any possible salad variation helps during winter—a season when garden meals become all too predictable. Most minor greens still resemble the weeds they recently were. They'll require little or no extra fertilizer nor special care beyond weeding and thinning.

Garden Purslane *(Portulaca oleracea)* is an oversized version of the common low-growing weed. The thick juicy leaves and strong upright stalks resemble a commonly grown indoor ornamental called the jade- or money plant. Purslane is not frost tolerant. It has a crunchy bland taste useful in salads *in small amounts.* Early in November, certainly before hot weather arrives, thinly sprinkle the fine seed in a shallow furrow, barely cover it with fine sifted compost and keep it moist until germination. Thin progressively to about 30 cm apart. Harvest by cutting stalks about 10 cm above ground; the plant will then regrow. If seed heads appear cut them off; they are inedible, while seed development will reduce future leaf growth.

French Sorrel *(Rumex acetosa)* is a refined version of sheep's sorrel, a common weed. It is a perennial that needs nothing more than weeding and a thin compost mulch applied once a year. In winter and early spring the leaves have a lemony sweet taste. Small quantities improve salads, particularly cabbagey salads. I find the flavour gets too strong to enjoy in hot weather. Sow seeds mid-September to mid-October. The minute seeds are thinly sprinkled into a very shallow freshly-scratched furrow and not covered, or perhaps given a very thin covering of sifted compost. Seeds will fall into cracks and crannies; this may be enough covering. Keep the row damp and they will germinate in a few weeks. I suggest starting the sorrel patch by first sowing a one metre row. Thin the row progressively to about 10 cm apart. Almost all the plants will put up inedible seed stalks a few months after emerging but plants do not completely go to seed—they continue producing useful leaves amongst the seedstalks. However, allowing seedmaking greatly reduces the formation of new leaves so I cut off seedstalks off as soon as they are spotted. During the first summer try to find at least one plant in the row that did not go to seed so fast, or so much—or best, not at all. Dig that precious non-flowering plant up and use it to start a new patch. Now you're set for your lifetime. Sorrel transplants very easily. It allows crown/root divisions almost any time. I have started three sorrel patches and each time found a plant that did not make seed.

Arugula (Rocket) *(Eruca vesicaria subsp. sativa)* is very fast-growing annual brassica with a delicious peppery taste—in cool weather. In hot weather its flavour gets too strong for me to enjoy. My early spring and late summer rocket sowings occupy up to one square metre because I can make an entire salad of rocket. I thinly sprinkle seed in a 1 cm deep furrow across a raised bed, furrows 300 mm apart. I do not thin the rows except where I dropped way too much seed. Pick leaves as needed or else cut young plants off above the soil line. Best to cut where the stems turn to leaves because the stems are less choice eating. There is no way to keep rocket from going to seed (or from getting strong-tasting when it gets large). Don't fret: from mid-spring through mid-summer simply start a new row(s) every month. March/April sowings can occupy more space because they won't get so peppery during winter. Harvest late sowings by taking individual leaves as wanted. This patch will overwinter and may be allowed to make seeds in spring. Arugula won't cross with other brassicas.

Lately I've been using rocket as a short-term green manure crop. I scatter rocket seed and rake it into a just-harvested bed. Within six summer weeks a thick stand of rocket can be mid-calf high and putting up flower stalks. Rocket rots quickly if it is dug in before it starts opening flowers. Even when in full bloom and waist high it can easily be yanked out of the ground, roots and all. Of course, to be able to afford to use rocket as a green manure I must produce my own seed. A seed-making patch yields more than 250 grams per square metre.

Orach *(Atriplex hortensis).* Shallowly sow the (parsnip-resembling) seeds in early October, a time when natural moisture and sufficient warmth make germination certain. One metre of row will more than suffice. Thin progressively to about 30 cm between plants (and use the thinnings in salads). There are two sorts, green and purple; I prefer purple for the visual accent it makes. The leaves taste good until the plant begins to bloom; then they don't taste good. Orach can grow big. Once I had a volunteer come up near a compost heap; out of curiosity I allowed it to grow until it reached 150 cm tall and its many side branches came to occupy a circle 1.5 metres in diameter. If I didn't know better I might think that plant was cannabis. Orach seed matures late in summer. Even one seed-making plant will scatter seeds widely; if it likes the soil orach will come up all over but plants hoe out easily *when they are small.*

Anise Hyssop *(Agastache foeniculum).* Shallowly sow the minute seeds in early October when natural moisture and sufficient warmth make germination certain. One metre of row will more than suffice. Thin gradually to 10-15 centimetres apart and use these thinnings in salads. Then pick younger leaves, which have a strong anise flavour. Encountering only two or three leaves in a large salad is enjoyable. Too much of it ruins a salad. The plants put up pretty purple flowers that resemble mint and are highly attractive to bees. The flowers drop fine seeds in their vicinity that may form a self-sowing patch.

Vegetable Amaranth *Amaranthus tricolour).* Seed catalogues say this plant is useful in salads I'll give you that the colourful leaves are pretty but in my opinion amaranth is a summertime cooking green that tastes disgusting when raw. The plants get a metre tall and more. Shallowly sow the small seeds in early October when natural moisture and sufficient warmth make germination certain. Thin progressively. One metre of row more than does it.

Minutina *(Erba stella)* is useful in winter salads. The fine seeds germinate easily in mid-March. Sow them in a shallow furrow. Barely cover the seeds with fine compost. Until they germinate, water in the morning after any day that the sun had been bright. Then thin the tiny seedlings gradually until they stand 5-10 centimetres apart. During late autumn and winter the tough sour-tasting leaves, when finely cut, add interest to salads. Minutina goes to seed in spring and may naturalize. I have found it growing like a weed in lawns on sand soil.

Brassicas

Annie and I especially depend upon coles during autumn and winter. Brassicas are nutritious: F.C. King said in *Farmers of Forty Centuries,** that the labour that built the Great Wall of China was fuelled more by cabbage than by rice. The crop yielding the most protein per acre is not lucerne or soybeans, but chlorophyll-rich kale. Chlorophyll, a complete protein, is as nutritious as fish, red meat or eggs.

Brassicas include kale, cabbage, cauliflower, broccoli, brussels sprout, kohlrabi and collard. All these derive from wild cabbage, a weed that especially thrives on limestone soils. Wild *English* cabbage is unusually morphable. Scottish kale most closely resembles the wild ancestor. Breeding greatly enlarged the terminal bud while the main stalk was compressed—a cabbage. Axial buds (which are dormant on the kale stalk until the plant blooms in spring) became brussels sprouts. The stem became kohlrabi. Wild *Italian* cabbage makes larger flowers than the English variant. It became broccoli and cauliflower. Unfortunately, the more inbreeding amplifies one aspect of the plant, the less vigour the variety has.

The least inbred brassicas like kale, collard, swede, field kohlrabi (for stock feed) and purple- or white sprouting broccoli are low demand crops with strong root systems like their wild ancestor. These vegetables tolerate dry gardening better. Cabbage, garden kohlrabi, brussels sprout, cauliflower and broccoli have been highly inbred and grotesqued. They require loose airy soils, lots of soil fertility and moisture.

"Low," "medium" or "high" demand mainly refers to the amount of nitrogen the crop requires but all brassicas require high levels of available calcium. Not only will a calcium deficiency stunt them but with cabbage and brussels sprout lack of calcium can cause browning on internal leaf margins. Lime prevents this.

Cabbage grubs can turn brassica leaves into lace; they can wreck the crop. These larvae appear mid spring and continue through summer. You can count on them arriving. Their destructiveness diminishes after Christmas, diminishes even more after mid-February; they will be pretty much gone by the end of March. Fortunately, the damage can be greatly reduced with Bt, which is a non-toxic organically-certified biological pesticide. Bt does 90% of the job; combining it with another OG approved pesticide called spinosad gets every grub. See Chapter 8, "Pests." As you might expect, kale, sprouting broccoli and swede are less bothered. Probably that's why kale's name in Hollandish is boorkol—peasant's cabbage.

Broccoli, brussels sprout, cauliflower and cabbage form many pairs of opposing leaves along one main stem before making their edible parts. The main stem of cabbage and cauliflower has been so compressed it's hard to see that there is one. With kohlrabi there is no trace what happened to the main stem. No side branches appear on any these vegetables, including broccoli, until the plant goes into bloom. The size of the terminal flower (broccoli/cauliflower) or of the cabbage head or of the brussels sprouts depend upon how large the plants got before they head up or flower. Late-maturing varieties have more time to grow large before the edible part forms so the flower or cabbage head will be larger too. Late varieties always need more growing space than earlies.

The gardener's task with most brassicas is to help them make rapid vegetative growth until the edible part starts developing and then stop pushing. All brassicas can usefully be side-dressed in the seedling stage and one or two times more. The final side dressing for summer harvests should be applied three weeks before flowering or heading begins. Brassicas for late-autumn and winter harvest stop growing fast late in April; these should be side-dressed for the last time late in March. They'll develop maximum cold tolerance that way. Overwintering brassicas—purple- and white sprouting broccoli, cauliflower and spring cabbage—should be side-dressed early in April so they grow larger over the winter and side dressed again when rapid growth resumes early in spring.

A great many brassica transplants appear on garden centre sales benches. I think that's why most gardeners believe that cabbage, cauliflower, broccoli and brussels sprout *must* be raised from transplants. But if decent seed had been sown when weather conditions are favourable—not too early—and if the seedbed is right, then directly seeded brassicas equal or outproduce transplants. Brassica seedlings of most varieties are delicate during their first month; they absolutely require airy fertile moist soil. If their seedbed doesn't resemble a fine textured container growing medium then make a teamug sized hole at every intended position and fill it with container medium made to my recipe. Sow a pinch of seeds in that and side-dress the seedlings as soon as they start forming their first true leaf. I can't figure out why anyone goes to the bother of transplanting coles.

Tasmanian farmers grow brassica seeds for international vegetable seed producers. This wouldn't happen unless Tasmania's climate was near perfect for this species. However, with the exception of kale and swede (both can be maintained for many generations from a small plant population) and maybe garden kohlrabi (where 50 seed-forming plants could be crammed into 20 square metres), conserving heirloom brassica varieties does not work for the backyard gardener (see Chapter 6, "Seeds").

Brassicas are bee pollinated. There are two species: *B. olraecea* includes broccoli, cauliflower, cabbage, brussels sprout, collard, kohlrabi and scottish kale. Swede and Siberian kale are a different species called *B. napus.* Olraecea freely crosses with all other olraecea but not with napus; napus only crosses with napus.

Napus is biennial. All olraecea that originated from *English* wild cabbage are biennial. Seed growers should destroy any of these that bloom before overwintering; this plant is an undesirable rogue. Broccoli and Cauliflower are from *Italian* wild cabbage; most varieties will go to seed their first year if sown in spring. But to make *fat strong* seed in Tasmania they too should be overwintered. Purple sprouting broccoli derives from Italian broccoli crossed with kale. Like kale, if it is started in September/October it grows all summer, autumn and through winter, becoming an enormous plant that flowers next spring. Varieties of cauliflower that have been bred to overwinter do the same thing. If spring sown they can make huge plants yielding gynormous heads after growing nearly a full year. And then they make seeds.

The backyard gardener can not avoid catastrophic inbreeding of a fancy brassica variety when they try to produce seed through many generations but there is a way we still can produce useful brassica seed. It is essential to make seeds from fully grown near perfect plants that survived winter. It is essential to involve at least six such plants to avoid an immediate massive loss of vigour due to inbreeding. Big brassicas may be dug and transplanted to a convenient spot late in winter or left to make seeds where they grew. By October they'll put out enormous sprays of seed stalks covered with yellow flowers. Most types should be on at least one metre by one metre centres when they're blooming. Cease irrigating when the first seed pods start drying out. Soon the majority of the pods will contain dry or nearly dry seed and a few pods will have released their seeds. At this stage, cut off the huge sprays close to the ground. Spread them on a tarp under a roof where there is plenty of air circulation so they dry completely. Once the straw has become crisp, thresh and then winnow the seed.

I suggest that you never use your own (Gen_1) seed to make a second generation (Gen_2) unless you have enough space and passion to involve at least 100 near-perfect plants in every generation or else you'll soon have a non-productive variety. Still, given good storage conditions the first generation seed you grew from a handful of plants will provide enough for you and the whole neighbourhood for many years. Less refined brassicas—kale, swede, collard, maybe purple sprouting broccoli—can be kept going through several generations of seed making by involving 20 or so plants in each production. I have so far successfully produced ten generations of NZ Butterswede using approximately 20 individuals in each generation.

Hybrid brassica varieties have dominated the commercial market since the 1970s because farmers find hybrids to be more productive. With hybrids nearly every seed makes a good plant, every plant grows at the same speed. The whole field may be harvested in one day. Hybrid seeds cost much more but the farmer must use them to remain in business. Open-pollinated varieties found on picture-packet seed racks and sold in some home gardener catalogues are usually produced by low-priced growers specializing in cheap home garden seeds that are of such poor quality that no farmer would ever use them. Lacking ongoing plant-breeder attention (which is costly) these shonky varieties no longer perform like they once did. "Heirloom" brassica varieties offered by alternative garden seed sellers either are the exact same stuff found on cheap seed racks or else they really are produced by backyard amateurs from only a few plants, in which case they will grow a high percentage of non-productive plants. I don't know about you but for me I'd prefer to harvest a useful cabbage or broccoli than take pride in appearing to be politically correct.

Commercial quality cauliflower, cabbage, broccoli and brussels sprout varieties range from early- to late maturity. Starting several varieties at once allows the harvest of main heads of broccoli and cauliflower to go on for up one month from a single sowing date, or in the case of brussels sprout and autumn/winter cauliflower, from early autumn through late winter from one sowing. However, Tasmania's small population does not allow our local seedsmen to inventory the full range. Thus I feel compelled to import brassica seeds and to mention specific varieties that are available abroad. As of January, 2025 there is no quarantine restriction on brassica seed imports.

Brassicas may be wrecked by a soil-borne disease called clubroot. I have never seen a clubroot infected plant or even heard of anyone in Tasmania whose garden has the disease but the DPI says clubroot exists here so I feel honour bound to alert you. Infected roots swell into twisted irregular knobs that can't assimilate nutrition. Stunted plants with swollen, knobbly roots are proof. If clubroot is present in your garden don't let any visitors with gardens of their own walk in it. Do not compost infected brassica wastes; instead, send them to the tip. Clubroot is not easy to eliminate; to achieve that the garden must be kept entirely free of all brassicas for seven years. However, even three or four years without brassicas will greatly reduce the fungus's effect. Online, there is a detailed fact sheet about clubroot; Google: "Pacific Northwest Plant Disease Handbook." Read the section on "Cabbage and Cauliflower—Clubroot" A few varieties carry genetic resistance to one or more strains of clubroot but resistance to one strain does not necessarily mean resistance to your strain.

Broccoli

(Brassica oleracea italica)

Culture: Prepare the bed for a low demand crop. At each intended position place four to six seeds in a shallow depression made by pressing the thumb or fist one cm deep into recently hoed/raked soil. If the surface inch isn't yet first-rate then make a small hole the size of a 250 cc jam jar, fill that hole with potting mix made to my recipe and start a cluster of five seeds in that. If your soil tends to become crusty then cover the seeds with fine compost instead of with soil. Gradually thin each cluster to the best plant. Direct-seeding like this also works with cabbage, brussels sprout, cauliflower, kohlrabi and kale.

In my opinion, *minimum* spacing for most broccoli varieties is 60 cm x 60 cm. Dwarf varieties and Gai Lan (broccolini) make smaller plants; use positions 45 cm x 60 cm. To harvest bigger heads and more- and larger side-shoots too, grow late-maturing varieties on positions 75 cm x 60 cm.

Side-dress soon after germination. I thinly spread one- or two tablespoons of COF in a 50 mm wide band around the seedlings. Side-dress again (with considerably more material) after the cluster has been thinned to a single plant (at the four- to five leaf stage) and side-dress for the last time when the plants are about half grown.

Purple Sprouting is extremely vigorous, like kale. There is no absolute need to side-dress Purple Sprouting before the end of winter unless you want huge plants. The earlier Purple Sprouting is sown, the more uncontested root zone provided, the more often it gets side-dressed, the larger the plants will grow before blooming and the larger the flowers and the total harvest will be. I prefer to start Purple Sprouting mid- to late-January and provide 90 cm x 90 cm spacing. Plants sown on this date can be pushed to grow over 120 cm tall by spring and will form very large flowers. The outcome is almost as good from sowing mid-February on 75 x 75 cm or mid-March on 60 x 60 cm. I think regular (Italian) broccoli tastes better than Purple Sprouting and because of that I have discovered that most Italian varieties will survive winter and produce in spring if they are sown late in March to early April. If you're attempting this please know that if the plants are sown too early they end up blooming late in winter and their flowers will be small.

Garden planning: I can harvest Italian broccoli most of the year. Early spring harvests come from overwintered plants sown late March/early April. If you're super keen then start seedlings indoors mid-August and transplant them mid-September. These may head by November. Direct seed after mid-September. Depending on variety the plant grows for 60-90 days and then makes the main flower. If the bed provides enough growing room then many varieties produce large side-shoots for another four to six weeks.

Hybrid varieties reduce the farmer's harvesting cost by heading up all at once. The old commercial open pollinated varieties that once allowed the harvest of beautiful heads over several weeks now have degenerated so much they no longer are productive. I think it disgraceful and reflects poorly on the human race that these seeds are still sold to gardeners. My harvest-period-extending strategy has long been to grow two plants from each of several hybrid varieties with different maturity times sown at the same time. That way the main flowers form over three or four weeks and then large side shoots develop for yet another four weeks. After that the side shoots on most varieties get progressively smaller and less desirable. So every six weeks from September through the end of March I start another patch. The last sowing overwinters and produces early in spring when there is little else to eat. So for this one I overwinter a dozen plants.

Insects and diseases: Three practices compensate for damping off and the mysterious disappearance of small seedlings—sowing several seeds in each position; side-dressing soon after emergence; and thinning gradually. Cabbage moths are strongly attracted to Italian broccoli so best to spray Dipel every week or so from the time miniscule diamondback moths start flitting about your brassicas until the end of March. If you'll put weak foliar fertilizer in the spray tank with the Dipel the plants will grow much faster. If when you foliar feed you'll use something that provides lots of trace elements and balanced NPK—like NTS 10-10-10—the plants may become so healthy that grubs can no longer chew through the waxy coating brassica leaves can develop when the plants enjoy near perfect nutrition. It should be a weak solution because you're going to spray it so frequently. Purple Sprouting isn't bothered so much.

Harvest: The main flower should be harvested at it's peak of flavour, which is just before the beads swell in preparation for opening yellow petals. Side branches emerge from each leaf-notch soon after cutting the main flower. Later-maturing varieties form more leaf pairs so they make more secondary flowers. After harvesting the first set of side shoots the plants will produce many small side branches. Often these make very small flowers. But if you'll remove every small flower where it emerges from a side branch (even if you discard them), and if the plant still has growing room, then it probably will form new large side-branches from its base that make even more large flowers.

Saving seed: A broccoli flower quickly goes past the point of being prime eating and opens yellow blooms. However, in our climate it may be impossible to achieve strong broccoli seed of a late variety from a spring sowing. Also, this approach unavoidably selects for quicker opening of blooms, which results in less time to harvest the edible part. I opine it is far better to overwinter Italian broccoli when producing seed.

Fancy brassicas require constant plant breeder attention that vigilantly eliminates deviations in order to remain productive. These expensive efforts are now directed at hybrid varieties. No matter how gorgeous the catalogue image or packet photograph is, these days almost all open pollinated varieties—with the exception of Umpqua—produce small, highly variable, low-quality flowers. This includes Waltham 29, DeCicco, Calabrese and Italian Sprouting.

Varieties: The only open pollinated variety I know of that is worth its space and your time is Umpqua. Almost all hybrid varieties perform well in Tasmania. You may have believed propaganda from the alternative seed community asserting that hybrid broccoli is flavourless, lacks nutritional content, makes no side shoots. In my trials hybrids always taste far better than degenerated OPs; only one hybrid variety out of ten I recently trialled failed to make a great many medium- to large sized side shoots. In fact most hybrids produce side shoots that are larger—and far better tasting—than the main flowers of degenerated OP varieties. My suggestions for superior early hybrids are few because buying abroad is so inconvenient—Belstar, Green Magic and especially Amadeus (JSS), which makes an unusually delicious large main flower followed by extraordinarily large side shoots that keep appearing over many weeks after the main head is cut. In terms of having yield go on for a long time, Amadeus has done better than starting several early varieties at once. Dependable late-maturing varieties include Marathon, Ironman, Diplomat, Tahoe, Decathlon, Shogun and especially Arcadia (SH) which also makes better side shoots than most.

I do not sow late varieties between September and mid-December because their flowers usually have leaves emerging through them when they form during long days. I buy many hybrid varieties from North American catalogues and focus on the latest ones.

Purple Sprouting originated as Italian broccoli x kale and White Sprouting came from cauliflower x kale. Both were bred for overwintering in England. Sprouting broccoli's main flowers are not as large as Italian broccoli but it tastes good and it feeds the family early in spring when there is little else. English seed companies provide early- and late maturing PSB varieties; growing both kinds results in a longer spring harvest period. The English hybrids also produce double what the OP varieties yield. My preferred source is Moles.

Chinese broccoli, or Gai Lan, also known as broccolini, is the latest fad. It forms a smaller plant that makes many small flowers with elongated stems that are reminiscent of asparagus. It may be grown on 450 mm centres. I've had the best results from hybrid varieties.

Dry gardening: Early varieties will produce if the gardener provides twice the usual growing area per plant *and* sows before September 15 *and* sprays frequently against diamondback moths. Hopefully the main heads will have been cut before the soil gets too dry. Fertigation gives more side-shoots.

Purple Sprouting broccoli slots neatly into a dry garden. Prepare and fertilize the bed intended for this crop by the end of September. Keep the bed entirely bare during October to preserve soil moisture. Sow the seeds in November while there remains a fair amount of subsoil moisture. Give each plant heaps of elbow room, in Oregon I used 120 cm x 120 cm. Spot water the positions to germinate the seeds and continue to spot water them until the seedlings are 150 mm tall. From that point their roots should be down far enough to cope. Then spread a thin mulch. Provide just enough summertime fertigation that the plants don't get severely stressed. No need to make them grow fast—just survive. Side dress them when the rains return and by next spring they'll be huge and produce abundantly.

One more water-saving approach: start Italian broccoli about March 1st in seedling trays, pot them up a size or two as necessary, transplant them out mid April and spot water as necessary until the rains keep the soil moist. These provide a harvest that starts in winter or early in spring. Do not let these seedlings become pot bound! Or they'll prematurely make small flowers.

Brussels sprout

(B. oleracea gemmifera)

Brussels sprout first grows tall (resembling uncurly kale) and then the plant forms miniature cabbages at every leaf notch along the central stalk. Early maturing varieties usually are short with sprouts packed tightly. Earlies start forming sprouts in March. Their harvest would be mostly done by the end of May. However . . .

Aphids cluster on developing sprouts. I can't prevent this from happening by making the plant healthier. There are plenty of aphids around in March and they're superfond of newly forming brussels sprouts. Every sprout that starts forming before the second week of April is ruined completely, which amounts to most of them on early varieties. Some midseason varieties start forming sprouts early in April; only ones near the bottom of the stalk will be aphid damaged. I remove them after the first week of April and feed them to chooks. The remainder of the plant will make good sprouts. Later varieties start forming sprouts *after the aphids have completely vanished.*

Mid-season and late varieties always survive our winter. The harvest goes on until mid- late August.

If you sow a late variety way too soon, like mid-October, one of two things happens. If the variety is primarily influenced by photoperiod it starts forming sprouts mid-April (which is totally okay) but having been given so much growing time it has become overly tall and may topple when the winter winds blow. With some varieties sprout formation begins after the plant grows a certain number of leaf pairs. This kind sown too soon starts yielding when aphids are still numerous. If you sow later maturing varieties after mid-January the result will be a short plant with a thinner stalk that forms fewer leaf notches; it will make fewer- and smaller sprouts. The bottom line: *use later maturing varieties and sow them between 15 December and January 1.*

Hard frosts raise the sugar content so inland-grown sprouts taste better. Coastal market gardeners enjoy more autumn and winter sunshine and milder temperatures so they end up with larger, better looking sprouts that don't taste quite as good.

Culture: I position brussels sprout plants 75 cm apart in the row with 60 cm between a pair of rows lengthwise down a 1,200 cm wide raised bed. The plants *totally* shade the bed by the end of February and grow ever taller through March and into April. Brussels sprout is a medium-demand crop until sprouts start swelling. Supplying too much nitrogen whilst the sprouts are forming can make them loose and bitter. Side dress enough to keep them growing fast; provide their final dose mid-February. Gardeners with sandy soil where anchorage against winter gales is poor might tie their plants to stakes or else start them a few weeks later so they don't grow so tall. In that case use positions 60 cm x 60 cm.

Garden planning: I want to start harvesting mid-April and continue harvesting through winter. Market gardeners could harvest abundantly all winter from mix of midseason, main season and very late varieties. However, only six plants of one midseason variety produce more than enough for the needs of us two oldies. Brassicas do well following alliums. The garlic crop is always lifted between late November and 10 December; my brussels sprout patch goes into that space.

Insects and diseases: Aphids form colonies on half-developed sprouts. There is no need to fight; the chill of autumn wipes aphids out. I find that cabbage grubs have less interest in brussels sprout, not no interest, less.

Harvest: Sprouts near the bottom of the stalk enlarge first. They are snapped off a few at a time before they get too large. Oversized sprouts lose eating quality so I harvest twice a week. A plant usually yields heavily for the first six weeks and less after that. Commercial growers sometimes pinch off the growing tip to encourage all the sprouts to fill out simultaneously. This practice does not suit the home garden. Unopened flowers make a delicious broccoli substitute in September.

Saving seed: It's a brassica; produce seeds from high yielding near-perfect plants after they overwinter.

Varieties: At one time Catskill and Long Island Improved were widely used productive open-pollinated varieties bred for autumn harvest in eastern coastal North America. They have deteriorated exactly like Waltham 29 and DeCicco broccoli. English seed houses still offer a few productive OP late and midseasons varieties. A new very late maturing open pollinated variety called Red Bull (ADA) actually is uniform and productive. Red Bull is a trendy foodie-approved red-coloured vegetable with a bitter flavour, supposed to be more nutritious because of that. But me no like eating it.

When I went into the seed business (1979) there were around one hundred OP varieties available in England. Some of them were named for the district they were best adapted to; many of them were Roodnerf strains with specific harvest slots. Moles sells two *inexpensive* OPs plus Red Bull. I haven't done a trial but I don't trust these two to be productive because Moles says they're for the commercial seedling raiser (who knows that the gardener rarely appreciates why that pretty bedding plant failed to produce much).

Every hybrid variety I've trialled has proved productive and almost every one was excellent eating. The differences mostly concern maturity. Diablo (SH) is a proper midseason hybrid that makes more than half of its gorgeous sprouts by mid-June, with fewer in July and August. Find many choices from Moles.

Dry gardening: Sow December 15, position seed clusters on 1 metre centres; thin progressively. Fertigate every few weeks until it starts raining.

Cabbage

(B. oleracea capitata)

Culture: Cabbage yields nearly as much food as root crops do. Cabbages are grown just like broccoli. There are three maturity types: (1) *early* also includes "mid-season," which is a later-finishing larger-sized early; (2) *late;* and (3) *overwintered,* also called spring cabbage.

Early cabbages quickly form supermarket-sized heads in 65 to 80 days. Earlies may be directly-seeded between mid-September and mid-February. Do not count on early varieties to withstand months of winter weather whilst headed up. Especially quick varieties make small plants; position them 45 cm x 45 cm and give them quite fertile soil that is kept moist at all times. Most earlies do better on 60 cm x 60 cm. Small sized red and small savoy cabbages are early varieties.

Midseason varieties are harvested 90- to 120 days after sowing. They make a larger head; use positions 75 cm x 60 cm. They're often not winterhardy.

Late cabbages grow for 120- to 180 days before harvest. Sow lates mid-December through mid-January. A quicker finishing late variety like Savoy King may be sown later, but not after mid-February. Late varieties do poorly if sown before mid-December because: round heads become pointy and loose inside; they split instead of standing a long while after heading up hard. Late cabbages need positions at least 75 cm x 60 cm. There are red, green and savoyed lates, as well as late varieties for making sauerkraut.

Overwintered cabbages (spring cabbages) are a gambler's crop in the UK: will they make marketable heads in early spring or will they produce only seed stalks— which happens to most varieties if they achieve too much size before winter. But if started too late they may make disappointingly small, loose heads. I depend upon Spring Hero, a totally reliable Japanese-bred hybrid of this sort. If sown mid-February on stations 60 cm x 60 cm it forms its first head in winter and does not go to seed in spring. Instead it'll make another head if the first one was harvested correctly. If sown mid-March through mid-April it makes slightly smaller heads early in spring, long before there are any cabbage grubs. Side-dress lightly during winter.

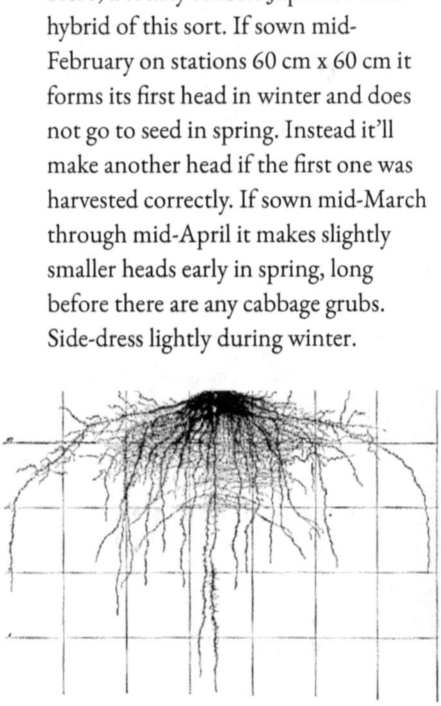

Midseason cabbage 75 days after transplanting

Garden planning: You may harvest cabbage every month of the year. From August through November eat Spring Hero. In order to harvest the soonest from a spring sowing start an early variety indoors the first half of August and transplant in September. About that time directly seed earlies and repeat that about a month later. These mature December/January if you'll fight grubs.

I love to eat coleslaw in high summer so I start a few Savoy Kings about November 1st. I have to spray them with Dipel many times until mid-January when grub pressure lessens. I sow a few more December 15th and more than a few around the end of January because this last sowing feeds us during Autumn and winter.

Maximally cold-tolerant savoys are found in English catalogues. Sown early- to mid-January, the earlier varieties mature April/May. The latest head up June/early July and hold in the field through August without rotting or splitting.

Insects and diseases: Grubs can ruin cabbages. Thoroughly spray Dipel every seven to ten days.

Harvest: Cut earlies promptly. Some earlies can hold for more than a week after heading up hard but most varieties soon burst. Tightly headed-up lates may hold for several winter months but may burst in autumn if sown too soon. But if started too late the heads will be small; and if started way too late, will fail to head up before going to seed in spring.

Saving seed: Grow seeds only from true to type plants that survived winter after heading-up. When contemplating how to overwinter early varieties for seedmaking, consider this: if a few basal leaves are allowed remain attached to the stem after the head is harvested, the stump starts regrowing, the plant probably survives winter and seed stalks appear in spring.

Varieties: A few open pollinated cabbage varieties are still available but most of them have degenerated to the point of worthlessness. When early maturing OP varieties were productive most were named Golden Acre or else the catalogue compared the variety to Golden Acre. Birdland has an extraordinarily good tasting Golden Acre; from it I get proper heads on three out of four plants. Southern Harvest sells Copenhagen Market.

I see little point in reviewing early hybrid varieties because they always seem to fall out of fashion within a few years of release. Most early hybrids are for market gardeners who wish to harvest an entire field at one go. The gardener does better with an early hybrid that the catalogue praises for holding in the field without bursting.

Early-maturing red cabbages grow just like early green ones. Late reds tend to be fibrous, as they must be to hold for months in harsh Dutch or English winter weather.

Tasmanians need a late cabbage that withstands rain and frosts for months after heading up without splitting or rotting. Varieties like this come from Holland, the U.K. and Japan.

In my opinion the best late for the home garden is savoyed, meaning with blistered, bumpy leaves. Savoys make superior salads and slaws and hold longer without bursting. Savoys can be cooked or krauted. European savoys are absolutely the most freeze-tolerant of all cabbages but they achieve that by being fibrous. Tough. Chewy. Japanese-bred savoys are tender enough for salad but winter-hardy enough for Tassie. Savoy King is Japanese-bred and grows a large head. Savoy Ace (STK) is very similar but a little smaller, slightly quicker to mature and better for market gardeners.

January King is a slow growing traditional English home garden very late variety. It is semi-savoyed, extremely frost tolerant. It resembles ordinary green supermarket cabbage with some purplish tints. Quite pretty! But many J. King strains have degenerated. A hybrid version called Deadon is reliable and tasty.

In regions where the earth freezes solid in winter people used to make the entire winter's sauerkraut supply in autumn from large late varieties and store it in a root cellar. I'm sure it got soft and mushy before spring. I prefer making small quantities frequently from almost any kind of cabbage and eating it half-fermented and still crisp.

English garden seed companies offer many overwintering varieties. Spring Hero (SH) is a ballhead that *never goes to seed prematurely.* Spring Hero is the best overwintering variety I've ever grown. It forms extraordinarily thin tender leaves that make excellent salad. Spring Hero does something unusual. If most of the basal leaves remain attached to the stem when the head is (carefully) cut, then the plant immediately resprouts. Each new leaf cluster could form another excellent cabbage five to seven weeks later, but they won't make proper heads unless *all but one of them are removed.*

Dry gardening: If you agree with me that eating cabbage in winter is important to health then producing a dozen big heads should be worth some precious water. Sow a late variety mid-January. Spot water the germinating seeds. Fertigate through the summer. Stop fertigating when it starts raining.

On a tiny irrigated nursery bed start spring cabbage early in March on positions 20 cm x 20 cm; dig them in autumn and transplant on 60 x 60 cm.

Chinese cabbage

(B. rapa pekinensis, B. rapa chinensis)

Chinese cabbage goes to seed when days are long. In our latitude spring- and early summer sowings put up seedstalks before they are big enough to make proper heads. Chinese cabbage for autumn harvest is easy.

Culture: Chinese cabbage *requires airy fertile soil that always provides lots of moisture.* Improve clay soils by spading in a layer of compost 25 mm to 50 mm thick. Sow four seeds in a circle the size of a fifty cent piece are on stations 60 cm x 60 cm. The seeds larger than other brassicas; the seedlings start out large and grow fast. Thin to one plant before there's any competition.

Do not transplant! Directly seeded Chinese cabbage forms a very helpful taproot; transplanting destroys the taproot. *Do not buy Chinese cabbage seedlings from a nursery.* They usually are started with cheap seeds of degenerate OP varieties that I've seen described in commercial seed catalogues as being "offered for the nursery trade."

Keep the plants well watered because they have shallow feeder roots and must make rapid growth to head successfully. Any check in growth may trigger seed formation. *Side dress frequently!* This is a high demand crop. Side dress the first time immediately after positions have been thinned to one plant.

Garden planning: Sow in February in order to harvest from mid-April through May. Sow earlier and you'll probably get seed stalks. If you sow in March the heads will be too small.

Insects and diseases: Slugs usually do no damage and can be washed out in the kitchen. The cabbage grub has less interest in Chinese cabbage than it has in most other brassicas; if you're spraying Bt anyway, give it a light touch.

Harvest: Full sized heads that aren't harvested promptly soon release *delicious* flowers with long tender stalks that are excellent in stir-fries or good raw in winter salads if taken before the budlets open yellow flowers. When harvesting, if you'll preserve a few large leaves at the base then the plant will regrow small, tender leaves and then flower stalks; both are good in salads and stir-fries during winter.

Saving seed: If *might* be possible to grow decent seed in our climate by selecting true-to-type heads at full size in autumn, keeping the plants or regrowth alive through winter after cutting the heads . . . under plastic? However, I did a Chinese cabbage variety trial in the 1980's involving every open pollinated variety still available. Even that long ago I discovered no productive open-pollinated strains.

Varieties: Hybrids go in and out of fashion so rapidly that there's little point in naming the ones being sold as this is written. Make sure you're using a hybrid that isn't for summer harvest.

Cauliflower

(B. oleracea botrytis)

The tastiest cauliflowers form in cool weather. Although it is possible to harvest in summer I no longer aim for that because cauliflowers forming in hot weather usually leave a bitter aftertaste and too often aren't crisp. Success requires using high quality seeds bred for heading up in the season you're using them in.

Culture: Grow cauliflower like broccoli. Position cauliflower on stations 60 cm x 60 cm. With late and overwintering varieties you can harvest really big ones by using stations 75 cm x 60 cm. Side-dress lightly and quite close around the plants shortly after germination; side-dress generously at least once more.

One way to achieve a November/December harvest is to raise indoor seedlings of an early variety—sow early in August for transplanting outdoors mid-September—because soil will be too cold to direct seed until mid-September. For autumn and winter harvest sow mid January through mid-February.

Almost all cauliflower varieties make compact root systems. They require always moist soil to grow really well.

Overwintered varieties are strongly biennial and strongly controlled by photoperiod. No matter when they are started they'll form heads around the same date in spring but the larger they grow before heading up the larger

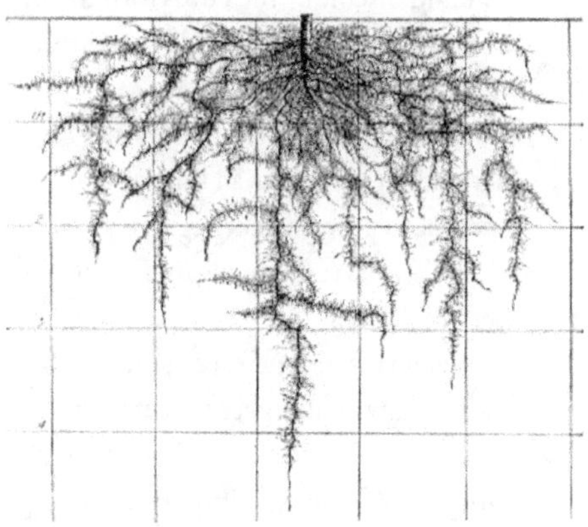

Cauliflower root system at harvest time. Note that most of the roots are located in the top 30 cm. Caulis remove topsoil moisture rapidly.

the head will be. I start them mid-February, provide generous spacing and correspondingly generous side-dressing—and harvest huge heads. They'll make supermarket sized heads when started early in March. Keep well weeded over winter. Side-dress enough to keep them growing slowly in winter. Side dress generously when growth speeds up early in spring.

Garden planning: The year's harvest begins in September from the earliest to finish overwintered plants. The latest overwintering varieties head up in November. Overwintering varieties make the best-tasting cauli of the year. September/October bring vegetable scarcity so overwinter at least 12 plants using several varieties.

Setting out seedlings of earlies in September or direct seeding earlies about September 15 makes for a harvest before hot weather arrives if you successfully fend off grubs.

Direct seeding October and November yields lower quality cauli late December through February.

Direct seeding mid-December through mid-February brings harvests March/May, potentially lasting into June/July if you sow very late varieties. Hybrids make a concentrated harvest of large handsome heads. I use many varieties with different growing times.

Insects and diseases: Cabbage grubs prefer cauliflower. Dipel usually is enough to get them through. Slugs and snails are thick in spring; they can badly scar and discolour the curds forming on overwintered plants. For this I put out snail bait early in spring.

Harvest: To be crisp for eating raw harvest before the small bumps that will become yellow flowers begin to swell. Certainly harvest when gaps first appear between curds.

Varieties: Garden seed sellers don't move many cauliflower packets so most don't offer a wide choice. But I strongly fancy cauliflower so I import seeds. Very few open-pollinated sorts remain productive. Amazing (JSS) is an open pollinated main crop variety of excellent quality. All Year Round makes delicious solid heads, except that more than an occasional plant doesn't. Birdland's Snowball works in spring, autumn and winter but is not Amazing. Only Amazing is amazing.

Every hybrid variety I've ever grown (a great many) has been excellent. To achieve a long autumn/winter harvest start an assortment with maturity times ranging from 64 days to 90 days. I can recommend Snow Queen (SH). I especially like Denali (JSS). Most winters I study Stokes', Johnny's, Territorial's and Moles' online catalogues. When I find a new-to-me late-maturing variety I usually import a few years worth of seeds for it. I invest because my seed inventory is stored properly; old seeds almost never die before they are used.

British winter-heading varieties can become huge plants before finally making an enormous cauliflower in June, July and August. Give them extra growing room. Territorial offers a blend-packet containing a mix of high quality English overwintering varieties that head out over several spring months. Southern Harvest would do that too if it served a population of seven million.

"Purple cauliflower" tastes like broccoli but looks like cauliflower—I disparage this harder-to-grow broccoli variety that doesn't make side shoots.

Dry Gardening. Not likely, except for overwintering varieties, which could be started in an irrigated nursery bed and transplanted out late April/early May.

Collard

(B. oleracea capitata)

Collard, called colewort in England, is a loose-leaf cooking cabbage that does not form a head. Collards are grown like kale but with one advantage—collard doesn't require frost to develop better flavour.

Kale

(B. oleracea acephala
B. napus pabularia)

Kale is the easiest brassica to grow. The leaves of oleracea varieties are usually cooked but can be included in salads—in moderation and if finely cut. Half-developed leaves of napus varieties are excellent in salads.

Culture: Kale is a low demand crop. In hot weather the taste of oleracea kale is too harsh for me to enjoy but it develops sweetness after frost. So I sow kale in January and start harvesting in April. Place four of five seeds in a thumbprint-sized depression 1 cm deep on stations 60 cm x 60 cm apart. Progressively thin the positions to a single plant. Side dress if you want high production.

Garden planning: Kale is more nutritious than cabbage because its dark-green leaves are loaded with high-protein chlorophyll. With each passing year I more enjoy kale's intense flavour and chewy texture in salad. And then there's colcannon, a delicious traditional Scottish protein-fortified carbohydrate food. Cut potatoes into chunks. Coarsely chop kale leaves until you have four volumes of chopped kale for each volume of potato. Newbies to kale might strip out the mid-rib before chopping. In a large soup pot add water one cm deep. Put spud chunks on the bottom, kale on top of them. Cover and steam on medium-low heat until the potatoes are tender enough to mash easily. Then generously add butter and mash everything including any water that hasn't yet steamed away. Mixing kale with spuds significantly ups the protein and mineral content. The flavours compliment. New gardeners might grow only one or two kale plants until your dietary sensibilities expand.

Insects and diseases: Cabbage moths lay far fewer eggs on kale than on cabbage, cauliflower or broccoli; this is especially so if the crop is not started too early. Losing a bit of summer leaf to grubs may seem of little consequence if the patch is growing vigorously but if soil conditions are not good then the loss can seem catastrophic, in which case use Dipel or next year delay sowing until early February.

Harvest: Snap off individual leaves starting at the bottom; half-developed leaves near the top are less tough and milder tasting. I prefer to not eat the mid-rib. With *oleracea* kale take care not to break off the top growing point. Should that happen formation of new leaves will cease until spring regrowth begins. Late in winter little leaves resembling loose brussels sprouts form along the stalk; they are especially delicious in salad. Unopened flowers appearing in September fend off starvation if you're hungry.

Oleracea kale toughens rapidly after harvest. If you tried supermarket kale and didn't like it, try growing it yourself and eating it immediately after harvest.

Saving seed: Both species of kale can be reproduced for many generations from a small number of plants in an amateur's back yard.

Varieties: Oleracea hybrids dominate all commercial growing; you can expect open-pollinated oleracea kale to be variable and somewhat less vigorous—that doesn't matter much in the garden. The common sorts are usually called Blue- or Green Curled, or Scotch. Southern Harvest also has several notable heirlooms. If you go shopping world wide, know that Euroland uses excellent hybrids like Winterbor, Redbor and Darkibor.

Napus kale variety names usual associate with Russia. The plants are smaller with a rosette growing habit, the half-developed leaves are tender (compared to oleracea kale) and without oleracea's strong flavour. Every garden seed company sells Siberian and/or Red Russian. Sam Bayley says his Siberian (green leaves) has thicker leaves and more "bang for the buck" compared to his Red Russian. Birdland's Red Ursa is especially nice.

I have been especially impressed by Nero di Toscana (oleracea). It has long narrow blistered leaves with superior flavour for salads.

Dry gardening: If water is short and the soil is deep then sow oleracea kale early in October when there is a good deal of subsoil moisture. Start clusters of seeds on stations 1 metre x 1 metre apart. Thin and weed carefully. Fertigate if and when you can. Each plant benefits greatly from 10 litres of fertigation twice a month through summer and side-dressing whenever the rains start, usually in April. You may end up with giants 120 cm in diameter and 150 cm tall. If they didn't get more than the bare minimum of moisture during the summer, look stressed and gnarly be comforted: as soon as it begins raining side dress and they'll burst into growth and provide lots.

Kohlrabi

(B. oleracea caulorapa)

Culture: Kohlrabi is a low- to medium-demand *cool season crop.* With somewhat irregular open-pollinated varieties, sow 1 seed per cm, 1 cm deep, in rows 45 cm apart. As the seedlings become established thin gradually and carefully so that in the end the plants stand 12 to 15 cm apart in the row; *keep firmly in mind that crowded kohlrabi fails to develop properly.* Hybrids form compact plants. Sow hybrids on stations 12 cm apart in rows that are 30 cm apart. Hybrid kohlrabi seeds germinate strongly! I carefully place exactly three seeds at each intended position in the row. Thin clusters to one plant by the time they have three true leaves. Side dressing COF after the seeds have sprouted makes faster growth and sweet, tender bulbs.

Make sure the plants never experience moisture stress because the edible part remains tender only while the plant is growing rapidly. Should the plants become stressed, should the weather get hot, then kohlrabi becomes dry and fibrous.

Garden planning: Kohlrabi gets large enough to use 60 to 70 days after sowing. Sow a small patch about mid-September to start eating mid-November. The harvest ends when hot weather arrives. I never plan to harvest kohlrabi in summer. I sow several times during the month of February. The harvest starts late March/early April. Given space and fertility that encourages winter growth they may retain good eating quality until August.

Insects and diseases: Cabbage moths show less interest in kohlrabi. My biggest problem has been with rats and mice. I've deterred them by spraying neem or quassia. This makes the skins too bitter to gnaw upon but the skin is peeled before eating.

Harvest: *When crowding slows growth kohlrabi become woody.* This happens in cool weather too. Consequently, harvest by taking every other plant in the row so the survivors continue growing. High quality varieties may remain tender when they've gotten to the size of a very large grapefruit *if they have been growing steadily.*

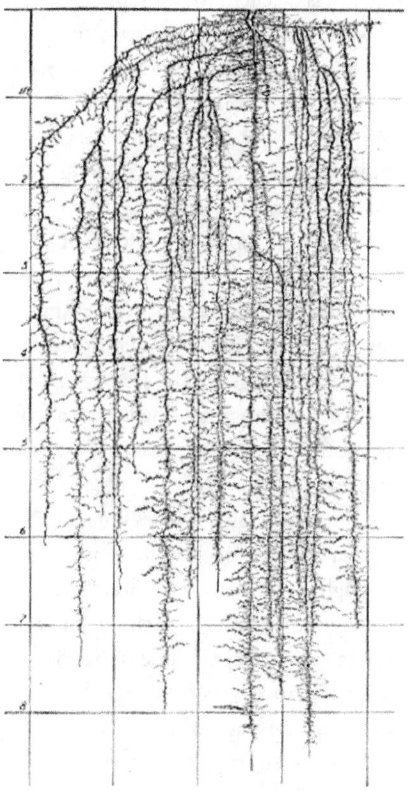

Root system of a mature fodder kohlrabi. The garden vegetable developed from this farm field fodder crop, as evidenced by the nature of the root system. Kale's root structure is similar.

Saving seed: Kohlrabi overwinters and then makes seeds. Maintaining quality requires careful selection of a large plant population in every generation. Garden kohlrabi are smaller than most brassicas when in bloom so during winter a home gardener could transplant 50 near-perfect seed-making specimens into 10 square metres on stations 40 cm x 40 cm. I point out that to find 50 near-perfect ones you'd probably have to grow at least 200.

Varieties: Open-pollinated seeds are cheaply produced for the home garden trade. They often are called Purple Vienna, which has purple skin and white flesh, or White Vienna, which is pale green-skinned with white flesh. I avoid both. When I see a seed company offering these sorts I doubt that company's ethics.

I look for catalogue verbiage stating the variety "remains tender longer." I've also noted that purple-skinned varieties seem to retain good eating qualities longer in winter. Kolibri, a purple hybrid, is excellent for most purposes. It has fewer leaves that are attractively confined to the upper portion of the bulbing part so the skin is smooth, thin and velvety. Market gardeners find Kolibri easy to sell. Delicacy Purple (SH) is a new OP variety. It is larger than Kolibri, in my opinion it tastes better, stays tender a lot longer than Kolibri. I coarsely grate kohlrabi into something resembling coleslaw with a vinaigrette dressing. I refrigerate the excess. Kolibri becomes unpleasantly smelly after a few days but Delicacy Purple keeps in the fridge for weeks.

There are giant varieties similar to fodder kohlrabi but with flavour good enough for humans. They'll enlarge slowly and remain edible through the entire winter. Superschmeltz (SH) is excellent. Space giant kohlrabi plants as though raising medium-sized cabbages—60 cm apart in rows 75 cm apart—and start it a month earlier than you'd start the small-sized ones.

Dry gardening: I've never done it but I'd try sowing Superschmeltz in December, spaced 90 cm apart in rows 120 cm apart and fertigate enough through summer to allow slow growth.

Swede

(B. napus rapifera)

Lately I've been growing more swedes than potatoes because swedes hold in the soil all winter, because they are nearly as satisfying as potatoes yet are not a carbohydrate food, because the cabbage grub has little interest—and because *I grow a home garden variety with wonderful flavour.* I hope you doubters are now curious enough to read what else I have to say about this much disparaged vegetable.

Culture: Swede is a low demand crop. Best to sow between mid-January and mid-February. Place the seeds one-cm-deep in furrows 60 cm apart. Hope to see one seedling emerge from every cm in the row. Thin progressively until they stand 30 cm apart in the row. *Thinning to adequate spacing is essential. Crowded swedes make small bottoms.*

Garden planning: A family like ours, using swedes like others use potatoes and aiming for a full winter's supply, could easiliy consume 10 square metres of swedes. When the crop is done the bed makes a good place for peas or spring greens. Swedes that fatten in cool weather taste better.

Insects and diseases: Cabbage grubs show little interest in my swedes. The minor damage they do makes no problem. However, I have seen cabbage grubs ruining swedes in other peoples' gardens so my supposition is that the cause almost certainly was poor plant nutrition.

At the first sign of mice gnawing on my winter food supply (not just of swedes, but sometimes carrot, parsnip and beetroot too), using a long-handled tablespoon I put a small mound of rat-and-mouse food into a 30 cm long section of 100 mm white plastic downpipe (to prevent rain from ruining the pellets), placed on the earth near whatever is being gnawed upon. The feeding stations are promptly refilled until the local rodent population loses its appetite for them.

Harvest: You can harvest swedes until seed formation begins at the end of winter. Eating quality collapses as soon as they start going to seed. Swedes sit mostly on top of the ground. If a few consecutive days of continuously subfreezing weather is possible at your location, then do what I did in Oregon where winter is harsher than it is in Tasmania. Late in May bury the roots by hilling up several cm of soil against them. Make sure the crowns are well covered but the leaves should remain exposed. When our swede patch first shows signs of going to seed my wife Annie digs them all and stores them in a big restaurant fridge (not self-defrosting! which desiccates what's inside) where they remain edible for another two months.

Saving seed: Swede crosses with Siberian kale; do not allow that to happen. Make seeds from carefully examined individuals selected because they are smooth globes, not footballs, form a single tap root and a compact crown (where the leaves attach). If some of your swedes taste much better than others then select for better flavour by cutting out a small wedge and tasting it raw. Try to save seed from at least ten swedes in order to avoid the rapid onset of inbreeding depression of vigour.

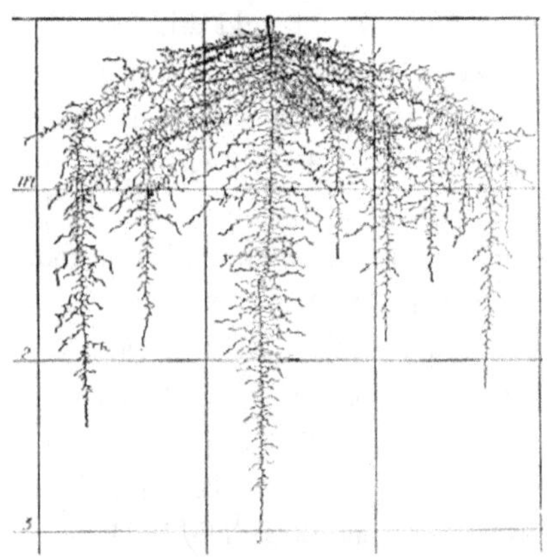

Root system of a half-grown swede. This drawing suggests that unirrigated swedes could benefit from being as much as 600 mm apart.

Involving at least 25 individuals would be smart. When replanting selected swedes, give each one ½ square metre of ground if they are large roots. Swede seed lasts a great many years (7-10) if it fully ripens under dry conditions and is stored in a dry unheated room in the house.

Varieties: Most Purple Top and Laurentian varieties are uniform and productive. But I don't like their cow-fodder flavour. Best Of All (FOT) is an English home garden variety that to me does not taste best by a long shot. The Tasmanian (aka New Zealand) Butterswede (SH) has not a hint of bitterness that many people find objectionable. Perhaps the Butterswede is called that because the taste is so rich it hardly needs butter.

Dry gardening: This method will only work in *deep open moisture-retentive soil.* Dig and fertilize the swede bed in spring. Keep the bed and an extra metre of ground on all sides entirely bare of vegetation so in late January/early February the subsoil will still be moist when you sow. Hopefully some of the fertilizer will have been leached into the subsoil by spring rains. Make the between-row space one metre. By hand wet down a narrow band along the row. Keep irrigation up until the leaves are about 10 cm to 15 cm tall (and the roots have reached damp soil). *Thin to 30 cm apart in the row and weed carefully.* In the right soil they could grow steadily without further watering until rain returns.

Turnip

(B. rapa rapifera)

When people think "turnip" most of them also image "livestock food." But there are great tasting varieties that should be tried at least once. You turnip-doubters should be informed that the flavour improves enormously when soil gets into balance and even more if they are foliar fed something generously supplying trace elements.

Culture: To end up with delicious turnips you must provide plenty of moisture and schedule them so the bottoms form in cool weather. Turnip is a low demand crop. Sow twice; once in September and again from mid-February through mid-March. Make furrows one cm deep and 45 cm apart. Sow the tiny seeds thinly; try for about one per cm. After the seedlings develop their first pair of true leaves, progressively thin so the seedlings stand 8-10 cm apart. We eat young white skinned Asian varieties raw, like radishes. Anytime the soil even begins to approach being dryish, irrigate them.

Garden planning: If the spring sowing hasn't been entirely harvested before hot weather arrives they will turn woody or pithy and/or become strong-flavoured. If you really like turnips I suggest making several small spring sowings between the first of September and the middle of October. This many attempts are in order because the earliest sowing may run into severe weather that stunts the crop (it usually grows well); the latest sowing may experience hot weather that ruins their flavour. But at least one of these attempts should come right.

Turnips sown in spring are usually harvested within two months. Turnips intended for autumn and winter harvest will hold in the garden for a long time, especially if they still have room to continue growing whenever the weather permits. For the autumn/winter harvest sow two or three times between mid-February and mid-March. Thin progressively.

Insects and diseases: Not usually a problem in fertile moist soil; however, I always give the leaves a light touch when spraying Dipel on other things.

Harvest: In spring take them before the root is more than 6 cm in diameter. Turnips in autumn will grow to twice that size or more (like swedes) if given time and room to expand but most varieties taste best if picked medium-sized. Harvest every other plant to give the survivors room to keep growing.

Saving seed: Much like swede. Turnip is biennial and less winter-hardy than swede. If a spring sowing goes to seed in summer, eliminate the plants. Grow seed only from overwintered plants. Turnip is reputed to cross with mustard and also with Chinese cabbage. Select for compact crowns (where the leaf stalks attach to the bulb) and thin single tap roots. You can cut out a thin wedge to taste them immediately prior to transplanting for seed-production.

Varieties: Purple Top, sometimes called Purple Top White Globe and its hybrid offspring, are not, in my opinion, nearly as good for munching raw as are the all white Asian hybrids like Hakurei and White Cross. When company comes to visit I may put out a nibble plate with a curry-ginger flavoured mayonnaise dip, turnip wedges, kohlrabi sticks and cauliflower chunks instead of the usual unhealthful salty snacks. For greens, any variety's leaves are edible but Shogoin was specially bred for this purpose.

Dry gardening: No way.

Root Crops

Root crops taste much better when the subsoil abundantly holds balanced mineralization and allows root penetration. Consider the carrot: at first the seedling expends more energy extending a taproot than it does growing leaves. Then the plant fills the subsoil with roots. Much less feeding occurs in the topsoil.

Root crops produce a great abundance of nutrient-undense food when the subsoil is inaccessible or is devoid of plant nutrients, which is the usual case in Tassie. I learnt that the expensive way, through experience. Maybe you can learn it second hand, which costs less. My previous garden on red krasnozem soil needed five years of full remineralization before the subsoil began to loosen. I didn't know root crops could taste so good until that happened.

Some deep sands are wide open; balanced compete nutrients applied to the topsoil soon leach into the subsoil; root crops grow great in this situation. Lush vegetable crops growing on deep alluvial sandy soil along the Forth river demonstrate this. Root crops do not develop brilliant flavour when an inhospitable clay subsoil lies below a sand or loam topsoil.

Parsnip and carrot need loose topsoil to develop properly. If the topsoil tightly compacts, if the plants are crowded there will be many mishapen roots.

If the subsoil gets dry, then the leaves will still look okay because root crops sustain themselves on stored water but the edible part develops irregularly, gets woody.

If subsoil is inaccessible or subsoil fertility is chemically out of balance but the top soil is loose, moist and fertilized then the vegetables may look okay but they'll taste like shop carrots. Repeated applications of lime and gypsum will eventually open subsoils that can be opened. Eventually. Foliar feeding moderate NPK with luxury levels of trace elements (like Nutri-Tech 10-10-10) noticeably (in the mouth) compensates for subsoil deficiencies.

For root crops to produce as well as they can in clay soil requires loosening the topsoil but not providing too much nitrogen—this makes a problem because feeding clay a lot of rich compost can provoke too much top and too little bottom. Better would be a moderate amount of compost and also balancing calcium and magnesium; then clay may loosen without so much organic matter. Another strategy for clay begins the previous year. Dig in 50 mm layer of compost and grow a nitrogen demanding crop. Next year use that bed for root crops. Another solution for heavy clay: make a special raised bed by covering the clay with loam topsoil 30 cm deep. After growing root vegetables there rotate into potatoes, cauliflower, celery or melons; all these species do much better in loam.

I've grown tasty root crops entirely without irrigation on deep alluvial silty clay loam. Root crops might be dry gardened in a loam topsoil above a clay subsoil, also known as a duplex soil. Only a trial will show if it works in your garden. Root crops store water so when the plant is under moisture stress it shows no sign except that it grows slowly or not at all and loses eating quality. Increased interplant spacing may allow unirrigated root crops to access enough moisture to grow steadily (and taste good). I suggest dry gardening root crops in rows that are one metre apart. Sow late in September whilst there remains sufficient topsoil moisture to sprout the seeds. Thin the row carefully; carrot, parsnip and beetroot should stand 150 mm apart in the row by the time the leaves are 100 mm tall. Keep the area perfectly weed-free. Harvest every other plant through summer such that the remaining roots stand 300 mm apart. A crop grown this way may still be good to eat next winter. Or else the plants may become inedible before the rains return. Anyone exploring this possibility should do variety trials.

There are hybrid beetroot, hybrid carrot and recently, hybrid parsnip varieties. Hybrid uniformity greatly increases the percentage of the crop that can be sold—and that *was* profitable at first—until all the other farmers used hybrids too. And now they all must use hybrids or else they fall behind their competitors. Without commercial demand, seeds of the old open-pollinated varieties have become far less productive.

Root crops rot in the ground after the surface inch freezes solid and then thaws. If that much cold is possible at your location then bury the crowns under a few centimetres of soil late in May.

I include potatoes and radishes in the root crop section because they're equally sensitive to soil compaction, can succeed as low-demand crops and don't show much when they are under moisture stress. Also, potato prefers to be a subsoil feeder. I did not include turnip and swede in this section because they behave like brassicas, which they are.

Timely and careful thinning is essential to harvesting straight smooth roots. Too much competition greatly lessens flavour and makes for tough chewing.

Beetroot

(Beta vulgaris)

Clayey soils can grow acceptable beetroot because the edible part forms at the surface. Still, the finest roots develop on deep open soil. Intermittent moisture stress causes white rings (zoning) that do not change the flavour. Reduce zoning by always keeping the topsoil moist. Zoning is much less likely when the subsoil is open to root penetration.

Culture: Beetroot is a low demand crop with a larger need for boron than most vegetables have. Almost all Tasmanian soils are deficient in boron which is why my COF recipe includes it. Beetroot seeds will usually germinate by September 1 in milder microclimates but there are several good reasons to delay sowing for a few more weeks: there will be fewer mysterious seedling disappearances; low light levels make the seedlings grow very slowly until the end of September; a sowing done 15 September will start being harvested only a few days after a sowing made 1 September. Seedlings that experience less weather stress will prove more productive. Make spring sowings 1 cm deep in furrows 45 cm apart. Beetroot seed usually is inexpensive; home-garden-quality beetroot seed often germinates weakly so it is best to put one seed per cm in the furrow.

Like spinach, beetroot seeds shoot well in cool soil but germination can be poor when the summer sun shines and air temperature exceeds 25°C. When sowing in summer place seeds half again deeper and put more seeds in the furrow to compensate for an inevitably lower germination rate. If air temperature approaches 30°C before emergence the seeds may fail altogether.

Thin progressively. By the time leaves are 100 mm tall what are called "baby" varieties should stand 3 cm apart. Canning varieties (uniform maturity for once-over harvest) should be 5-6 cm apart. Most varieties lose eating quality when they enlarge to over 8 cm in diameter.

Garden planning: Around mid-September I sow two rows across a 1,200 mm wide bed. This patch provides plenty for two oldies from early November until after Christmas. I start another patch mid- to late November (before hot weather starts) that feeds us the rest of the summer. This sowing is also only two short rows because we don't eat as many beetroots when there are French beans, cucumbers, zucchini and tomato. For harvesting late March through mid-May I start three rows in mid January and try to slot that into a week of mild weather. For winter use I start three or four rows in mid February.

Insects and diseases: I've had no problems after 25 years gardening in Tasmania except with rodents in winter.

Harvest: Beetroot gets woody when plants can't grow due to crowding. So harvest by thinning the row. Beetroot is less tasty when oversize. Best to have another patch coming on when the previous sowing has become large.

Saving seed: Beetroot is wind pollinated. The pollen has a musky odour; it drifts two kilometres on a light breeze. Beetroot crosses freely with silverbeet. Seed can easily last seven years in cool dry storage. Tassie's mild dry summer produces extremely vigorous seed with a long storage life.

Choose seed making roots as you harvest for the table during winter. Select for a tight crown, a single fine taproot, ideal shape and uniform deep red colour (unless the variety is white or yellow). You can taste each root by cutting a thin slice off one side. Immediately replant selected roots in a bed where the seed patch won't be routinely irrigated next summer. Position the crown 1 cm below the soil line, position roots 60 cm x 75 cm apart, even further apart if the beetroots are more than 100 mm in diameter. Allow the leaves to emerge above the soil. Overwintered beetroots put forth new leaves early in spring and then floppy seed bearing branches emerge that can exceed 2 metres in length if the roots were large.

Somehow keep the tangle mostly free of weeds. If forming seeds rest on the soil they will rot. You'll harvest much more seed by tying flowering branches to stakes or otherwise holding them above the soil. Pull the plant or cut individual branches when a generous half the seeds have become dry (light brown). Allow them to finish drying under cover on a tarp. When the branches have dried to a crisp, strip the seed from them by hand (wearing gloves); clean the dusty seed by pouring it between two buckets in a mild breeze.

Six large beetroots that are making seeds cover at least three square metres of bed and will yield several kilos. But if you save seed from a population of only six plants and repeat this inbreeding once or twice, the variety may collapse. Carol Deppe's book, *Breed Your Own Vegetable Varieties,* says involve at least 50 beetroot plants in a seed production. But what on earth could a gardener do with so much seed! And few gardens have that much extra space.

A better home garden strategy is to produce only one generation of beetroot seed and make the most of it. Start by growing a large patch of a high quality open pollinated variety for autumn/winter harvest. Make seeds from 6 to 10 of the most perfect roots. Store a half litre of the resulting seeds with a bag

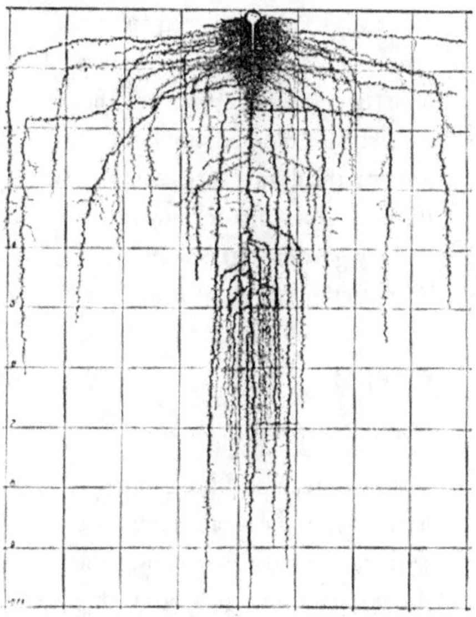

Beetroot at 3-1/2 months of age. Note the massive root development in the subsoil

of active silica gel in a truly airtight jar in a fridge so that it will still germinate strongly many years later; my intention is to use that jar when my big bag of unrefrigerated seed begins to weaken or gets close to being used up (I often gift beetroot seed by the handful). Eventually, buy another large packet of commercial quality OP beetroot seed; do another seed production with it.

Varieties: The most broadly useful garden variety happens to be a true heirloom, Early Wonder Tall Top. It matures irregularly, so that one sowing can be harvested for up to two months. EWTT handles all seasons and has excellent culinary qualities. Canning varieties like Detroit Dark Red, Ruby Queen or Red Ace hybrid are bred for uniform size and shape and lower fibre content (quicker to cook).

Most varieties first make a large top before even starting to form an edible bottom. "Baby" varieties make perfect roots the size of hens eggs whilst the plants are still small. If not harvested small then the babies grow on to achieve considerable size. Cylindrical beets are for canneries because they can be conveniently sliced into same-sized rings. They also are low in fibre so they're quicker to cook. Cylindrical varieties require very loose topsoil to form long straight roots.

There are white, yellow and internally striped (selected *for* zoning) varieties. White varieties were crossed with sugar beet; consequently they are sweeter than red beetroot but in my opinion the flavour lacks complexity. Burpee's Golden is delicious.

Dry gardening: See the introduction to this section, "Roots."

Carrot

(Daucus carota sativa)

Carrots can produce a huge harvest from the area involved. Carrot seeds germinate well in spring; they shoot faster in summer but there are difficulties in hot weather—the tiny seeds must be placed shallowly and take 8 to 14 days to shoot but germination will fail if the soil around the seeds dries out before they put roots down. Carrot shoots are weak and can't reach the light through crust or hard soil. Seeds started in spring usually shoot well because the soil stays naturally moist. After mid-November, raking compost into the seedbed before sowing keeps it loose and moister. This technique helps greatly when sowing most kinds of small seeds.

Culture: Carrot is a low demand mostly subsoil feeding vegetable. Only very small plants feed in the topsoil. When preparing their bed, deeply and *thoroughly* loosen topsoil to the full depth a spade's blade reaches (25 cm). This may seem hard work but the percentage of smooth shapely carrots will be higher—especially if you're growing a long variety. If the first digging did not result in a fine loose seedbed I suggest preparing another spot because the previous crop strongly influences the current soil texture.

Sow in furrows one cm deep, two seeds per cm, rows 30 cm to 45 cm apart. Choosing between-row spacing depends on how much top the variety makes. Placing seeds carefully one-at-a-time takes more patience than I have but when seeds are hand-sprinkled into a furrow the result usually is a tangle of crowded seedlings that requires a long time to correct. Chapter 6, "Seeds," suggest a simple and fast sowing technique that greatly reduces thinning.

Thin progressively, *carefully and thoroughly so that by the time the seedlings stand 15 cm tall they are far enough apart in the row that when the roots are mature they will not quite touch.* Some varieties have strongly attached tops that allow carrots to be hand pulled; in this circumstance the final thinning can be delayed until the roots are large enough to eat as baby carrots. Some varieties just won't be tugged out; the tops break off when you try. Thin these to their final spacing before the tops are 15 cm tall.

Keep the bed weed-free. With less fibrous (tender munching) varieties it's prudent to keep the topsoil moist at all times because irrigation or rain may cause splitting if the bed was dryish.

It seems carrot seedlings barely grow during their first month. Actually, a hair-like taproot is descending much faster than the leaves ascend. If the taproot does not encounter an impenetrable clod, a stone or zones of high nitrogen concentration, then the carrot will fill out straight and smooth rather than be forked, bent or terminated abruptly. If the topsoil remains moderately soft and if the carrots don't overly compete with each other or with weeds, then the roots may fill in uniformly.

To grow decent carrots in clayey soil, dig in a 50 mm thick layer of (preferably old) compost the previous autumn and then grow blue lupins or tic beans over winter. Next spring the bed will behave much more like loam. If pre-preparation didn't happen and now it is spring, then dig in only 25 mm of compost, use a variety that makes short pointy roots and hope for a good result.

Garden planning: Carrots may be sown anytime between mid-September and early February; they will be large enough to start harvesting about two months after they germinate. Most varieties can be harvested over a two

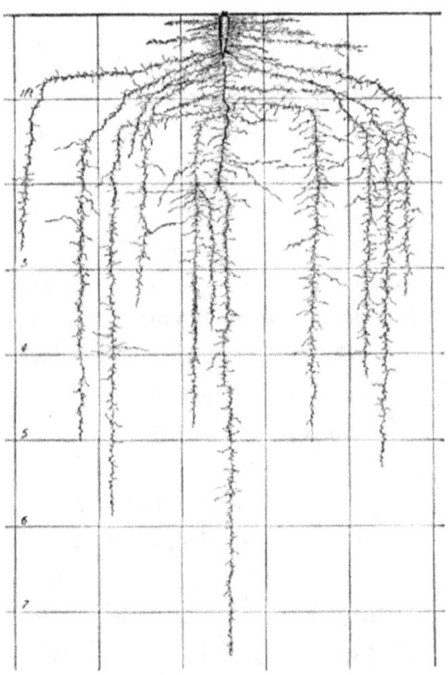

Carrot root system at harvest.

or more months but eating quality declines when they can't grow any larger. I start two-square-metres in spring. This patch will be harvested from late November into February. We sow two more square metres in mid-December (before the weather gets hot); these are eaten February through April. The final sowing early in February occupies several times as much area; this patch is for autumn/winter harvest. When fine roots start emerging from the carrots, usually about mid-August, we harvest everything and refrigerate them in plastic bags. These remain edible until thinnings from the first sowing of spring have become large enough to eat—I've just described how to produce a year round supply.

Insects and diseases: No problem.

Harvest: Some varieties make short- to medium-length carrots with strongly attached tops; in some soils you can harvest these by taking every other plant. Some varieties have weakly attached tops; these we must dig. Some varieties make long roots that must be dug.

Saving seed: Carrot is a bee-pollinated biennial that requires isolation of 1.5 km to get commercial level purity. Tasmania doesn't have wild carrot in its paddocks so it is not at all difficult to produce seed that is pure enough for the home garden as long as no nearby flower bed grows Queens Anne's Lace (a garden flower bred from carrot). During winter's harvest select perfectly shaped roots with a compact crown (where the leaves attach to the root). The carrot should neatly snub off or else smoothly taper into a single hair-like tap root. Select for smooth skin; good colour, etc. Select for flavour by tasting a slice taken off the bottom.

Replant selected roots with their crowns at the soil line, on positions 30 cm x 60 cm. Next spring they'll put up umbrella-shaped white flowers. Each flower approaches maturity in its own time over a span of a few weeks. Cut each flower with 10 centimetres of stem attached; do this when the seeds in it have turned brown but have not completely dried (too much seed will be lost if you wait that long). Spread the mostly-dried flowers on a tarp under cover to become brittle. Then rub between gloved hands until the seeds have separated. And then winnow out the chaff by first sifting out the large bits and then pouring what remains between two buckets in a light breeze. Carrot seeds form in pairs. If you want less thinning to do, wearing leather gloves rub the seeds firmly between the palms until the pairs separate. A dozen roots will make a litre of seed that might live ten years with decent storage. To reduce inbreeding depression of vigour involve at least 25 carrots in each seed production, better 50. Best a few hundred.

Varieties: Hybrids are extremely uniform. Because of that if hybrid varieties are not carefully and promptly thinned then overcompetition will cause many misshapen roots. Open pollinated varieties and especially heirlooms grown by amateurs exhibit huge differences in vigour from plant to plant; these produce more than a few misshaped roots no matter how expertly grown. However, when a crude variety is not carefully thinned the stronger plants still produce useful roots by overwhelming the weaker ones. Seed like this may be better for a gardener who doesn't thin carefully.

When the home gardener chooses a variety I think good flavour comes first and close after that comes considerations about fibre content (munchability raw) and lastly, shape. Cylindrically-shaped blunt-bottomed Nantes types and their modern descendants usually are tender because they develop less fibre; these are best for salads or munching raw. But very tender carrots often split when they get large. Nantes varieties differ in length. If your topsoil isn't soft then consider growing a shorter variety.

Southern Harvest (and Steve Solomon for his own garden) once conveniently imported excellent carrot seeds from England and USA. In the year 2015 Quarantine imposed expensive-to-comply-with carrot seed import restrictions. My best guess is the new rules assist commercial vegetable seed producers that made multi-million dollar investments in a carrot seed processing facilities here. These import barriers financially benefit farmers that get seed production contracts but small scale importers like our garden seed companies have been sacrificed.

Of Southern Harvest's varieties, Baby produces a good yield of slender, flavoursome Nantes type roots. And their Early Nantes is similar in quality but makes shorter roots. Mokum F1 is an excellent Dutch hybrid that tastes great. I mostly grow Mokum.

Birdland's Purple Dragon has been carefully selected for improved flavour, good visuals and strong tops that attract buyers at Saturday markets.

Mr. Fothergill's provides a wide choice. Their carrot seed packets are amply filled. Their hybrid varieties are uniform and far more productive compared to their open pollinated ones.

On clay soils best use short pointed varieties, like Chantenay.

Parsley / Parsley Root

(Petroselinum crispum)

Many people unnecessarily purchase seedlings when parsley is easy to direct seed *if started after the soil has warmed up but before summer arrives.* Parsley is rarely appreciated for its delicious root that tastes like parsnip and holds in the ground all winter. Parsley root can be roasted, steamed or whizzed to soup.

Culture: Parsley can be a low demand crop similar to carrot but it forms a less aggressive root system than carrot, which means that in order to harvest leaves in abundance parsley requires irrigation. Abundant leaf formation also requires nitrogen; give it moderate side dressing.

Leaf parsley: early in October sow 1 seed per cm, 1 cm deep, in rows 45 cm apart. Don't crowd the rows!

Keep seeds moist until germination; that may take two weeks. Thin progressively to 15 cm apart. Side dress if production of new leaves declines before March. Side dressing in autumn may trigger leaf diseases.

Root parsley: The slow-growing plants should be started the first half of October. In order to harvest smooth unforked roots the soil must be loose, friable and without clods. So if your soil tends to form clods don't prepare the bed until the soil is at the correct moisture content. Parsley roots develop acceptably in heavy soils that parsnip won't tolerate. Progressively thin to 15 cm apart. Finish thinning by the time the plants are 15 cm tall.

Garden planning: Two 1,200 mm rows of leaf parsley sown in early October produce a gracious plenty for us from December until next October.

Insects and diseases: There are wintertime leaf diseases that ruin some varieties. The cures are conducting a variety trial, balanced soil fertility and possibly strengthening the plant through foliar feeding during summer.

Harvest: *Leaf varieties:* in December and January harvest no more than half the leaves; leave half to feed the plant. Starting February old leaves turn yellow; these should be removed to increase air circulation. That's probably why later in summer Annie efficiently harvests all but a few plants with a complete haircut, taking everything above 100 mm tall. These plants soon regrow all new leaves. Less hardy varieties die back during winter, especially in frosty districts. If the crowns didn't rot then the root may resprout in spring for a second round of cutting. Dig *root parsley* from March until it starts making seed in spring.

Saving seed: Parsley is biennial and bee-pollinated. Seed is grown and harvested much like carrot. Allow the plants to overwinter and then make seed. Leaf varieties do not require digging and replanting because there is no reason to select for root shape. Off-type plants should be culled before they flower. Cut each branch after a few seeds on it have shattered. You'll harvest for more than one week. Fully dry the flowers under cover spread out on a tarp. Then rub the crisp flowers between (gloved, if tender-skinned) hands, and winnow.

Seed for root parsley should be produced from at least 12 carefully hand-selected near-perfectly shaped roots—50 perfect roots would be better. Involving several hundred roots prevents inbreeding depression of vigour. Select the finest as they are dug during winter and then promptly replant them on 30 cm x 60 cm.

Varieties: I've conducted variety trials involving as many as a dozen fancy European curly leaf varieties and noted subtle flavour differences; some varieties make longer stems; leaves on some varieties are more finely curled. These variations make little difference to most people. But the ability to resist leaf disease during winter also depends on variety, and that does matter.

Flat-leaf or "plain" types are stronger tasting than curly varieties. They're best for drying. They also tend to be more winter disease resistant.

Be aware—root varieties *might* be high-quality uniform selections (parsley root is a popular vegetable in Euroland) or it may be cheap stuff produced entirely for the home garden trade. Look for Dutch varietal names and high priced seeds. Quality stock will produce 95% near-perfect roots; cheap stuff may produce 15% smooth unforked roots. If you want to taste root parsley without the bother of growing it, then dig up a curly leaf plant and steam its forking rough root. The taste will be the same as root parsley; main difference involves how much trouble it will be to clean them and how little yield they'll bring.

Dry gardening: Grow like carrots, although parsley needs occasional fertigation if it is to do more than barely survive long rainless summers.

Parsnip

(Pastinaca sativa)

Parsnip *requires* deep loose topsoil to form long straight smooth roots. The seed is not long-lived; even when it is fresh less than half of it germinates. The biggest obstacle to success with parsnip is buying seed that will shoot so there's much gardener's lore about coaxing weak parsnip seeds.

Culture: Parsnip is a low demand subsoil feeder. Deeply dig in a full dose of COF. An early October sowing may get woody by summer's end. A January sowing remains choice eating through winter. A sowing before mid-February yields smaller roots that still are useful. Getting good germination in hot weather requires daily watering.

Sow seeds 1.5 cm deep, 2 seeds per cm in rows 45 cm apart. Consider covering the seeds with finely sifted compost if sowing in hot weather. Before reticulated water was the usual thing the parsnip seed row was covered with a plank that was lifted daily to check for germination. When the first seedlings pushed through the surface the plank was removed.

Thin the row carefully. Crowded tops fail to develop proper bottoms. The *minimum* final spacing should be 8 cm apart in the row. Thin before the tops are 150 mm tall! After that it becomes impossible to tug out plants. Crowded rows make *much* smaller irregularly formed roots.

Garden planning: Sowing early in October provides from mid-December through March. Roots sown in January will reach eating size before April and will hold through winter. If the subsoil is welcoming the leaves stay green and the bottoms size up slowly through winter. If the subsoil is infertile the leaves may get diseased and die back during winter but the roots will probably be fine.

Insects and diseases: Parsnip seems invulnerable to every Tasmanian pest except field mice. To reduce mouse damage use a hoe to pull up 5 cm of soil over the crowns with leaves still exposed to light. Do this in April.

Some varieties develop reddish-brown skin rust. And some roots adjoining the one attacked don't get the disease. If the rust has not penetrated deeply then peel it off and use the root. After I grew a few generations of seeds from roots that were free of rust I no longer saw the disease. Did I breed a better variety or did my subsoil improve?

Harvest: Dig as wanted. Early in spring they'll start putting out fine feeder roots marking the start of seed making; immediately dig the lot. Ours store for several more months in a fridge.

Saving seed: Like carrot. During winter when harvesting for the table transplant perfectly configured roots on positions 30 cm x 60 cm. Select for smooth skin, uniform taper, no forking, no side-branches and a tight tidy crown. If you have loamy soil select for long roots. If you have heavy ground, select for shorter roots. It is okay to cut off some of the bottom to make the root easier to replant, allowing selections to be made for better flavour and lack of a hard core.

Parsnip seed stalks grow two metres high and may fail to self-support in windy positions. I put tall garden stakes at the seed-making bed's corners and then stretch a chest-high restraint of haybale twine. Ripe seed readily shatters so cut each drying flower (with 100 mm of stem attached) when the seeds have turned light brown but before more than a few seeds have detached from that flower. I check every morning during the two week harvest period by giving the stem of every flower that looks like it might be done a sharp tap with my finger. If doing that makes a few seeds fly I take that flower. If no seeds detach I wait until the next day and check again. I spread out drying flowers on a tarp in the garage. The seed is liberated by rubbing dry flowers between the hands. Parsnip seed is too light to clean by winnowing. The best way to remove almost all the unwanted flower parts is with a coarse mesh sieve that catches the large bits and passes seeds through. That is clean enough for home use.

Parsnip seed can germinate well for three years but only if it starts out with high vigour and is stored cool and in low humidity air. High vigour is caused by excellent nutrition and achieving full ripeness. King flowers make larger seeds that shoot faster/stronger. To have the most vigorous possible seeds is to only use seeds from king flowers.

To prevent inbreeding depression of vigour, involve at least 25 roots in each seed production. It would be better to grow seeds from fifty roots. In my garden 25 roots produce 20 litres of seed that is dry, clean and ready to sow late in January, which is an excellent time to establish the winter patch. For many years I provided these fresh seeds to Southern Harvest. You could too.

Varieties: Achieving seed that produces smooth attractive roots requires *expensively* growing it from carefully chosen perfectly-configured full-sized roots. It costs a primary grower enormously less if plants just overwinter and then go to seed without ever being dug, selected and replanted. Combine that with short storage life, add in a dash of shonky business ethics and you'll see why I say that buying home garden parsnip seed is risky. Best you do the painstaking by-hand selection and the harvesting of one flower at a time yourself.

Melbourne Whiteskin improved considerably over the generations I grew the seed—until too many roots formed hard cores because I failed to choose seed making roots carefully enough. Now I produce Lancer that originated from Johnny's in Maine. Gardeners with brown rust problems might get better results from Gladiator F_1 (FOT). Birdland's Melbourne Market is good!

Dry gardening: Parsnip suits water-short situations if you plant in spring.

Potato

(Solanum tuberosum)

Potato is a solanum. So are heat-loving tomato, pepper and eggplant. But spuds thrive in cool weather. Tasmania provides plenty of that. You might think that potatoes are not worth your time and garden space. Think again. When spuds grow in fully remineralized soil their flavour is remarkably better than what the supermarket offers. My potatoes don't need sour cream, vinegar, salt, pepper or tomato sauce. Proper potatoes won't leave a bitter aftertaste; they are not treated with anti-sprouting chemicals.

Potato produces much more food from the space involved than any cereal crop. A fertile acre can produce enough wheat to feed six egg-laying chooks and generously supply the daily bread for an entire year. An irrigated eighth acre produces over two tons of potatoes if the crop starts with virus-free seed. And in case you did not pay attention to what I already said about bread making in the chapter about compost, wheat grown in Tasmania's humid climate usually produces a crumbly heavy loaf.

Culture: If your aim is to grow a family-sized nine month potato supply I have a method to share that gives you a high yield of large potatoes for the least work. Achieving maximum yield requires more than abundant balanced nutrients and plenty of soil moisture. It is essential to grow potato in always loose airy soil that allows tubers to swell easily. Farmers do everything possible to avoid compacting the potato field. These days they keep wheeled vehicles off the field by using centre pivot irrigators that also apply soluble fertilizers and chemicals.

Before there were herbicides, weeds in the potato field were eliminated by flipping loose soil up and over the forming spuds with a plow. This old fashioned technique can easily be imitated in the backyard garden with a common garden hoe.

Spring frosts kill potato vines to the soil line. New shoots will emerge but this setback lowers the final yield. So exercise patience. Start the *main storage crop* well after frost danger has passed. There'll still be plenty of time for it to mature. In fact, way too much time. I suggest mid-November as the best time for planting the main crop. Starting later than this reduces yield; starting earlier makes the crop finish before mid-March—and in consequence of finishing in warm soil you may dig sprouting tubers that don't store as well.

I put a single potato row down the centre of a 1,200 mm wide raised bed. I avoid compacting the soil by standing on the paths along either side of the bed. This much width for a single row may seem wasteful compared to what you may have seen driving by farm fields but my vines will thickly cover the entire bed and half the paths on both sides as they photosynthesise every erg of solar energy hitting that space. The yield of large potatoes will be enormous. Farmers can't sell large potatoes; they grow smaller ones.

Spread a full dose of COF plus an extra half dose over the entire 1,200 wide area and dig- or rotarycultivate it in. I increase the amount of fertilizer because I want the largest possible yield. I dig the fertilizer in deeply because potatoes feed well below the surface. After digging I spread compost over the bed 15 mm thick and shallowly hoe that into the surface. This makes for looser soil over the potatoes.

The very best seeds are small whole potatoes weighing 60- to 90 grams each because these don't have to be cut. Seed potatoes weighing more than 120 grams should be cut into pieces weighing at least 60 grams, better 90 grams. Ideally, each cut piece contains at least two eyes, three eyes at most. Carol Deppe depends on home grown spuds. She says it is unwise to plant a seed piece containing more than three eyes because every eye emits shoots; too many shoots emerging from one spot result in harvesting a larger number of smaller potatoes instead of fewer large ones. Carol says this precaution especially applies to finger varieties that normally form a great many eyes.

Many opinions exist about the best way to cut seed potatoes. Some say cut them a few weeks before planting and then hold the cut pieces in a cool place and in bright indirect light to let the surfaces heal over as the chunks start turning green. Greening-up encourages potatoes to sprout. When I tried cutting weeks before planting my seed pieces dried out so much that many of them failed to sprout. Some people plant immediately after cutting the pieces but first treat the cut surfaces with fungicide or natural rot suppressants. I think this is unnecessary bother in our climate. I plant immediately after cutting seed pieces, but I cut up *chitted* potatoes and almost never have a seed piece fail to shoot.

Chitting seed potatoes before they are planted encourages seed pieces to shoot before they rot. Commercial growers can't chit because sprouting seed potatoes demand gentler handling than machine planting allows. You on the other hand are going to plant by hand.

I urge you to buy seed potatoes mid-winter; the garden centres will have plenty then so you won't have to substitute a less desirable variety. Store seed potatoes in a cool completely dark place with air exchange (not in a plastic bag)—such as in a cardboard box in a shed. Even better in the fridge. Four weeks before planting spread them out in bright indirect light where it is cool but not cold (ideally 10°C). After a few weeks they'll green up and buds will appear at the eyes. If you've timed it right and it wasn't too warm during greening up these buds will not be shooting vines before you plant, or if they have started emit vines they will only be a few millimetres long and far less likely to be broken when planted.

Cut large potatoes immediately before planting. Take great care to not break off any emerging vines! If you started greening them up too soon or if storage conditions were too warm then there'll be a great many brittle sprouts. These will not cause any loss if they are not broken by rough handling.

Using a common garden hoe excavate a V-shaped furrow lengthwise down the centre of the bed that is at least 10 cm deep, better 15 cm deep. Gently place seed pieces in the bottom of it spaced 30 cm apart. If there's sprouts take care that the majority of them face up or at least are not pointing down. Use the hoe to pull a little soil over them. Do not completely refill the furrow.

Each action I suggest contributes toward putting *very loose* soil over the forming tubers and never stepping on the bed. Avoid compacting the bed!

Potatoes form along the vines close to the seed piece. They must be kept in the dark before harvest or else they'll turn green and become poisonous. After the vines have grown about 15 cm tall, place your feet at least 50 cm away from one side of the row, reach over the vines with a common garden hoe, press the blade lightly on the ground and pull it towards you, scraping up loose soil, depositing it against the vines. Do this from both sides of the row. This action, called "hilling up," also eliminates weeds. Now loose soil more deeply covers the base of the vines whilst the crop's rapidly expanding leaf canopy prevents rain and irrigation from compacting that soil. Hill up once a week; this gradually builds up a low mound over the bed's centre and also eliminates weeds. The first time you hill up only move 25 mm of soil over the row leaving plenty of vine still able to photosynthesize.

The vines grow taller and eventually they can no longer stand erect. This makes it impossible to hill up any more soil without damaging the vines. At this point there should be a long, low mound of loose soil that is at least 30 cm high and over 45 cm wide at the base. The soil you pulled up will be well protected by the vines so that irrigation or rain will not compact it. Consequently the yield will be larger. One more advantage to Steve's method: digging spuds out of loose soil takes far less effort. Synchronicity, eh?

After hilling up has finished there won't be many new weeds appearing. When an occasional weed makes its way through the vines and finds sunlight, hand pull it. It'll lift easily from the soft loose soil.

During its first weeks the potato only grows vine and leaves. Then flowers appear. Tubers start forming at the same time, not before that. Blooming goes on for some weeks. When flowering ceases new vines stop appearing, existing vines stop elongating and no more potatoes are set. The plant then concentrates on enlarging the tubers it has already started. While the plant was growing vines it needed lots of nutrients in order to make chlorophyll. During the time it fattens existing tubers it needs much less nutrition because tubers mostly contain starch, which is made from sunlight, water and carbon dioxide gas. The abundant fertility put into the bed before planting is also fading.

Summer is ending, light intensity lessens, sugar production slows as chlorophyll ages and loses photosynthetic efficiency, the leaves deteriorate, the potato skins thicken. The crop will store better if the spuds finish in dry soil. Then either frost kills the vines or they die back on their own. It's time to put the main crop into storage.

New potatoes. If you aim to enjoy new potatoes as soon as possible and have a good supply all summer then 10 days before the last usual frost date plant a few row metres of Pinkeye or Bismark. If a late frost blackens the emerging vines they'll soon reappear but the yield will be less. No big deal if that happens; this isn't the main crop that'll hopefully feed you through autumn and winter. Here's an occasion to cover the row with frost cloth; it also speeds up early vine growth. The fabric must be removed to hill up but after each hilling up I suggest putting it back over the row to accelerate growth. A few repeats and the (probably tattered) fabric will no longer be needed. By using frost cloth you'll dig new potatoes sooner.

Garden planning: One week before the tomatoes go out I plant five row metres of Bismark under frost cloth. This supplies us from December until we dig the main crop in April. I start the main storage crop mid-November. For this five row metres provides plenty for two oldies who try to avoid carbohydrates—most of the time. Our main crop stores until October—two sowings, a nine- to ten month supply. Grow spuds my way on anything except clay soil and you'll find that 10 row metres yields 100 kilos.

Immediately after digging the main crop I plant the ex-potato bed to garlic and shallot; I also could sow a green manure or overwinter broad beans.

Insects and diseases: Scab is a disease that attacks the potato's skin. It makes rough corky patches that have to be cut away before cooking. Scab is often said to be promoted by high soil pH so many garden writers oppose liming the potato bed. But the species actually has a high need for calcium. For a great many years the potatoes I grow with COF have been entirely free of scab. Perhaps that's because the amount of aglime in one dose of COF is small but the gypsum in COF makes a great deal of calcium available. Rotation does prevent scab so grow potatoes only once in four years in the same bed or row. However, the year after harvesting there will be volunteers coming up from tiny overlooked tubers. Destroy every one of them and do it right away before *they* form small tubers. And during that long rotation out of spuds do not grow tomatoes, peppers or eggplant. These solanums host the infection. And vigilantly yank nightshade, which is a wild solanum.

Aphids spread potato viruses. There are over 20 potato virus diseases. Viruses reduce plant vigour and lower yield. Potato viruses do not make their presence obvious. Once a plant has been infected the virus is carried ever after in its tubers. Each additional year that last year's potatoes become this year's planting seed the number of viruses in them increases—vigour and yield decrease accordingly. You might not experience a 50 percent yield reduction by planting your own small spuds grown from certified seed. Not the first year. But by the third year of sowing self-saved seed you'll pay a big price from reduced yield.

I don't know how many Tasmanians trade in certified seed potatoes. Most of them must provide farmers with the genuine article because most farmers that still are in business honour this proverb—*fool me once, your fault. Fool me twice, my fault.* Some seed potato sellers may provide garden centres with nothing but the genuine article. But from the erratic results I've had there must be some who misrepresent what looks like last year's below-market-grade eating spuds as being certified seed. The presence of infected seed soon becomes obvious when vines from some varieties more than cover the full width of the bed whilst other varieties form vines half that length and then yield very little. Yes, there are varietal differences in how long potato vines get but not this much difference.

Harvest: New potatoes eaten the day of harvest are a delicious treat. Three weeks after flowering begins dig the first plant in the row. Although only the size of hens eggs at this point they'll be the most delicious potatoes of all. But try to restrain yourself from digging another plant; the spuds you haven't harvested yet are getting larger by the day. Many Tasmanians bandicoot new spuds. When I've fished around with my fingers to grab a few I've caused so

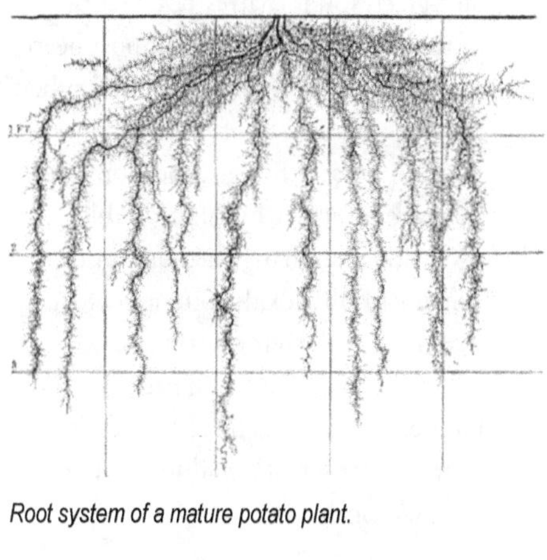

Root system of a mature potato plant.

much damage that the overall yield was reduced. I conclude it is better to just dig a plant. If you can't grow enough plants to dig a few early ones then I suggest creating a larger garden.

Best not to irrigate the storage potato crop in its last few weeks. Dry soil at the finish helps toughen the skins and improves storage. Ideally, dig potatoes after the vines have died, browned off. My vines have deteriorated but are still green in mid-April; I harvest anyway before it rains very much. Be gentle; do not bruise them. Do not wash potatoes before storage; washing greatly shortens storage life. Instead, try to dig when the soil is dry enough that the spuds come out of the earth fairly clean.

Potatoes could be left in their bed to be dug as needed through autumn and winter. But spuds may not keep as well in your ground as they do in mine; that depends on drainage and location—here's one circumstance when gardening in a higher elevation interior district advantageously produces a lower wintertime soil temperature. Why not try it for yourself; don't dig the last few row metres. Then lift one plant every few weeks. See what happens.

Green potatoes have become toxic throughout; they should not be eaten. Peeling off the green outer flesh does not eliminate the toxin. The green colour is not the poison; it is chlorophyll that formed because light was present. That light also induced the manufacture of solanine, a toxic alkaloid that now permeates the entire potato. Don't feed green spuds to livestock. Get rid of them—and not in the compost heap where they'll grow and make little tubers that . . . .

Ideal potato storage conditions are 90 percent relative humidity, stable 4°C with air exchange because spuds exhale carbon dioxide. But not colder than that. If the temperature goes below freezing, they're ruined. Should temperature go much below 4°C then potatoes convert starch into sugar and taste wrong.

Industrial potatoes are stored under ideal conditions and are treated with sprouting inhibitor chemicals. They can last until December. At Grindelwald I stored my harvest in a dozen cardboard citrus fruit boxes stacked one box wide and three boxes high, kept in a protected covered outdoor storage area with one open side—a dimly lit shallow cave. The boxes were not put hard against a wall so that every box had free air movement on at least two sides to facilitate air exchange. This worked fine at Gindelwald. It might not be protected enough in the interior. At Grindelwald potatoes in storage began sprouting around the end of August but remained acceptable eating through the end of September. At Chudleigh where winter nights are colder they remain edible through October.

Any spuds that get cut or otherwise damaged while being dug should be eaten within a few weeks. Spuds showing diseased spots should be discarded. If stored they may rot and then induce rotting in adjoining spuds.

Potatoes planted before mid-November mature before it has gotten cool enough to put them in storage. Spuds that finish early keep better in their bed. Dig them after mid-April.

Saving seed: I already explained why not to plant small potatoes from last-year's harvest. The exception would be an heirloom variety with such extraordinary flavour that a low yield doesn't matter.

Certified seed starts in a tissue culture lab where the most recently formed cell at the very tip of a growing shoot is sliced off microsurgically before that cell has been invaded by viruses. This clean cell is put into a nutrient/hormone solution and held under temperature and light conditions that induce the cell to morph itself into a plant. When that plantlet has grown large enough to be picked up with a tweezers it is placed in a tray of very fine potting mix and grown in a thoroughly screened greenhouse so that no aphids can be present. The small handful of tiny potatoes this plantlet eventually produces will be the size of quail's eggs and are properly named "first generation certified seed," often called minitubers in the trade.

Next year the minitubers are planted in high-elevation fields where aphids are naturally very few to none. Certified seed potato crops are increased there for several generations before there is enough to sell. Third generation certified seed has a very very low level of infection and would be too expensive to sell to farmers, who mostly use fourth generation seed which is still nearly virus free. Seed potatoes should no longer be called "certified" after the fourth generation of increase.

Varieties: I think there is a far better chance of getting genuine certified seed from varieties used by market gardeners—including Dutch Cream, Bismark and Pink Eye. Seed potatoes should be near perfect looking, free of scab, no rot spots and small. A small seed potato is called a "single drop" in the trade because it does not need to be cut. If the seed spuds resemble commercial culls that's probably what's offered.

Earlies. Bismark is the best early variety for the North. Southerners prefer Pink Eye. In my garden Bismark forms tubers before Pink Eye does. Bismark grows really big ones that store well. When Pink Eye grows large it forms deep hard to clean creases. Both varieties make great potato salad. My wife and I opine that Pink Eye tastes slightly better.

Main Crop. When I last grew Bintje the vines grew weakly and the yield was very low. Dutch Cream is the same general type of yellow-flesh all purpose potato but it yields abundantly.

Kennebec does well in many soils and situations; it bakes, mashes, roasts and fries. But it hasn't yielded much in recent years (virus?). King Edward is a multi-purpose heirloom still popular with many Tasmanians including the Solomons. Up To Date is also excellent for baking/roasting, but not for boiling because it self-crumbles into mush. Finger varieties are usually great boilers and good for salad.

Dry gardening: Potatoes were domesticated high in the Andes Mountains of what is now called Peru and Bolivia—a semi-arid cool climate. Consequently most varieties are still able to forage for water. In the early 20th century many tens of thousands of acres of American spuds were dry-farmed in regions getting around 500 mm of annual rainfall. When dry farming the yield is mostly determined by the amount of subsoil moisture at planting time. To dry garden spuds that taste good there must be deep, fertile, moisture-retentive soil. Make the row centres 1,500 mm apart and place seeds 45 cm apart in the row. The yield can be quite respectable if the crop gets any meaningful rain in summer. There's a classic book that details dry farming potatoes in the Soil and Health Library called *Dry Farming** by Widstoe.

Radish

(Raphanus sativus)

Salad radishes require always moist airy soil if they're to come out tender, crisp and mild. They grow poorly in clay. Winter/storage varieties are more forgiving.

Culture: Radish is a low demand crop that stores a great deal of water. Plants with even an half-developed edible part *survive* dry topsoil but become sharp-flavoured and spongy rather than mild, juicy and crisp. The light loamy soils that grow salad radishes the best don't naturally hold a big moisture reserve. Salad radish does much better in beds that are kept damp at all times. Specialist radish growers invest heavily in irrigation gear. We home gardeners make do. To keep my life simple I grow salad radish for spring and for autumn and we eat other things when the weather is warm.

Please consider the root system drawing on this page. Most of the roots of this salad radish form in the top 10 cm. So it might seem that a thin mulch placed shortly after germination would be highly beneficial to this crop, but maybe not—yes, mulched radishes grow better but the mulch also breeds slugs and shelters snails that will feed on the radish before you do.

Salad radish varieties reach full size three to four weeks after emergence. The seeds will germinate in September. One sowing provides around 10 days of harvest; then the radishes become pithy, strong flavoured and/or split. I sow one or two rows across the bed every two weeks from early September through mid-November. If you bought high quality seeds then almost every seed will sprout and nearly every one is capable of making a near-perfect radish. Carefully place one seed at a time every 10 mm along the bottom of a furrow that is 1 cm deep, the furrows need to be only 15 cm apart if you accept not being able to use a hoe between rows. It is easier to place radish seeds precisely than it is to thin crowded seedlings later on. *Radishes will not bulb properly when competing with each other;* they make the best bulbs when they've never ever been crowded. The plants should stand 2 cm apart in the row by the time the first pair of true leaves is fully developed. Be always mindful of the shallow root system—keep the hoe blade close to the surface.

Winter radish is best sown mid-February through mid-March. They can grow huge; the plants should stand at least 100 mm apart in the row. Black Spanish needs 150 mm in-the-row spacing. Between-rows spacing should be 45 cm—60 cm for some very leafy varieties. I usually plant a row or two of salad radishes at the same time.

Garden planning: Salad radish can be grown between rows of other vegetables that get sown at the same time. The radishes will be harvested and gone before the adjoining rows need the space. If you do this you also forego using a hoe between the rows.

Winter radish grows a little during mild sunny winter days. They go to seed in August. Once seed making initiates the radish would only be eaten to fend off starvation.

Insects and diseases: Slugs and snails disfigure the skins of salad radish.

Harvest: Salad radishes must be taken before they get large because they'll split and/or get spongy (pithy). Salad radish leaves make acceptable stir-fry or soup greens in early spring when there isn't much else to eat. Immature seed pods from blooming plants add a touch of mild radishy crunch to salads if they are picked before seeds develop.

Saving seed: Salad radish is an annual; seed production is easy and the seed yield per acre is high which is why seed grown without careful selection is super cheap. Radish is bee pollinated; to make pure seed it needs isolation of one kilometre or more.

In my opinion cheap radish seed should only be used for salad sprouts the same way lucerne sprouts go into salads. It's a heartbreaker to sow this junk expecting to get salad radishes out of it. Producing radish seed that mostly makes well-formed vegetables is not so easy and not so cheaply done.

To produce junk radish seed fertilize for a low demand crop, use a low plant density, like 30 cm apart in the row, rows 60 cm apart, allow it grow on, control the weeds and soon it goes to seed! The seeds form in pods resembling those of the cabbage family. Harvest the entire plant when most of its pods have dried; finish drying the plant on a tarp under cover and when nearly crisp, pull the tarp out into the bright sun of midsummer to dry completely for an afternoon, maybe more than one

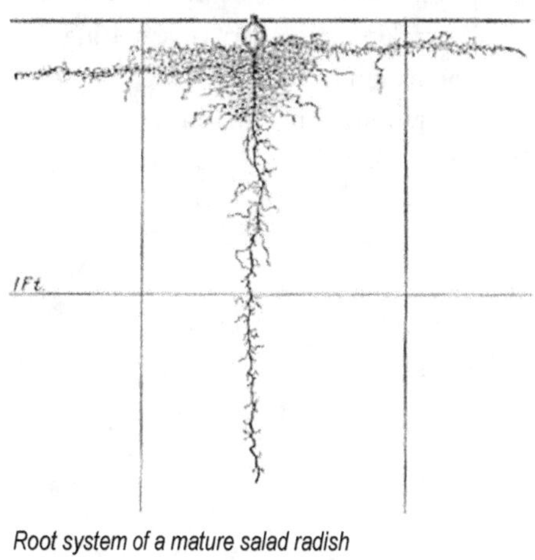

Root system of a mature salad radish

afternoon until all is crisply dry. Then thresh (scuffle dance on the straw). Then sieve out the sticks and large bits. Then finish the job by winnowing. The general method I have just described is termed "seed-to-seed" in the trade.

If you want seeds that produce a high percentage of useful salad radishes then select perfect roots for seed production when harvesting for the table. Choose a uniform shade of red (or what ever colour they're supposed to be), choose only perfectly round roots (or ideal cylinders with proper blunt bottoms if it is French Breakfast); select for thin tender translucent-looking skins, a single fine hairlike taproot and a tight refined crown. Go so far as to taste a thin slice off the side. I prefer mild, sweet and juicy, not mustardy hot and dry. Then remove the large leaves to reduce moisture stress (do not remove smaller developing leaves) and transplant. Bury them up to the crown, spaced 30 cm apart in rows 60 cm apart. Involve at least 25 individuals in a seed production (100 near-perfect selectees would be far better if you intend to repeat this through several generations). I suggest choosing perfect individuals out of a starting population at least ten times greater.

My advice—do not make seeds by starting with a low quality variety. If you make that mistake you'll be lucky if one plant in three or four makes a bulb vaguely resembling what the variety is supposed to be, much less find numerous perfect radishes. It is possible to restore a degenerated variety by working with a very large starting population carried on through many generations. But why bother. Start with quality.

Winter radish should overwinter before going to seed in spring. Perfect specimens are discovered one at a time whilst harvesting for the table; these are immediately replanted up to the crown at a spacing of 60 cm x 75 cm. Winter radish puts up enormous sprays of seed stalks in spring. Some varieties could use 100 cm x 100 cm. If the root is too long to conveniently replant, cut off some from the bottom. It won't matter.

Grow all types of radish seeds in positions where irrigation may be withheld while they are drying down. If English sparrows take interest in a radish seed patch they will harvest almost all the seed as fast as it ripens. Be prepared to drape bird netting over the plants when the seed pods begin to fill.

Varieties: Some winter radish varieties are pungent. They all have thicker skins than salad radish; most require peeling. Given good growing conditions, commercial quality open pollinated varieties yield a high percentage of near perfect radishes—like over 80 percent. Hybrid salad varieties should make 90+% perfect radishes. If a catalogue or seed rack offers you a few commonly found varieties cheaply and one or two selections at a higher price (these days, likely a hybrid), buy the costly seed.

Tasmania has no insect pests that seem to prefer eating radish leaves so we gardeners can use short-topped varieties that yield the most from small spaces. Tall-topped varieties, of which Champion is the old standard, work well in earlier sowings and for autumn but when days lengthen Champion and Easter Egg, which was bred out of Champion, rapidly become pithy.

Salad radish varieties may intentionally be pungent or they may be mild and sweet but all varieties are intended to be crisp, not pithy, intended to not split, not to make multiple tap roots nor get unpleasantly hot and dry. No salad radish variety should have thick, tough or rough skins. If the variety you grew did any of these things, try another variety next year; maybe try another seed company.

I've always had difficulties with White Icicle; it usually becomes hot and pithy despite all my efforts.

Some varieties of long white Asian radish are supposed to be for summer production but in my garden these bolt to seed before sizing up; autumn/winter varieties do fine. I especially treasure Black Spanish, a long-keeping black-skinned pungent white-fleshed winter radish that grows nearly as large as swede and holds in the garden from late April through August. After peeling the thick skin I grate them, mix in freshly-diced raw onion, olive oil and black pepper. Nero Tondo (SH) is an improved Black Spanish. And I heartily recommend those long red-topped white skinned winter radishes deriving from the heirloom China Rose. Where Black Spanish is rather dry-fleshed and pungent, these cylindrical winter radishes are mild, juicy, tender when eaten raw and are good in stir fries too.

Dry gardening: Salad radish is possible to produce without irrigation if sown early in spring; they finish before the topsoil dries out. For winter radish, absolute dry gardening is possible in the rare year that it rains enough early in March to make the soil damp. Or, reserve some water to start them off and keep them going until it does rain.

Cucurbits

Garden cucurbits—cucumber, melon, pumpkin, zucchini and other similar squash—are a plant family that makes annual fruiting vines. None of them withstand frost and all are poorly adapted to cool damp weather. Melon and cucumber (and possibly squash too) originated as semi-arid-climate plants that extend a tap root deep into subsoil moisture—many cucurbit vegetables still make strong taproots as well as *a network of surface feeding roots that can reach as far as the vine goes.* All cucurbits do best when they are directly seeded because confinement in a container terminates the taproot and cucurbit roots often get damaged during transplanting.

When stressed late in summer by humidity, less light energy and colder nights, cucurbit leaves inevitably will be covered with powdery mildew. This disease prevents photosynthesis and soon kills the plant. Foliar feeding aerated compost tea and/or a balanced complete foliar a few times during summer helps fend off PMD.

Please try foliar feeding zinc against PMD; this method works in my garden. Cucurbits are big users of zinc. I speculate that cucurbits may succumb more readily to PMD after they have assimilated the readily available zinc in their root zone. As soon as PMD appears on any cucurbit in the garden dissolve one scant tablespoon (15 gm) of zinc sulphate into three litres of water and spray that on all cucurbits until water drips off every leaf. Best do this in the morning before the sun gets strong. Any PMD already on the leaves will immediately die because you sprayed slightly salty water.

Spraying bicarbonate of soda at one tablespoonful per three litres also instantly kills PMD but with bicarb the disease returns the next day. If zinc shortage was the cause then the vine may remain PMD free for a few weeks. Eventually it will succumb anyway.

For my convenience I will use the American term "squash" to refer to zucchini, marrow and pumpkin. I rank cucurbits according to how well they handle cool humid conditions. Best is squash and then in declining order, cucumber, cantaloupe, and worst, watermelon. Most squash varieties do okay on Tassie although traditional mainland pumpkins may not get enough heat here to fully ripen, especially this is so in our cooler microclimates. Cucumber requires warmer conditions than squash so it must be started a few weeks later than squash. Melon is even less chill- and humidity-tolerant than cucumber. A very few hybrid melon varieties produce half-sized but still delicious fruit in the warmer parts of Tassie if they are encouraged with black plastic mulch. They are like eggplant in this respect.

Direct seeding cucurbits requires technique, patience—and most years, persistence. Sun Tzu's *The Art of War* defines patience as self-control over one's impulses. With cucurbits, restraining your desire to get the summer garden going is the key to success. All types of cucurbit seeds require warm soil to germinate. Don't even try to sprout squash seeds before the soil reaches 18°C five centimetres below the surface. Cucumber seeds need it a few degrees warmer, I'd say at least reach 21°C for a good part of the day. And I urge new gardeners not to guess when their soil does get warm enough. Any gardener that has not yet been educated by a soil thermometer definitely should be. Once a gardener has seen how weather conditions (sun/cloudy) (warm/chilly) change soil temperature then they'll know by gut feel when the soil has become warm enough. And when it isn't.

Cucurbit seeds are large; they should be placed deep enough in damp soil (not soggy) that they won't need

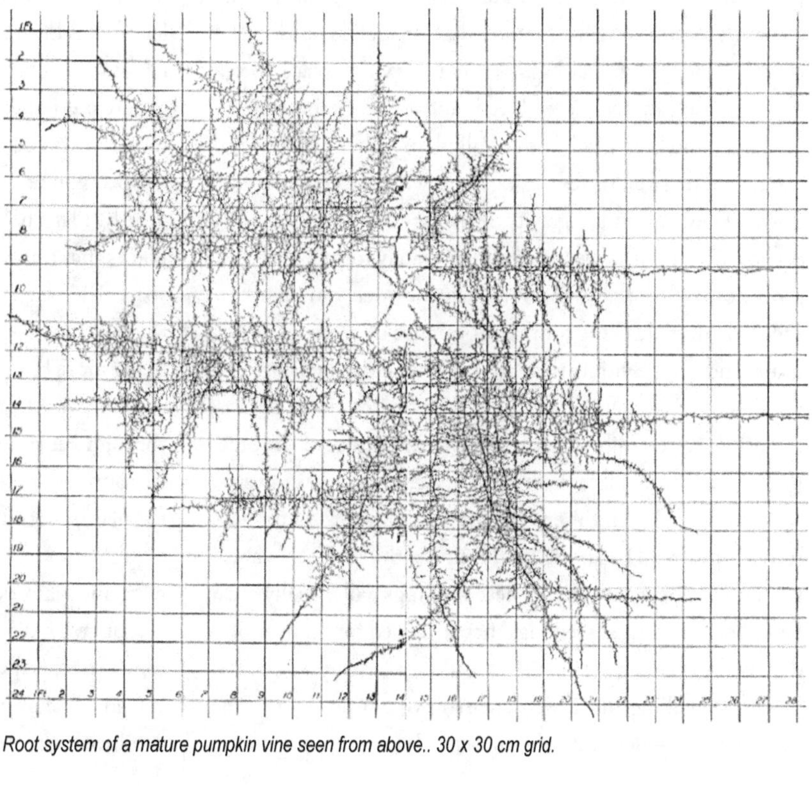

Root system of a mature pumpkin vine seen from above.. 30 x 30 cm grid.

daily watering. I'd say 25 mm under is enough. Gardeners who frequently water germinating cucurbit seeds often experience poor results. Pray the weather doesn't become rainy from sowing until seedlings emerge. Cucurbit seeds germinate very slowly—if they germinate at all—when the soil is chilly and wet. If they do start to shoot in chilly damp soil then the seedlings may catch PMD before they reach the surface. Ideally, the root enters warm damp soil while the shoot comes up through warm dry soil.

Spring usually brings some chilly, rainy days between sowing and emergence. The best thing to do when that happens is to sow again a few inches away from the first lot as soon as conditions stabilize. Some springs I've had to make three adjacent sowings on the same hill, each one a week after the previous. Whichever sowing grows best dominates the position; seedlings that grow less well are eliminated.

You'll get faster and far more certain germination by chitting cucurbit seeds. Chitting is wise practice every year but this technique really shines when spring weather is unusually unsettled. Cucurbit seeds must not be soaked in water. Instead, fold two separate squares of kitchen paper towelling into quarters. Sandwich a few cucurbit seeds between them. Position each seed carefully so that the ends of the seed from which the root emerges all point in the same direction. Moisten the paper until water drips out and then, holding the sheets between your palms, press them together firmly. Squeeze out as much water as will easily release; don't try make the towels too dry because even ten big seeds in the sandwich adsorb a lot of water. Then put the damp seed sandwich inside a small airtight container such as fast food comes in, or use a zipper bag. Put that in a warm place, ideally at 24°C. You can stack several seed sandwiches in the same container and keep track with small plastic labels. Position the container so all the emerging roots will point straight down. They respond to gravity. If a root doesn't emerge downward from the seed it will immediately form a loop and grow downward; that will not be helpful when you plant the seed. Start checking for the appearance of roots after 48 hours and every 8 hours thereafter. Plant all the seeds before the first root to emerge gets longer than the seed itself because the brittle roots easily snap off and this kills the seed. At each position carefully place three already sprouting seeds in very loose moist soil with the emerging root pointing down, the seed's top should be about 25 mm under the surface. Leaves will appear a few days later. These seedlings will initially grow faster than unchitted seedlings that struggled for many more days before finding light.

Before making any flowers cucurbit vines must first form a genetically predetermined number of leaves, often as many as ten. Suppose it is ten—the first flower develops from the eleventh leaf notch. The next five to seven leaf notches all emit male flowers; only then does the vine start alternating male and female flowers. Male flowers open at the end of a long thin stem, last for a day and then fall off. Female flowers attach to an ovary that resembles a miniature fruit. Obviously, no fruit can be set until female flowers appear. The appearance of the first female flower usually takes one month in Tassie. Achieving fully ripe pumpkins or very many ripe melons demands getting them to set sooner. The gardener can provide a head start by raising transplants, or far better, by sowing chitted seeds. Young vines grow faster in warm conditions. Best that melon grows above a sheet of black plastic spread over the surface—like eggplant.

All garden cucurbits may be fed like high demand crops; they'll yield much more and grow larger. However, early growth *must* be slow until conditions warm up. A slow-growing plant can not use many nutrients. In fact, intaking nutrients in excess of the immediate requirement soon makes a plant unhealthy. So start cucurbits as low-demand crops; then side dress and/or fertigate as soon as the vine begins growing fast. Side dress several times; stop side dressing around the end of January or a month before there is no more unoccupied bed space. I spread COF in a 30 cm wide ring atop bare soil where vines will soon be. The well fed vines soon cover that side-dressing and it is time to side-dress again.

Competition reduces the production of new fruit. This is especially true of bush summer squash including zucchini. The plant may appear to be a bush because the interstem length has been compressed by breeding but the root system of some varieties still resembles a spreading vine. Imagine a 10 square metre bed is assigned to zucchini. Most gardeners cram ten or more zucchini plants into that space. By December the bed will be terminally crowded; fruit production slows greatly. Plant health declines sharply. Suppose instead of 10 plants that only three zucchini plants were given that entire space. By the end of January these three will entirely cover the bed, have formed side branches and will have produced many more high quality fruit than ten crowded plants could have. Abundant production on this bed continues through February. These three plants may expand over the surrounding paths. If those paths were dug up and fertilized the plants would continue into adjoining beds.

To get more early production from bush squash, start with one plant per square metre. After they have produced one or two fruits each you can tolerate eating fewer zucchini for the next few days. So eliminate seven plants and lightly spread COF over the gaps. The three survivors soon will produce more than the ten plants did. The same principle holds true of maxima pumpkins. At Grindelwald two hills with only one maxima pumpkin vine in each were repeatedly side-dressed. These two rapidly covered 40 square metres and produced around 40 big pumpkins.

Most garden books say cucurbits often wilt during mid afternoon heat and that this is harmless. Incorrect! Wilting is a yield-lowering stress that can easily be prevented. Afternoon wilting happens because two or more plants growing from the same position must *compete* for moisture, not because the topsoil has become slightly dryish while sun is strong. Having two plants per position is smart strategy in much of North America, where one squash vine borer can collapse an entire plant in an instant. The borer is most destructive early in the season, leaving plenty of time for the surviving plant of the initial pair to fully occupy the space. Tasmania has no squash vine borers but we do have too many garden books from the United States.

Pollination is done by bees. Varieties that can cross should be separated by two kilometres. Fortunately, it is not difficult to keep bees out of cucurbit flowers and hand-pollinate them. Only a few intentional pollinations result in a great many seeds. With squash, *very early in the morning* before the bees are at work, remove a freshly opened new male flower and strip off its petals, leaving only the stamen with a coating of pollen on its tip. Then locate a female bloom that first opened that morning. Insert the stamen into the female flower and brush the pollen receptor with it. Then protect the female bloom from bees for a few days—twist the tip of the flower shut and secure it with a loop of string. The petals drop off by themselves after the ovary can no longer be pollinated.

Cucumber and melon flowers are too small to pollinate that way. For these, one day before a female flower opens put it into a small bag made of cheesecloth or spun polyester fabric tied to the stem behind the flower. The beeshield is removed to hand pollinate the flower and then it is replaced. Remove the bag a few days later to let the fruit develop.

Mark the ovary by tying a brightly coloured piece of yarn or strip of cloth to the stem and permit this individual fruit to get fully ripe before picking it. Be sure to avoid inbreeding; transfer pollen between different plants. Several cucurbit generations can be produced from only a few plants without noticeable loss of vigour.

Cucumber

(Cucumis sativus)

Culture: Impatient gardeners transplant garden centre cucumber seedlings at the same time they put in tomato seedlings but the weather is still too unsettled. All too often these seedlings die, or if they do survive they don't start growing fast for nearly one month because of all that stress—if they ever do grow properly again. Instead, make a cost-saving bet by sowing chitted cucumber seeds one week *after* the tomatoes go out; many years these will fail to shoot or if they do shoot then the seedlings likely will emerge with PMD or soon catch it. In that event immediately rechit and resow. I prefer to sow chitted cucumber seeds three weeks after the tomatoes go out. Starting later means harvesting sooner.

Position each plant in the centre of a competition-free root zone at least 1,500 mm diameter. In our polytunnel one cucumber vine has covered twice that much area by mid-February. To stay healthy the root system must occupy that much soil even when the vine climbs a trellis. Follow the general procedure for all cucurbits.

Garden planning: Two positions soon yield more than we can give away. In early January the harvest starts with one cucumber every other day. Then three. By February we pick 15 to 20 every other day. The vine starts failing around mid-March along with the fading summer. It would break down much sooner if it lacked growing room.

Insects and diseases: Other than powdery mildew I've had no troubles. Some varieties are said to be "mildew resistant." That usually means they'll survive a few days longer than varieties that aren't. Then again, "resistant" could really mean that they successfully make tasteless cucumbers when growing on depleted farm soils.

Harvest: Making seeds is a huge effort for the plant; it greatly reduces fruit set. So don't miss any fruit when harvesting and pick them when half of full size. Smaller is tastier.

Saving seed: Cucumbers do not cross with other cucurbit species. The Armenian cucumber, sometimes called Giant Serpent, is actually a melon that doesn't cross with other cucumbers. Incidentally, newly-pollinated rockmelon and honeydew that still are the size of a lemon taste like a cucumber.

The seeds within are mature when the skin has turned yellow-white. Remove the seeds with the pulp around them and ferment all this in a bowl at room temperature (20°C to 25°C), stirring daily. The pulp liquefies after a few days. Promptly pour the ferment into a strainer and wash the seeds thoroughly to remove all pulp. Fermentation also removes the sprouting inhibitor. Then spread the seeds out on a newspaper to dry completely at room temperature.

Varieties: Marketmore, an open pollinated supermarket-style slicer, works well. Southern Harvest has other varieties of this type and several productive pickling varieties. One of them is gynoaceous, meaning it makes only female flowers so it starts bearing sooner but only does that when there is another variety nearby that makes both male and female flowers.

What we call "burpless" varieties are intolerant of cool weather. On Tassie only the earliest burpless hybrids work outside of a polytunnel. Suyo Long is the traditional Asian burpless OP; in my experience it is not early and performs poorly outdoors. I checked every burpless variety offered in every Aussie seed catalogue and couldn't find anything I'd gamble on in Tassie. If I strongly fancied this type I'd pray for seeds of Tasty Jade (JSS) to unexpectedly arrive in my mailbox. Or grow burpless varieties in a polytunnel.

Apple, Lemon or Crystal are similar heirlooms that make lemon-sized fruit with a remarkably sweet flavour and crisp texture. The aggressive vines suit large gardens and dry gardening.

In my opinion, the best tasting cucumber by far is variously called the Middle Eastern, Beit-Alpha or Lebanese. This sort is small, crisp and sweet. The thin skins need not be peeled. Most Lebanese varieties grow where summers are hot-hot and humidity is low. On Tasmania most Lebanese varieties are late to form fruit and are relatively unproductive. This is especially true of open-pollinated varieties on seedracks. A few mid-eastern hybrids that are truly early can yield heaps. Southern Harvest has much interest in this sort and offers more than one variety. Craig RZ from Activevista works great in our polytunnel and is delicious.

Dry gardening: Make hills 2 metres apart in all directions, thin early to one plant per hill. Bearing vines are fertigated every two to three weeks. Crystal-Apple-Lemon especially suit dry gardening.

Melon

(C. melo, Citrullus lanatus)

Tassie's cool nights are difficult for melons. Only a very few hybrid varieties yield much, these must be coaxed and their seeds must be imported if Quarantine allows it that year. Watermelons are the diciest—usually succeeding only in the warmest districts on light soils growing over black plastic.

Culture: Melons do best in sandy soil that warms up quickly in spring. Less-gooey clay soils may barely grow them if heavily amended with organic matter. A black plastic mulch (see "eggplant") or a cloche provides melons with more heat. Even on dark-coloured loam, black plastic covering the bed makes a big difference.

During the last week of October chit a few seeds for every plant finally wanted. About a week prior to chitting, prepare and fertilize the entire melon bed for a low demand crop. Then make super fertile hills 1,500 mm apart along the centre of a 1,200 wide bed; blend 125 ml of COF under each hill and side-dress another 125 ml outside the base of the hill. Then spread a sheet of black plastic large enough to drape over the bed's edges. Anchor it with soil along the edges, leaving as much plastic exposed to the sun as possible. On the day the seeds are ready to plant, cut out a 15 cm diameter hole over each hill. That way the plastic will have heated the soil where the seeds go. Carefully plant three chitted seeds about 25 mm deep below each opening and when doing this scatter a few snail pellets under the plastic immediately around the hole because the plastic makes a slug- and snail haven where the only vegetation they'll have to nibble will be the emerging melons.

Gradually thin each position to one plant. In an average summer you'll start harvesting melons in February. If the year proves a hot one you may enjoy melons through mid-March. The first time you irrigate (or it rains) there'll be small puddles at every low spot. Make a small hole in the plastic at each low spot. I do this with a gutterspike (long fat nail) lashed to a broomstick.

Garden planning: Hope to harvest six small melons per position in a good summer. When the vines fall apart in mid-March, clean up the bed. Around mid-April sow a green manure.

Insects and diseases: Cooler nights and morning dews in early March weaken all varieties. Then the leaves get PMD, all ripening ceases and any immature fruit rots.

Harvest: *Cantaloupe/rockmelon* skins develop a yellow-orange tint as they ripen but colour doesn't determine when to harvest. Both rockmelons and honeydews (muskmelon) slip the vine (detach) easily when they are truly ripe. Push *gently* on the stem where attaches to the fruit. If light pressure separates melon from vine, it is ripe. If it doesn't slip the vine, try again tomorrow. Rockmelons and honeydews do not ripen after harvest. They only ripen when living leaves put more sugar into the fruit. Supermarket cantaloupes have been bred to appear ripe when they still are unripe because truly

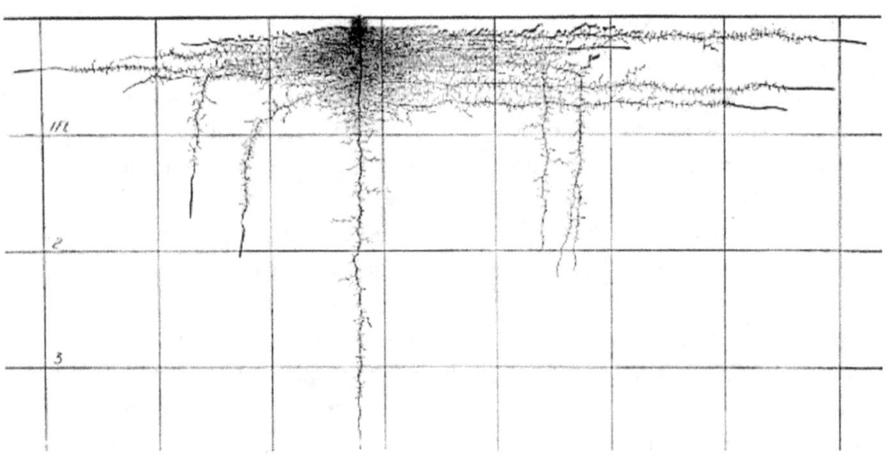

Root system of a half-grown cucumber plant. (Each square is 30 x 30 cm.)

ripe cantaloupes are too soft to ship inexpensively and have a short shelf life. Supermarket stuff may soften a bit if left on the kitchen bench for some days but it cannot become sweeter or tastier, only softer and rottier.

Watermelons do not ripen after harvest. They do not slip the vine when ripe; instead, the thumpy sound they make when knocked on with the knuckles must be knowledgeably assessed before picking. I lack the vocabulary to describe the sound. After harvesting a few you'll know too.

Saving seed: Rockmelons have netted skins; they do not cross with muskmelons such as honeydew, which has smooth skin; neither one crosses with watermelon. When the fruit slips the vine the seeds are mature. With watermelon I'd let the fruit start to rot in the field before taking the seeds. Extract seeds, put in sieve, wash until clean, spread on paper to dry. Sadly, even the earliest open pollinated melon varieties yield little in Tasmania. So I don't produce OP melon seed.

Varieties: The earliest open pollinated varieties at best provide a few small melons if grown above black plastic. A few early hybrid varieties do modestly well if grown above black plastic. In many years of conducting melon trials in Oregon I've seen dozens of supposedly early hybrids fail to ripen anything during cool summers. Sugar Baby does okay in warmer districts. Blacktail Mountain (BIRD) actually produces watermelons! Mountain Sweet cantaloupe (BIRD) actually produces too. Probably thanks to Quarantine, Sam Bayley (SH) seems to have given up on melons. He used to have several varieties but now only provides Hale's Jumbo, which I'd consider a wild gamble outside a polytunnel. Were I a melon fanatic I would be strongly tempted to scoff at Quarantine's restrictions and ask a North American friend to send seeds from Territorial, Adaptive or West Coast. *Anything* these companies offer would work on Tasmania.

Dry gardening: Like cucumbers.

Zucchini and Pumpkins

(Cucurbita spp.)

North Americans call pumpkins "winter squash." They call marrows and zucchini of all shapes and colours "summer squash." Fair enough.

Culture: Squash seedlings withstand conditions that ruin cucumber and melon. Squash seeds germinate when the surface inch has warmed to 20°C whilst the sun is shining on it. Very vigorous squash seeds manage to shoot (slowly) when the soil is a few degrees colder than that *if the soil is not too wet.* But because it took so long to emerge this exhausted seedling starts out growing so slowly that seedlings emerging two weeks later into better conditions outgrow it from the start and end up yielding sooner.

Fertilize the entire bed for a low demand crop. Sow seeds when or soon after you set out tomatoes, ideally at the beginning of a week-long period of sunny weather. To avoid lowering soil temperature *minimize watering until seedlings appear; if it must be done, do it in the morning and pray for a sunny day that rapidly warms the soil.*

Summer squash: Spacing depends on variety. For most bush varieties sow on positions 1,200 mm x 1,200 mm. Some varieties can use more space. (In a polytunnel I use 1,800 x 1,500.) Be prepared to sow again (and again) should the weather turn poor before emergence. Initially thin to the best two plants per position. These days hybrids get the breeder's attention; open pollinated varieties often throw off-type plants, so let these two plants grow on until they make their first fruits. Then allow only the best plant in that position to remain. I know this will seem like wasteful murder to many but the loss of yield will be very temporary.

Three pumpkin species are grown in Tasmania: Cucurbita *maxima,* C. *moschata* and C. *pepo.*

C. maxima makes aggressive vines and (usually) large hard-skinned pumpkins with large seeds that often taste good. Position C. *maxima* 2.5 to 3 metres apart on a bed at least 3 metres wide. When C. *maxima* varieties are given that much fertile root zone be prepared to find vines crossing paths and invading neighbouring beds and then some. I usually locate C. *maxima* at the garden's edge where vines can run over the grass or temporarily grow over a working compost heap.

C. pepo makes smaller vines that yield small pumpkins with smaller sized seeds that usually do not taste good (excepting some of the American jack-o'-lantern pumpkins). Pepo vining varieties cope when crowded at 100 cm x 120 cm but do better on 120 cm x 150 cm.

C. moschata produces butternuts. Their vines are intermediate in spread between C. *pepo* and C. *maxima.* Butternuts are heat lovers; I would only attempt them where a lemon tree will thrive—thrive, not just barely survive.

A short-season high-elevation Tasmanian garden can fully ripen pepo pumpkins if they have 100 consecutive frost free summer days. Maxima pumpkins make fast progress towards getting ripe only when the temperature is above 20°C and the sun is shining. Traditional mainland varieties are maxima, they need 120 warm sunny days to fully mature seed and develop full-flavoured flesh. Some years most of northern Tasmania gets just about that much heat.

Side-dress pumpkins and summer squash in rings 30- to 45 cm wide just beyond the plant's perimeter. Once that zone of fertilized soil has been covered (in sunny warm weather this much advance could happen every few days), side dress again.

Stop side-dressing squash about the end of January. If the plants run out of uncontested space before the end of February then next year consider giving them more root zone. Given enough growing room a zucchini may abandon its bush habit and start branching out like a pumpkin vine. I've more than once seen one summer squash bush branch out and cover a 3.5 metre circle.

Garden planning: Two zucchini plants given full sun, rich soil, abundant irrigation *and adequate competition-free space* will provide a family with more than they could ever want from Christmas through February, and then yield less through much of March. Because Annie and I thrive on zucchini, about mid-December I may start two more plants on close spacing (1,200 mm apart on a bed 1,200 wide) because they'll not grow so large before the season ends. These new ones still have the vigour of young plants when the first sowing declines.

One *C. maxima* vine given all the space, fertility and moisture it could use produces 50 to 100 kilograms. *C. pepo* pumpkin vines may yield ten to fifteen fruits weighing 1 to 2 kg.

Insects and diseases: I will reinforce here what has already been said in my introduction to cucurbits. Squash get powdery mildew when the weather becomes too cool and too humid to suit them. Squash seedlings can emerge with PMD if they manage to shoot in chilly wet soil. Diseased seedlings take a long time to resume proper growth if they ever do. Should the weather turn against you while squash seeds are germinating, immediately sow again in the same position or hill even before the first sowing emerges (or fails to do so).

Variety has a lot to do with susceptibility to PMD. One summer I tried growing Gem squash, a globe-shaped South African combination summer squash and pumpkin (pepo) with an aggressive vine.

I had successfully grown Gem in Oregon. Perhaps my success in Oregon was because Territorial Seeds imported the seed from South Africa. The strain of Gem I tried in Tasmania came from Queensland. It must have been selected to suit Qld. The vine grew vines rather slowly in my garden; it was a month later than ordinary zucchini to start flowering. By late January the first fruit were setting on those vines but the stress of fruit formation lowered resistance to PMD. And the plant died.

Sometimes pumpkin skins are damaged where the fruit rests on the soil. Storage life is reduced when this happens. It seems the damage is caused by slugs and snails or other soil animals. In the last few years I've seen much less skin damage. I think that's because I have steadily increased the amount of potassium in my soil. Potassium helps make harder skins. Side dressing an additional 250 ml of potassium sulfate per 10 square metres of root zone should be enough.

Harvest: Summer squashes are best picked small when they still have tender skins and the best flavour. Permitting a zucchini to grow into a marrow places a reproductive burden (seed formation) on the plant that reduces new fruit set.

In most parts of Tasmania, C. *maxima* pumpkins need every possible growing day to fully ripen flesh and seed. Almost-ripe pumpkins have pale orange flesh, thinner, less-vigorous seeds and less flavour. Fully ripe pumpkin flesh is usually deep orange; fully ripe seeds are plump after drying down. A completely ripened-on-the-vine pumpkin has a shrivelled brown stem that no longer transports nutrients. I have never seen shrivelled stems on Sweet Grey or on Queensland Blue but my wife's son has; he lives at St. Helens. Allowing pumpkins to remain on the vine for one week after powdery mildew has killed off most of the leaves helps them ripen a little more. However, leaving pumpkins out in the weather and frost also initiates skin damage that lowers storage potential. I've no certain answer about this conflict. I bring mine indoors when the deteriorated vine can no longer produce a useful amount of sugar.

To enjoy the longest possible storage life, sponge off pumpkin skins with disinfecting-strength bleach solution or fill the kitchen sink with it and then roll each pumpkin around in disinfectant for a few moments. Then cure the skins by drying them indoors at room temperature for a week or so. Pumpkins ideally store best at 12°C with low humidity air freely moving around them on all sides (and the bottom, too). Sweet Grey has lasted until early October lined up and tilted on their sides on a workbench in our garage. Why tilted? Because humidity tends to be trapped in the depression around the stem if the pumpkin sits flat, bringing about rotting. I've successfully held Sweet Grey over the winter in an unheated guest bedroom. I have stashed them under the sink in the kitchen where they soon formed rot spots. I have seen Sweet Grey stored on a covered veranda all winter; these were still in good nick when the tomato seedlings went out. Perhaps they kept so well because they had grown out of a heap of old compost that was rich in potassium.

Saving seed: There actually are four squash species, not the three I already mentioned. Each species will cross freely with other members of the same species. Fortunately for the seed saver, C. *pepo* (zucchini and certain small pumpkins) will not cross with C. *maxima* (big pumpkins), which is the other main group we grow here. C. *moschata* (butternuts) will occasionally cross with *pepo* or *maxima* but those crosses almost always yield seeds that won't germinate. The fourth species makes cushaw pumpkins, C. *mixta.* which are tropical and semi-tropical heat-lovers that don't work here. I do not know which squash species C. *mixta* may or may not cross with.

C. *pepo* includes all summer squashes, most jack-o'-lantern pumpkins and certain short-storing pumpkins such as Acorn, Delicata, Vegetable Gourd (aka Sweet Dumpling), Vegetable Spaghetti and Gem. C. *pepo* can usually be recognized by its smaller seeds. Pepo pumpkins have the shortest storage potential. However, gardeners in cooler districts can at least get fat, vigorous seeds and fully-ripe pumpkins from it.

C. *maxima* varieties usually make large hard-skinned pumpkins with long storage potential—Queensland Blue, Jarradale, Triamble and Sweet Grey are

C.*maxima*. I like munching seeds from some maxima varieties. Queensland Blue is the standard garden variety on the mainland because of its fine flavour and because, I speculate, its skin is almost impenetrable to wildlife. Sweet Grey tastes about like QB and stores well enough. On Tassie, Sweet Grey matures significantly sooner than QB.

C. *moschata* (butternut) typically requires a minimum of 130 warm days for full maturity of fruit and seed. Moschata needs more heat than *C. maxima.* On Tasmania, butternuts work best in banana belt microclimates.

If there is sufficient distance from neighbours to allow natural pollination, then the easiest seed saving system is to grow only one C. pepo summer squash variety and only one C. maxima pumpkin variety. In suburbia grow as many varieties as you wish to but hand-pollinate the flowers.

Squash is far less harmed by inbreeding than most other bee- or wind-pollinated species and the seed is long-lived. The gardener may produce squash seed using only two plants, intentionally crossing every flower that produces seed. Only one pumpkin contains enough seeds for more years to come in a home garden than the seeds will still germinate. If seeds are made with early setting fruit and if the weather has been favourable then they'll be fat, fully mature seeds. If that seed dried down fully and is stored cool and dry then it may retain good germination for seven to ten years. I suggest the gardener does not produce yet another generation from their own seed. When your Gen_1 seeds stop germinating strongly, do not produce Gen_2 from them; instead buy a new packet and do another Gen_1 seed production.

Remove the seeds (with strings and other plant material), wash clean by rubbing them in water, spread the wet seeds only one layer deep on newspaper and let them dry fully (two weeks in a warm room). Some people believe squash seed continues to ripen in the pumpkin after harvest. For sure there's no harm in storing seed-producing pumpkins for one month in a warm place before extracting their seeds.

Varieties: *Zucchini*: Costata Romanesco is a bush zucchini that makes ribbed fruit with the very best flavour of all in our opinion. It's our first choice even though Costata makes oversized leaves that don't tolerate wind well and it needs more growing room than most other zucchini. Many Tasmanians think Blackjack is the pinnacle of zucchini flavour; I suggest these folks try Dark Star (BIRD) which is highly productive and forms a strong, easy-to-pick bush.

I especially like Lebanese, also called Grey Zucchini (FOTH). Southern Harvest has a highly productive refined hybrid of this sort. All those other shapes and colours of what Americans call summer squash are basically zucchini in another costume. Except for Gem. These grapefruit-sized round fruit have thin hard skins resembling pumpkin. They are boiled, then the tops are cut off like a miniature jack-o'-lantern, and the meat scooped out with a spoon. Fully mature Gem squash become little pumpkins with orange flesh that will store a long time.

Pumpkin: Most pepo varieties succeed on Tasmania. Hybrid maxima pumpkins are more productive than open pollinated classics like Queensland Blue and are worth the extra seed cost. Maxima pumpkin varieties differ in size, earliness and keeping quality.

Youngs Vegie Shed in Launceston sells what seems to me to be an open pollinated derivative of hybrid Sweet Grey that is grown by a local farmer. I believe seeds from these pumpkins will grow true-to-type. I mention this because Sweet Gray probably is the best variety for Tasmania and because it is quicker to finish than traditional mainland OP varieties. Sweet Gray hybrid used to be sold by Yeats but for some reason has been removed from their seedrack—yet last time I checked it was still being produced for the commercial trade. The variety Yeats replaced Sweet Gray with resembles Sweet Gray but is not long keeping.

Australian pumpkins differ from American varieties. Americans prefer winter squash flesh to be very soft after cooking—almost pre-mashed—and want it much sweeter than Australians prefer. An American maxima variety called Sweet Meat (ADA, TSC) is very popular in western Oregon. It matures sooner than Sweet Grey and stores well. Sweet Meat may be the best pumpkin for Tasmanian short-season districts. This heirloom was recently reselected by Carol Deppe.

When it comes to pepo pumpkins I suggest Delicata or Sweet Dumpling which is similar in appearance to Delicata but with smaller fruit that serve one person.

Dry gardening: Increase interplant spacing. Position each zucchini 1,500 mm x 2,000 mm; grow pumpkins on stations 3 metres x 3 metres apart. Thin stations to a single plant. Fertigate every three weeks. When I did this, in order to avoid damaging the vines I left the fertigation bucket in place, let the plant grow around it. Romanesco, the best zucchini candidate for this form of culture, will sprawl close to three metres plus in diameter both above and below ground.

Alliums

Leek, shallot, onion and garlic are frost hardy members of the allium family. All of them grow vegetatively until bulbing or seed formation is triggered by changing daylength. Formation of new leaves stops completely when bulbing or seed making starts. The size of the top has achieved when bulbing starts determines how large the bulb becomes. *In order to harvest big bulbs, encourage vegetative growth.*

Spring sown onions start bulbing when daylength declines after the summer solstice. Depending on variety, bulbing begins anytime from early January through mid-February. Autumn-sown onions start forming bulbs after overwintering when daylength is increasing. Overwintering varieties that are bred for our latitude start bulbing mid- to late October. Autumn sowing a variety that should be sown in spring results in seed making in spring, not bulb formation. Sowing an overwintering variety in spring leads to harvesting very small bulbs. Overwintering an overwintering variety in Tassie that was bred for the daylengths of NSW leads to harvesting very small bulbs or else the seedlings may freeze out. From this complexity comes the saying "he knows his onions."

Growing large onions, large shallots or impressive garlic only happens if the tops grew large before bulbing starts; this requires abundant fertility. Side-dress! Whilst forming bulbs the plants store up sugar made by their existing leaves. Sugar manufacture requires fewer soil nutrients than making chlorophyll. Consequently, make the last side dressing six weeks before bulbing starts.

Alliums make a coarse inefficient root system. To compensate, they store water in thick juicy leaves, allowing alliums to survive periods of moisture stress while showing hardly a sign of difficulty other than making less (or no) growth. Moisture stress must not be allowed if you want to harvest big ones. During the onion seedling's first month its roots do not penetrate any deeper than the slow-growing leaves reach upward. So I water onion seedlings often enough to keep the top 100 mm of the bed moist; I keep this up until the seedlings have formed roots where the soil doesn't dry out so rapidly.

Wild alliums thrive in sandy soil because they store moisture—they're like cactus in this respect. Allium roots can't penetrate tight heavy soil. Prepare clay by first digging in a 25 mm layer of compost in addition to the usual fertilizer. After providing all that, if properly spaced onion bulbs fail to at least touch the next one in the row or if garlic heads are small then next year use tighter interplant spacing in hopes of harvesting more overall weight of smaller bulbs from the same space. If crowding on heavy soil seems to cause- or worsen leaf diseases then do a soil test and bring your soil into balance. If the soil is loamy or sandy but onions or garlic heads are small, then irrigate more often and/or feed them better and/or give them more growing room.

Allium seeds can germinate in chilly soil but their delicate shoots can't emerge through a hard or crusted surface. If that describes your garden please consult the germination techniques described in Chapter 6, "Seed." Allium seeds retain good germination for only a few years so weak seeds are often fobbed off on gardeners. I think ethically-challenged seed sellers shoot themselves in the foot when they make their customers fail.

Allium seedlings transplant with naked roots and do it best when their shafts are over 5 mm in diameter. Leek seedlings take little effort to grow to this husky size in outdoor nursery beds. Garden centres often sell onion and leek seedlings when they are too small. Shame on them! Transplanting these weaklings can fail.

Alliums can get leaf diseases when humidity is high, especially so when the plants are crowded. Allium leaves have an aerodynamic shape that shrugs off wind. Wind helps keep humidity down. So position the allium patch in the least protected part of your garden. Industrial onions are often grown on soils that lack trace elements; I think that's why they often require fungicides. But if you'll use COF and compost, follow my spacing suggestions and have free-draining soil, then you may never see an onion disease (garlic is another matter). Alliums need more sulfur than most crops. COF provides abundant sulfur from gypsum. If you don't use COF spread the amount of gypsum in COF on allium beds. Tasmanians have long depended on a local shallot variety they misname "potato onion" because this species better copes with heavy soil and resists onion diseases. I see no reason to settle for "near enough." Better to read *The Intelligent Gardener* and bring your soil into balance or just use COF.

Brassicas grow especially well following alliums.

Onion and leek are pollinated by bees. They are different species that do not cross. Varieties producing seeds have to be isolated by 500 metres (commercial seed fields are separated by 1.5 kilometres or more). Allium seeds can be vigorous and shoot strongly when they develop in balanced soil, warm (not hot) conditions and low humidity. But warm dry climates may present hot days when seeds are finishing, which can kill them, Ending up with weak, low-germ or dead seeds are common trauma in the allium seed business.

Gardeners can produce vigorous high-germination seeds by harvesting each flower stalk when the first seeds in it are ready to fall out of the cup they formed in. Leaving all of the still-green part of the flower stalk still attached to that flower, cut that stalk and place it on a tarp under cover where there is good air circulation. Be unconcerned if these drying-down flowers have been invaded by black aphid-like insects. They are harmless.

Before long the drying seed heads expose mature black seeds. Some fall on the tarp. At this point move the tarp into the sun during bright warm dry sunny afternoons and encourage the flower balls to dry to a crisp. Put them back under cover late in the afternoon. Achieving fully dry flowers usually takes me several sunny afternoons.

Then rub the crisp flower balls between your (gloved if your skin is tender) hands until all the seed has separated. Then winnow the mixture of seeds, desiccated black insects and dusty trash by slowly pouring it out of a bucket held about half a metre above a catcher bucket whilst a *gentle breeze* blows the dusty light stuff away. Allium seed often has little density so winnowing must be done in a gentle steady breeze. Allowing 10 to 20 percent of the seed to be blown away with the chaff while winnowing is to your benefit; this undense stuff would not germinate well in any case. Commercial onion seed is often put through a gravity separator to eliminate weak seeds and increase the germination percentage. Gardeners can accomplish much the same thing with wind.

Commercially-grown allium seeds usually hold three years in storage before germination percentage drops too much to sell them to farmers—who are a critical trade. My own seeds grown on fully remineralized soil germinate well for five years. To delay inbreeding depression of vigour involve at least 25 plants in each seed production. The Organic Seed Alliance specifies a minimum population of between 80 and 200 plants depending on the allium species.

Onion, shallot and garlic bulbs store longest when kept between 10°C and 12°C with abundant air circulation and moderate humidity. If you put bulbs in mesh bags then these should be hung with air on all sides. The very best storage comes from plaiting onion and garlic and hanging the braids. I even plait shallots. As with pumpkins, the best choice between cool but too damp or dry but too warm is probably warm and dry. Having bulbs losing some moisture is better than rotting or resprouting prematurely.

Garlic *(A. sativum)*
Shallot *(A. cepa)*

Garlic and shallot grow only leaves from autumn well into spring. Most garlic varieties start bulbing after mid-October. Early varieties finish bulbing mid- late November. The latest variety I've ever grown was harvested around Christmas. Shallot, aka potato onions, finishes early- to mid January.

Garlic does better when late spring is rainless because dryish soil when harvest approaches fends off root rot and also helps the outer skins cure better so the bulbs store longer. If you irrigate or if it rains much when garlic bulbs approach harvest their outer skins will soak up water, leading to damaged and/or discoloured bulbs and/or rotting. Getting significant rain at harvest time is unlikely—most years—but still, growing several varieties with different harvest dates lessens that risk.

Culture: Garlic bulbs form and mature just below the surface. If their soil gets compacted over the winter then the bulbs will be smaller. To prevent compaction in sandy or loamy soil hoe in 15 mm of compost and the usual amount of COF before planting. Clay soils will become airless and soggy in winter. Prepare clay and heavy loam by hoeing in COF and a layer of compost 25 mm thick.

Shallots form on the surface so they cope better than garlic does with heavy soil. Many Tasmanian gardeners don't know how to make bulbing onions perform so they depend on potato onions.

To plant garlic, first separate a bulb into cloves. Plant only the large cloves; eat the small ones. Each clove makes a bulb. Each shallot you plant multiplies into a cluster of ten or so. Plant both species root side down, the top of each clove or shallot just below the surface. Space garlic cloves from 10 cm to 12 cm apart in the row, the rows 40 cm apart. Position shallots 30 cm x 30 cm.

Reduce garlic leaf diseases by increasing in-the-row spacing to 15 cm apart; this lowers humidity. There is partial compensation; lowered plant density usually results in harvesting larger bulbs. In my garden problems with garlic leaf diseases greatly lessened as my soil became fully remineralized.

Local lore says start to garlic on the shortest day of the year and harvest it on the longest day. Late sowing like this might move the harvest a week later and does produces smaller bulbs with less tendency to split open if they stay in the soil for a few weeks after maturity. Another benefit: later maturity usually happens in drier soil. Those old timers did not know about remineralizing trace elements but they did know how to make the best of what they had.

I do know about soil balancing and

have access to plant nutrients that the old timers didn't so I start garlic and shallot in April because the size the leaves achieve before bulbing begins determines bulb size. To grow large tops both garlic and shallot must be encouraged to shoot quickly after planting. Dormancy in garlic declines during storage and eventually the cloves sprout by themselves even when they are not planted. But some varieties are still so dormant when they are planted in April that they do not shoot until late June, thereby missing the entire autumn growing period. Overcome dormancy by putting cloves for planting into a paper bag in the refrigerator in mid-March. Give them a solid month of chilling prior to planting out. This breaks dormancy.

Push winter growth by side dressing close to the row soon after the cloves shoot; generously side dress the isles when faster growth resumes in August. Keep the soil moist until a month before harvest and then let soil moisture decline so that the bulbs or shallots cure well.

Garden planning: We consume one or two garlic bulbs each week so I plant 100 cloves for the table, another 10 to make planting seed plus another 10 to provide a slim margin of safety.

Garlic and shallot fit neatly into a two year rotation. Alliums grow especially well following potatoes. Brassicas do especially well following alliums. So we dig our main crop potatoes by mid-April and immediately plant garlic and shallot there. Soon after the garlic harvest is the perfect time to sow brussels sprout. Other brassicas for autumn-winter-harvest like big late cabbages slot in neatly after lifting shallots. Potato, garlic, brussels sprout—it's a winner!

Insects and diseases: I've had no insect problems with garlic and know of none. Yield-reducing virus diseases do carry over from year to year in garlic much as they do with potato. I suggest starting with large healthy-looking locally produced bulbs found at a weekend market.

Garlic root rot is caused by *Sclerotium cepivorum,* a fungus whose ungerminated spores persist for 10 years in soil. It makes some plants rot during winter. After winter even more plants rot. The disease spreads from one plant to the next in the row. Increased interplant spacing slightly reduces infection. So does dryish soil as harvest approaches.

Root rot fungus forms seed-like sclerotia that look like tiny black dots. Long-lived sclerotia are spread by garden tools, by shoes, by your own compost. Once your garden gets garlic root rot you got it forever. Many folks new to homesteading have great results with garlic—at first. They envision its income potential per square metre involved and conclude it'll be a great cash crop. They continue getting great results for a few more years as they increase planting stock but then root rot appears and crashes their hopes.

I recently discovered an effective, non-toxic organic treatment that almost completely eliminates root rot fungi. This material is not found at garden centres. The smallest package of Nutri-Tech Trichoshield contains enough to supply a family garden for more than a few years. It is a dry powder concentrate of a predatory fungus called trichoderma that aggressively eats root rot fungus.

Trichoshield must be applied several times. Before planting mix a few tablespoons of Trichoshield with just enough water to make thick soup, like house paint. Stir in the water slowly, almost drop by drop; do not make the soup too thin. I mix it in a kitchen bowl or one litre plastic container. This much Trichosheld treats 100 + cloves. Roll garlic cloves in Trichoshield soup; some of it must adhere to every clove. Plant them immediately. Then immediately mix a generous tablespoon of Trichoshield into a 9 litre watering can and drench the bed. Two- 9 litre watering cans drench the area I use to grow 120 plants. Treat the patch again with Trichosheld early in July and yet again early in September. If you see any plants that are not growing in late September assume there still is root rot present. Drench the bed yet again. Trichoshield stores in a refrigerator. I've had some that worked after three years in cold storage. Order it direct from Nutri-tech.com.au/

Reduce garlic leaf diseases with foliar sprays and by increasing plant spacing which lowers humidity. Use something rich with trace elements like NTS 10-10-10 or Maxicrop Liquid Seaweed Plant Food Concentrate which comes in several variants. Use the version with the most trace elements. Trichoderema eat many kinds of fungi. You can mix Trichoshield into diluted liquid fertilizer. Spraying activated compost tea during autumn and winter also boosts disease resistance. Full soil remineralization helps fend off allium leaf diseases but not root rot.

Harvest: An occasional shallot plant puts up a flower stalk as the bulbs form. When I grew the local potato onion only one bulb out of 50 put up a flower stalk. Bulbs that go to seed do not make useful shallots.

At the same time hardneck garlic varieties begin bulbing below ground tiny bulblets start forming on a tall stalk that emerges. Bulblets could be used as planting seed but probably shouldn't be. If you plant a bulblet in autumn next spring it makes one unsegmented bulb that can reach 25 mm in diameter. Plant this *rondelle* the next autumn and after overwintering it forms a full-sized fully segmented bulb. However, allowing the bulblets to develop reduces the final size of the main bulb so when growing hardnecks *pinch off the bulblets as soon as the stalk emerges.* The lower part of the flower stalk remains like a brittle stick in the bulb's core—forming a hard neck. When softneck varieties mature no flower stalk emerges, the leaves brown off and wither like bulbing onions do.

The cleanest and longest-storing garlic is dug from crumbly dryish topsoil. Harvest after all the layers of skin over the cloves have fully developed but before the wrapper skins crack open. The harvest window can be as brief. Don't delay. If the wrappers break open then soil enters. This shortens storage life and makes the bulbs unmarketable. Bulbs harvested this late also have shrivelled leaves that do not plait.

Leaves of both hardnecks and softnecks begin to brown off as the bulbs develop but they should not have withered before it is time to harvest. Deciding when to harvest is always agonizing. Do this: dig one bulb as soon as there are signs of maturity. Peel off the outer layers. If the bulb has not yet segmented use it in the kitchen like an onion that tastes like garlic. Wait one week and try again. If the bulb has segmented, is forming cloves but has not yet fully developed internal skins around each clove, eat it and inspect another bulb in a few days. Keep checking every few days. If significant rain is forecast (or should you need to irrigate and can't avoid wetting the garlic bed), the harvest may be done when skins have fully formed around each clove but the whole thing is not quite ready. Better to wait a few more days or another week, but be mindful that wet soil at harvest time degrades the bulbs. Like I said, deciding when to harvest is agonizing.

Harvest garlic by first loosening the row with a spade, then gently lift the plants. Shake off or rub off as much soil as possible (this is much easier to accomplish when the earth is dryish). Spread the plants out neatly under a roof such that each plant enjoys good air circulation. After drying for two to four days, *before the outer leaves have become brittle,* a few outer leaves are peeled off by tugging down on them—and away goes any soil clinging to the bulbs. The clean bulbs are again laid out neatly and allowed to dry until the leaves and stalks have withered enough to plait. Be alert though; allow the leaves to dry too much and they'll become too brittle to plait. I immediately hang just-made braids so the still-damp leaves don't rot.

Braids store best when hung in a cool but not cold place with good air circulation. Garlic stored cold sprouts prematurely. We hang ours in the kitchen where it is a lot warmer than it ideally should be. Still, in-the-kitchen storage keeps our garlic in fine condition over the winter. Our hardneck variety usually starts sprouting in August; a late-maturing long-storing softneck variety I've grown doesn't shoot by itself until November. Garlic bulbs *whose necks got totally dry* before putting them in a mesh bag keep well if they are given good air circulation.

Shallot leaves behave like bulbing onion tops. All the bulbs should be lifted when most of their tops have weakened at the neck and fallen over. If the soil is dry and the sky is overcast, temperatures moderate, spread them out for a day or two on the (dry) bed they grew in, then spread them out under cover until the leaves have shrivelled enough to plait. We have kept shallot braids through the winter in an unheated covered outdoor shelter without them rotting or sprouting but I am sure ideal storage would be like other albums, moderate humidity, stable 15°C. We have experienced rotting shallots when they were stored in mesh bags; our fault because we did not dry the necks to a crisp before packing them away. Plaiting makes sure every neck is exposed to the air. And if an occasional shallot does rot in a braid it doesn't rot the others. Plaiting shallots, garlics and onions makes long keeping a lot more certain.

Saving seed: Garlic bulbs usually contain a mixture of clove sizes. One year I used the tiny ones for cooking, separated all the larger cloves by size, "large" and "medium," and grew each size in separate sections of the bed. I found that the large cloves made bulbs 25 percent bigger than the medium-sized cloves produced. Varieties of garlic do not cross nor does real garlic make onion-like flowers that form viable seed. An odd shallot does go to seed although shallot should only be propagated from bulbs because when seed formation happens the bulb becomes inedible. If you start shallot from seeds most of the plants may go to seed.

Varieties: The best way to get garlic for planting is to know someone already growing a fine variety or else buy the best looking locally grown garlic you can find at a weekend market.

Softneck varieties store longer than hardnecks but have milder flavour. Softnecks are easier to plait.

Elephant "garlic" may thrive where real garlic fails. It actually is a leek that makes enormous garlic-like cloves and also leaves behind a nuisance—gladiolus-like corms that emerge later. Elephant makes seedballs on top with real seeds in them, like leeks do. Foodies disdain elephant although the flavour of it is similar to the real thing.

Dry gardening: Garlic can be productive entirely without irrigation although a dryish spring lowers yield and a very dry spring causes crop failure. Prepare the bed as usual but arrange the bed with 60 cm between rows and 15cm between plants in the row. Unwatered garlic may mature magnificently given careful weeding. It may help to spread a thin mulch between rows in spring.

Shallots need irrigation during November and December.

Leek

(Allium porrum)

My wife requires plenty of onions. She also opines that alliums are nature's health food. But the only unsprayed nutrient-dense onions available at any price come from my garden. So I do whatever it takes to keep us well supplied. If my soil or circumstances or personal temperament or gardening style didn't favour growing bulb onions then leeks would be the most useful substitute to supply the kitchen during autumn and winter. Leeks do okay in heavy soil where bulbing onions barely grow. Leeks do not have to be pushed to grow as fast as possible. They are amongst the most cold hardy of all winter vegetables.

Culture: Leek is a medium demand vegetable that does best in light loamy soil. When they must be grown in clay, deeply dig in a larger than usual amount of compost and half again more COF.

Leeks grow slowly. Seedlings need three months after sowing before they reach transplanting size. Young leek seedlings only grow well when their soil is like always-moist potting mix. For these reasons it is best to coddle them in an especially prepared outdoor nursery bed located close to the garden tap.

My leek nursery is 1,200 mm x 1,200 mm, which is three times larger than necessary. Before sowing I transform the surface 100 mm into potting mix by hoeing in a 25+ mm layer of my best compost and 1 litre of COF per square metre. A layer of sphagnum moss 25 mm thick could substitute for compost, or better, be used in addition to compost because the lighter and looser the nursery soil is, the more roots will still be attached to the seedlings when they're transplanted. Then I rake out a level seedbed and make furrows 10 mm deep. A 1,200 x 1,200 nursery holds 3 parallel furrows that are 300 mm apart. This produces enough seedlings for three leak-loving households.

The best time to sow leek is when most gardeners put out tomato seedlings. My homegrown leek seeds rarely germinate as strongly as commercially produced seeds that were grown in an ideal climate. Consequently I sow 10 seeds per centimetre and thin out clusters soon after germination; my target is three good seedlings per centimetre. The rows will be crowded from the get-go but there's lots of rootzone in the isles and the seedlings will be transplanted before they get stunted. This much competition also makes them stretch, which you'll soon learn is desirable for producing the highest quality leeks. Side-dress a small amount of COF close to the row when seedlings are 50 mm tall. Side dress the isles generously when the seedlings are 125 mm tall.

The most useful part of the leek is the blanched (white) underground portion of the stem. The deeper the leek seedling can be positioned when it is transplanted then the longer the white part will be—so I grow leggy seedlings.

Dig and transplant the seedlings when their shanks have achieved pencil thickness; try not damage the roots when separating the seedlings. Washing the earth away from the roots with a jet of water doesn't destroy nearly as many roots as trying to do this with your fingers. Then grasp a neatly arranged bundle of bare-root seedlings in one hand and cut off the top one-third of their leaves (not counting the stem). This reduces transplanting shock. Temporarily store the clipped seedlings in a bucket, roots down. Until transplanting them keep the roots moist but not underwater. Best to transplant immediately although putting a sealed plastic bag of seedlings into the fridge for a day or two won't harm them.

You'll probably transplant in mid-January. Try to do it in the morning of what is forecast to be a cloudy day. If sunny weather is forecast then transplant an hour or two before dark. Two long rows barely fit on a 1,200 mm wide raised bed; a 1,500 mm wide bed would be much better for two parallel rows. If the bed is less than 1,200 wide make only one long row in the centre.

Spread a full dose of COF and generous compost. Then, dig the bed to the full depth a spade blade permits. Then, using a common garden hoe, excavate a very deep furrow down the entire length of the bed; 100 mm deep would be good, 150 mm deep would be best. If the bed is wide enough make a parallel pair of furrows 600 mm apart centre to centre. Position seedlings 100 mm apart in the furrow. Spread out the roots as best you can, cover the roots 25 mm deep whilst holding the stem upright and then gently compress the soil around the stem.

Then side-dress more COF close to the seedlings. Then with a common hoe gently push enough soil against the stems to bury them up to the first leaf notch—*not any deeper than that.* Finally, thoroughly water in the seedlings. If the weather becomes hot during the next week, water every few days. After that, water the leek bed whenever the rest of the garden needs moisture.

I suggest putting in so much fertilizer and compost because leeks will respond by getting much larger, sooner and also because side dressing becomes less effective after more soil gets hilled-up against the stems.

Does it seem doing all that would take a lot of time? Preparing, growing the nursery, preparing a 10 square metre production bed, digging and then transplanting seedlings, the whole thing combined takes me less than one full morning's work. In exchange we'll have all we want for the kitchen from autumn until spring and a great many more big leeks to gift.

Ongoing, eliminate weeds much like you hill potatoes—pull a little soil up against the stems and kill the weeds at the same time. Take care not to get soil into the leaf notches. As the leeks' height increases continue to scrape up soil against them with hoe. Because I crowd two parallel rows into a 1,200 mm bed, by mid-March the leaves so completely cover the bed that I can't hill up any more soil. If the rows had been further apart I could pull up more soil and harvest longer white stalks.

If you want to produce the longest possible white stems then start out by digging a ditch that is 300 mm wide and 200 mm deep. Pile the soil along both sides. Then generously spread

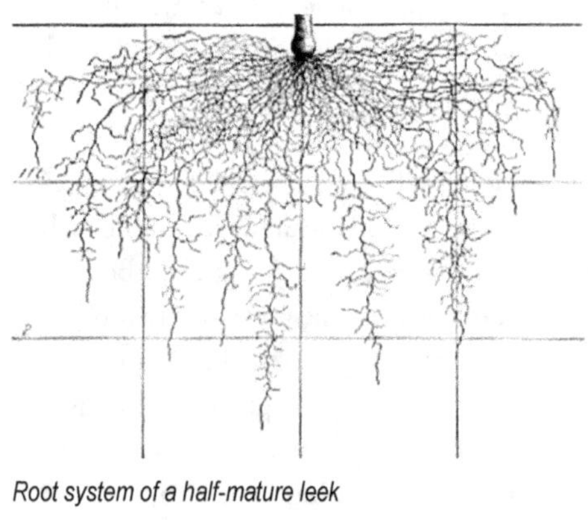

Root system of a half-mature leek

COF and compost in the ditch and deeply dig that in. With a hoe excavate a deep furrow down the centre of the ditch and transplant into that. Once the seedlings are in, side dress them and bury the seedlings to their first leaf notch. Gradually pull soil back into the ditch. When it is full continue hilling up against the stems.

Garden planning: One 1,200 mm long nursery row easily makes enough leek seedlings to transplant into the 10 square metre bed that generously supplies our kitchen during autumn and winter. I grow three nursery rows because I enjoy gifting leek seedling bundles.

Tasmanian home gardeners shouldn't depend on a variety bred for late summer/early autumn harvest. Autumn leek grows faster but lacks winter hardiness and will be the first to bolt to seed in spring. I have tried this type for April and May harvest but prefer to grow winter and "spring" varieties for early autumn harvest, even though they'll be slightly smaller. Most varieties for winter harvest go to seed in September. What are termed "spring leeks" don't bloom until October.

Insects and diseases: I've grown leeks for 40 years and have seen no insect or leaf disease. In microclimates with especially rainy winters I'd improve air circulation by spacing them a bit further apart.

Harvest: Begin digging them in April. Many people waste the leafy tops but these are useful when making soupstock. When flowering initiates the core becomes woody; soon the entire leek is woody.

Saving seed: Leek doesn't cross with onion. Select seed making plants as you harvest in winter. Choose plants with longer shanks from the bottom to the first leaf joint and without bulbous bottoms (illustration on previous page shows an undesirable individual). Transplant selected leeks 300 mm apart in the row, make the rows 600 mm apart. You may transplant straight back into the bed they were dug from.

The seed patch needs irrigation during summer. Around the end of February the balloon-shaped flowers will, irregularly, one at a time over several weeks, reveal the still moist black seeds they contain, indicating that harvest is approaching for that particular flower. The first exposure of black seeds in any plant indicates it's time to stop watering the entire patch. One way to check if a seed stalk is ready to harvest is to try to pull it from the soil with a gentle tug. If it lifts easily then it was ready. If it resists the tug there still are active roots; tug it again in a few days. This test doesn't work on all varieties. Stalks that won't easily pull out must be cut off as far below the flower as possible so that nutrients can be moved into the maturing seeds as the stalk dries out. Retain as much green stalk attached to the flower as possible.

Seeds continue ripening for many weeks after the stalk was cut. Spread the stalks out under cover on a tarp or sheets of newspaper to catch shattering seed. Even after the entire stalk has dried out, getting the seed heads themselves completely dry can take two months. For many years I grew seed for Durabel. This spring leek is so slow to go to seed (and so slow to mature that seed) that I've had to cut the flower balls off their dried-out stems and bring them into the heated part of our house to get fully dry. When the flowers have become *well and truly crisp,* rub them between your hands. I stress the word crisp because if there is moisture present at this time some seeds will get wrapped up in moist flower parts. I keep the mixture of seeds and very dry chaff in a woven plastic feed sack over the winter, intending to winnow it on a warm sunny day next spring. But having the seeds mixed with chaff helps reduce thinning. Usually that big bag never got properly cleaned.

Varieties: Europeans depend on leeks. Naturally, the world's supply of high quality leek seed is produced by northern European primary growers; the varieties offered there suit Tasmania.

Autumn leeks are tender, faster growing and less pungent than winter varieties. In exchange they are less likely to survive winter. North American seed merchants call them summer leeks. Bulgarian Giant (SH) is an autumn variety that Sam Bayley says handles Tasmanian winter well enough. King Richard (BIRD) works fine too.

Winter leeks are bred to resist cold, strong frost, constant humidity and rain; they're pungent. All seed sellers offer one or more winter varieties. Blue Solaise is excellent.

Spring leeks are winter varieties bred to go to seed later in spring. For many years now Southern Harvest has grown seed for Durabel after I gave up doing it for him. I thank Sam Bayley for realizing how important this variety is. Sam says his Blue Solaise also holds a long time in spring, like Durabel.

Dry gardening: I see the possibility of semi-dry-gardening leek. Start an irrigated nursery the end of October; use a winter or spring variety. Seedlings in this bed will need more growing space because they will be kept in the nursery a longer time. Make the nursery rows 450 mm apart, sow fewer seeds and thin so they stand 10 mm to 20 mm apart in the row. Give the nursery just enough water to keep it struggling. Transplant when the rains return. You'll harvest small ones June through September.

Onion

(A. cepa, A. Fistulosum)

Our climate suits onion. Tasmania's farmers grow many acres of pungent storage onions. There's no commercial market for Tasmanian salad onions but gardeners can grow them. Salad varieties make large soft sweet bulbs with little pungency. Most varieties store for only a few months; Southern Harvest sells one that keeps through half the winter. A full year's supply of unsprayed nutrient-dense onions is possible.

Bulbing onions may be directly seeded or else seedlings may be transplanted. I choose to direct seed because raising seedlings and transplanting them make unnecessary work; direct seeding produces large onions. I've never had an onion seed germination failure by direct sowing if that lot of seeds would sprout acceptably in a germination laboratory. Beware: weak or outright dead onion seeds often get sold to gardeners.

Before sowing onion seeds first blend a generous dose of compost into the surface inch of the bed to help keep the seeds moist and assist the emergence of delicate shoots. Having a loose surface inch also allows teasing spring onions out of a row of bulbing onions without damaging its neighbours. With open pollinated seed assume that less than half the seeds will shoot and many that do emerge will not grow vigorously. Therefore sow six to eight OP seeds for every onion ultimately desired. Better to overseed and thin because redoing a failed attempt will yield smaller onions.

Now I will restate some of my introduction to the allium family. The wild onion thrives in sandy positions by storing up moisture. It survives dry soil by using its moisture reserves but grows fast only in moist soil. The bulb will only be as large as the tops became before bulbing begins. So if you want to harvest big ones G-R-O-W the leaves! When the bulb is nearly mature the stem emerging from the bulb narrows at its base and the stem falls over just above the bulb. Then the outer skins toughen; the bulb starts to cure. Curing happens far better in dry soil. So stop watering when first tops fall over and pray for no rain.

To harvest very large bulbs sow as soon as strong germination is possible and then assist seedlings to grow as fast as possible. Stop pushing before bulbing starts because forming new leaves will stop. Sometimes onions divide (double) and make two (or sometimes three or four) bulbs joined at the base in the same way shallots multiply. Doublers don't store for long and there's more waste when peeling them. Most doubling is caused by using cheaply produced seeds that lacked attention from a plant breeder.

Onion varieties are bred to suit the daylength pattern found in a narrow band of latitudes. So a variety that works in NSW or is for QLD won't do well in Tasmania. Internet garden seed sellers and picture packets on seedracks rarely provide accurate information, making it seem that the variety being offered suits all circumstances. The domestically produced onion varieties that Quarantine so graciously allows Tasmanians to use are all sown in spring. They grow vegetatively whilst days are lengthening. They initiate bulb formation on declining daylength after the summer solstice. These varieties are harvested mid-February. Varieties that mature later than that here could be highly productive in Victoria. Shortly I will describe how to cure onions; this will illuminate why late finishing varieties may do fine in VIC.

Seed rack packets usually hold varieties that suit the daylength pattern and climate of New South Wales. These varieties are meant to overwinter or else to be spring sown but grow much faster in NSW than Tasmania's spring climate permits. Consequently they don't get nearly as large in Tasmania as the propaganda promises and will be more pungent than the catalogue suggests. The bottom line: I don't use most onion varieties offered in mainland seed catalogues or on seedracks no matter how wonderful the verbiage.

Storage/cooking varieties have considerable pungency, they make hard fibrous rings and many-layers of thick strong outer skins. All these traits contribute to long storage. Varieties that suit Tasmania should start going tops down by the end of January so they can cure in low humidity conditions. Well cured Creamgolds can hold past Christmas if they are stored properly. We are doubly blessed with 12 months of onions because by early December the current crop has grown large enough to use as spring onions.

Tasmanian onions should be directly seeded from mid August in the warmest districts until the end of September in harsher places. Early sowings usually produce larger onions but germination can be poor if the soil is too cold. When sowing early make sure the seed is very strong and put twice as much seed into the furrow.

Spring Onions come in three types: One kind forms bulbs but is very late to start-bulbing. It has translucent tender outer skins. It is harvested before bulbing begins. This type provides a relatively short harvest period. It is for market growers not for the home gardener.

Lisbon onions may be sown September through January. Early sowings half-way bulb around Christmas as they multiply like shallots, and then they resume growing. They make seed the following spring after overwintering. However, after multiplying they are not as pretty and take longer to prepare for the kitchen.

When the same variety is sown around the summer solstice it grows without multiplying, overwinters and goes to seed in spring. Thus with one variety and two sowings you get a 9 to 10 months supply. I have tried sowing Lisbon in February but they

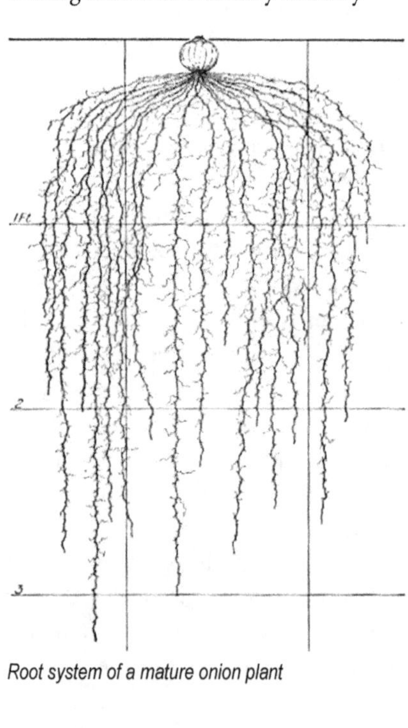

Root system of a mature onion plant

end up very small in winter. Yeats and Mr. Fothergill's sell a similar variety called "All Year Round." Welsh onions (*A. fistulosum*) do not bulb. They are pungent and fibrous. This very hardy species survives winter in northern Japan. Sow Welsh onions any time from September through January. They will overwinter and put up seed stalks in September, ending their usefulness. Welsh onions may divide/multiply if sown in spring. They grow faster than *A. cepa* and tend to become very large. You'll see them in supermarkets.

Culture: Bulbing onions are a medium demand crop that greatly benefits from side-dressing. Before sowing prepare the bed as for a low demand crop.

Bulbing onions should be sown as early in spring as strong germination is possible. That's mid- to late August in milder microclimates, mid- to late September in colder positions. Sow in a furrow 1 cm deep, 1 seed per cm in rows 45 cm apart. Side dress a small amount of nitrogen-rich fertilizer (COF) close to the row soon after seedlings emerge. Thin progressively until the seedlings stand 5 cm apart. Crowded onions may end up with harmless dents and flat spots and the average bulb size will be smaller but the total weight harvested may be greater. However, if they're seriously overcrowded then size and total weight harvested will be reduced. I don't think small onions are desirable because a lot more time is spent peeling them and there is proportionately more waste. So I ultimately thin my rows 8 cm to 10 cm apart and harvest lunkers.

Side dress again close to the seedlings mid October; place the fertilizer close to the row because the root systems are still scant. Don't use a great deal of fertilizer this time. Side-dress for the last time about November 15. This time generously cover the isles between rows.

There's a good reason to not thin to the final spacing when the seedlings are still small because you can use the thinnings as spring onions once they get a bit of size. Especially pay attention to maintaining abundant topsoil moisture when the seedlings are less than 15 cm tall because their roots at this point will be less than 15 cm deep. So keep the bed moist and keep the weeds out. Onion roots are shallow; damaged roots mean smaller bulbs; so keep the hoe blade near the surface. Cease all watering when the necks start to narrow as the tops prepare to fall over.

Spring onions: Sow from September through January. Arrange their bed as though growing bulbing onions but put more seeds into the furrow. When the seedlings have become well established, thin the rows so there remain two plants per cm. Give the surface inch twice the usual amount of compost because loose soil allows harvesting by gently tugging out the larger plants, encouraging the less vigorous ones to fill the gaps. Side dress if they are not growing fast or if growth slows. If you side dress spring onions after mid-March you'll induce winter diseases.

Garden planning: Bulbing onions cure better if they finish in dry soil so try to locate their bed where irrigation may be withheld starting when the first tops fall over. Five square meters produces enough salad onions to supply us until mid-winter when the few we haven't yet eaten start sprouting. An equal area given over to storage onions supplies the kitchen after the salad onions have been finished. Our storage/cooking onions resprout late November/early December. After harvest the bulbing onion bed is planted to brassicas or salad greens.

A single 1,200 mm long row of spring onions sown in September should provide plenty through summer but the quality of spring sown Lisbon declines after Christmas. So I start another row in January for autumn/winter harvest.

Insects and diseases: Covered in the introduction to alliums.

Harvest: Doublers that went tops-down should be the first ones eaten because these won't be good keepers. Onions that put up a seed stalk instead of going tops down never do form a proper bulb. When a flower stalk first appears the plant should be taken from the garden straight to the kitchen. If you started with high quality seed there won't be any bolters.

Well cured onions store longer. On soil that holds some clay cease all irrigation just before the first tops fall over by themselves. On sand stop watering when half the tops have fallen over. And in either case pray for no rain for the next few weeks—which is what we usually enjoy in Tasmania at that season. When a generous half of the tops have fallen by themselves push over the ones still standing, wait a week to ten days and then lift the onions. You may spread them out on dry soil for a few days if the weather is overcast or hazy and then bring them undercover to finish drying. If rain is forecast or if the sun is hot and strong, just bring them straight in.

Provide plenty of air circulation whilst the tops are drying. To achieve that I carefully arrange the onions in neat rows on the shed's concrete floor.

How to store onions? One way is to let them continue to cure until the necks have thoroughly dried all the way through, then trim off the shrivelled leaves and put the bulbs into mesh onion sacks. Hang the bags where air circulates freely. However—and this is a big however—onions will rot if their necks are have not totally dried before being put into sacks. *Totally dry.* Plaiting them into braids that weigh about 5 kg each works much better. Make plaits before the drying leaves become brittle. We built an insulated storage closet against a south-facing exterior wall of our house with a door to the outside. This part of our house is not heated. The design facilitates passive air exchange by drawing in cool but low-humidity air from the unheated room through a small opening near the floor and allowing warmer air to pass through an opening in the ceiling. It is especially set up to store hanging onion and garlic braids, as well as holding pumpkins and boxes of potatoes.

Harvest *spring onions* by thinning the row. The plants may seem battered in winter but the onions will look okay after the outer skins have been peeled.

Saving seed: Onions cross; they are bee pollinated so grow only one variety for seed. During winter take closely-inspected carefully-chosen onion bulbs from storage and plant them outside on a 45 cm x 45 cm spacing; bury them such that the necks are at the surface. Salad onions will sprout in storage as early as June, usually it is July with the variety we grow. When they start to sprout, plant them out. Storage onions should be put into the soil mid-August so that outdoor conditions make them sprout. Both sorts make seed the next summer. The only way to get highly productive seed is to grow it from carefully chosen near-perfect bulbs. Choose bulbs with narrow necks; usually these are better keepers. However, later-sprouting may also be linked to pungency; if you're growing a salad variety consider cutting out a small chunk (with a very sharp knife, not harming the core of the onion, which is where the shoot develops from) and taste each onion before setting them out; reject the most pungent ones.

I've observed that the mildest onions tend to be flat on top; globe-shaped bulbs tend to be more pungent. Knowing this can prove useful when choosing loose onions at the supermarket. Onions that double or worse, that bolt before bulbing should not be allowed to make seed because after a few generations most of your onions will have the same trait.

Varieties: Open-pollinated varieties have been out of industrial vogue since the 1980s—except on Tasmania, where Creamgold (SH, BIRD), also called Pukekohe, is still grown by farmers. Sheffield Red (SH) is a productive long-storing OP. Dominica Sweet (SH) is an extremely mild, very sweet spring-sown salad onion that grows large bulbs that often are flat topped. It is highly productive and keeps without sprouting into July in our storage room.

Pickling onions are bred to form thin tender translucent skins; these are planted on very dense spacings so that their bulbs don't grow large. Picklers aka "pearl onions," can be direct-seeded later in spring when creating excellent soil conditions is easier.

Tassie seed racks sell Creamgold or Pukehohe. Be cautious—there are at least three Creamgold strains in commercial use. Fothergill's once sold me a strain that is early maturing and not especially long keeping. I've heard of a Creamgold strain that is sown early in autumn, overwinters and forms bulbs before Christmas but I haven't found it for sale. The usual strain is a typical spring sown long keeping onion with very hard thick brown scales. Our onion crop is important to us so I get my seeds from either Southern Harvest or Birdland.

Soon after settling in Tasmania I did trials with every available "odourless" variety and also Hunter River Brown. These varieties are used in NSW. They are sown in autumn and make bulbs in spring whilst daylength is increasing. I point out that "winter" in NSW is not cold enough to make onions temporarily stop growing. An onion breeder told me that if a seedling achieves more than a pencil-thick stem before winter *and* its growth is checked by cold, it *will* go to seed in spring; it will not make a bulb. My trials also revealed that the "odourless" varieties have become much more pungent than they probably once were before hybrids took over commercial production. All these varieties proved to be highly variable and threw many off-types. Of the few varieties that actually bulbed there were many doublers and no variety was highly productive. Yeats Odourless had the mildest sweetest flavour and in it I saw the most potential to be reselected for Tasmanian conditions. Spring sown Dominica Sweet is far better than any of them.

Spring onions with Japanese names are almost certainly Welsh onions. These tend to be fibrous and pungent. Welsh onions are also far more cold hardy than Lisbon. They have straight shanks that present well in the supermarket.

Dry gardening: I don't think so unless Quarantine changes its seed import rules. In other parts of the world where the climate is similar to Tasmania people overwinter bulbing onions. I have long wished to do that in Tasmania but can't obtain seeds. These varieties would be sown mid- to late March whilst the soil is still warm enough to germinate the seeds. Their sowing date is critical; the seedlings must grow large enough to withstand winter frosts but if they get too large before winter they will not form bulbs in spring but will instead make seed stalks. This sort of onion probably could be grown without irrigation on Tasmania because they go tops down in October. Overwintered varieties usually produce the mildest, sweetest onions of all, although they rarely keep past the end of summer.

Asparagus

(Asparagus officinalis)

The size of our asparagus patch sometimes astonishes summertime visitors because it is 1,200 mm wide by 8 metres long by *2,400 mm tall.* It grows that tall because the soil is rich and I maintain good soil moisture. The bed is that large because we depend on asparagus from mid September through mid November. Establishing that patch could have cost us a lot because mainland-grown asparagus crowns are made unnecessarily expensive at the garden centre because of the harsh sterilization required by Tasmania Quarantine because our garden centres bring them in from big nurseries in VIC. Fortunately it is just as easy, maybe easier all things considered—and a lot less costly—to start your patch with seeds. The first harvest is just as quick to arrive and just as abundant starting from a seed as it is from crowns. And by starting with seeds an all-male bed is possible.

Asparagus plants are either male or female. Males only make pollen. Females only make seeds. Conventional wisdom says that an asparagus bed produces well for about ten years and then yield and spear size greatly decline. However, an *all male bed* produces larger harvests with a higher percentage of very fat spears and does that for many more years than a mixed sex bed because: 1) making pollen burdens the male plant far less than forming seed burdens the female. Consequently, male spears are fatter on average and males produce more spears than females. And 2) The most desirable spears are as thick as your thumb. But female plants drop a great many seeds on the bed that sprout and soon cause severe competition which hugely reduces the size of all spears and shortens the productive life of the bed.

All male hybrid varieties exist. Their seeds are pricey. All-male hybrids can not be counted upon to produce 100 percent males—I'd expect to see an occasional female. This section describes how to establish a for sure 100 percent male bed starting with inexpensive open pollinated seed.

Culture: Consider asparagus grown from seeds to be a high demand crop during the bed's first three years. Dig in a very generous 25 mm layer of compost and a standard dose of COF. Side dress more COF several times and irrigate generously through the first summer. In early spring of the second and third years spread a double dose of COF over the entire bed and mulch it with compost 10 mm thick. Do this early in spring before the crowns start shooting. In its fourth year and thereafter consider asparagus a low demand crop that gets a basic dose of COF and is thinly mulched with compost early in spring.

Gardeners have been misinformed yet again. The impression we are given is that transplanting so called "two year old" crowns brings about the first harvest at least one year sooner than had you sown seeds. The subliminal is that crowns are more reliable and easier to succeed with. The real story is this: what the garden centre calls a dormant two year old crown actually is not yet one year old reckoning from the time it started life as a germinating seed. It is ready to begin its second growing season when you buy it. If this were a human child, it would be having its first birthday a few months after you bought it. The act of digging the crowns destroyed a great deal of their root system; the act of sanitizing them to pass Tasmania Quarantine's import restrictions set them back even more. So the first harvest starting with crowns happens no sooner than from seeds.

Seeds are better for two broad reasons: (1) they cost much less than crowns so you can afford to destroy female plants and end up with an all male bed. (2) There are extra-productive hybrid seeds although you may have to import them from abroad.

If you intend to have a patch that produces abundantly for 20 years I urge you to make the bed 1,200 mm wide even if the other beds in your garden are not that wide. Sow seeds about the time tomato seedlings are put outdoors, when the soil has become reasonably warm but won't rapidly dry out. It's essential to soak asparagus seeds overnight before sowing them (the soak time not to exceed 12 hours). Drain the seeds and remove surface moisture by blotting them between sheets of paper towelling. Do this because slightly damp seeds are much easier to handle than slippery-wet ones. Then immediately sow them.

Be absolutely precise about this next step! If the variety is open pollinated or a regular hybrid (not all male) it will produce 50% females; you are going to eliminate all the females as soon as they are recognized. Carefully place only one seed every 100 mm in a 15 mm deep furrow made along the bed's centre. Take your time. *Do not put more than one seed in each position* because if two seeds germinate in the same spot it will be impossible to eliminate one plant and leave the other. Keep the row moist until the seeds shoot about two weeks later. In a cold wet spring emergence could take three weeks. Expect around 50 percent germination.

Thin the row to *at least* 300 mm apart by mid-January. Especially eliminate weak plants. If you end up with 400 mm gaps in the row, this will be okay. Even very young asparagus plants are hard to kill so thin the row with a trowel; entirely remove/destroy unwanted crowns. By the end of the first summer most of those young plants will have already divided into several connected crowns. Ending up with positions that are *at least 300 mm apart in the row* is essential. If plants are closer than that you will damage males when removing females. If there are gaps larger than 300 mm don't fret—it won't matter two years later if there are gaps 900 mm wide.

Asparagus grows slowly when it is moisture stressed. In order to eat a few spears in the second spring without setting the plants back I suggest pushing them go grow as fast as possible in their first year. Hope they get mid-thigh high. Keep the young plants well watered and side-dress close to the row a few weeks after germination; generously side-dress again mid-December. Keep the bed thoroughly weeded. Always! Weeds will be fewer in future years if the bed is kept clean. The plants soon form fat storage roots that gradually extend under the entire 1,200 mm wide bed. Many of them will be close to the surface. Deep hoeing can cause great damage. Mulching with compost every spring makes hand weeding much easier. Keeping a bed weed-free is the most difficult aspect to growing asparagus without using herbicide.

Around mid-summer in the bed's first year *a small percentage* of the females might make seeds. Most likely not. The flowers on male plants release pollen and then fall off. Flowers on female plants become small red berries but that usually doesn't happen in the first year. Males can not be easily distinguished from females until the plant either makes small berries or it doesn't. *Before any seeds drop on the bed, including green unripe berries,* dig up female crowns as soon as you spot them; immediately bin their ferns and unripe berries. Do not allow green berries to fall on the bed; do not put them in the compost heap; the berries might ripen viable seeds.

Asparagus ferns brown off and die in winter. Then cut them off 100 mm above the soil line. Compost them. In spring the crowns shoot up spears that in the second year soon become leafy ferns that will grow 1.5 metres high. Ferns may top out at 2.4 metres in the fourth year. All summer the plants store sugar and nutrients in fleshy roots. This reserve is used the following spring to make the spears you eat—so GROW those ferns for the first few years—make sure the bed stays moist and fertile; keep after the weeds.

Most directly seeded females will form seeds in their second summer, by which time each cluster of crowns may be 125 mm across with fat surface roots extending 300 mm to 400 mm from the centre. And that is why it is crucial to have the plants separated enough that you can thoroughly dig one out without damaging its neighbour very much.

Open-pollinated varieties occasionally make plants that produce a great many thin spears. Even if these undesirable plants are males, they should be dug out and destroyed as soon as they're spotted, even if that leaves gaps in the row.

By the end of the bed's second summer *almost all* the females will have been discovered and destroyed; my previous asparagus patch revealed one more female in its third year. If you started with an all-male hybrid variety then there still may be one female to dig out. Probably none. Because of that, all-male hybrid seeds could be placed 300 mm apart in the row and being hybrid, probably 2 out of 3 seeds will germinate. If you started with an open-pollinated variety or a regular (not all male) hybrid and thinned the row to 300 mm apart in the first year then the males will average 600 mm apart.

When destroying females I've occasionally found an underground stoloniferous runner (like some grasses make) extending as much as 150 mm from the parent crown. Be alert for this possibility. So dig meticulously.

After entirely purging the bed of females if there should be any gaps greater than 900 mm then dig up one of the most productive clusters of male crowns during winter dormancy, cut that cluster into a few chunks and transplant these into gaps.

One other thing you might do: each spring spread a measured cup of coarse sea salt over each 10 square metres of bed. This much salt will do no harm. Nineteenth century market gardeners spread salt on asparagus and spread a lot more than one cup per 10 square metres. I think putting more sodium into the soil adds flavour.

Garden planning: In its third year, an 8 metres long x 1,200 mm wide bed should yield two generous serves every other day over a month's time. By year four the same bed should yield two dinner plate-covering serves every other day for two months.

When choosing the bed's position keep in mind that asparagus ferns grow tall. My previous patch peaked out at 2,400 mm tall in year four. Asparagus ferns frequently fall over and lie on the earth. If I allowed that to happen the ferns of a four year old patch would cover the ground nearly 2 meters beyond its bed on both sides. I do not wish to give over a 5+ metre wide strip to asparagus. So I support the ferns in an upright position between two rows of star pickets, one row along each edge of the 1,200 wide bed. The pickets support two strands of wire or baling twine—the top one is 1,100 mm above the soil and another is stretched about 400 mm below it. I can reach under the lower wire to weed or harvest the bed. If the ferns were allowed to fall over it would be impossible to keep the patch weed free without stepping on the ferns, damaging them. Because tall upright ferns shade adjoining beds I think the best position for the asparagus patch is where it intercepts sprinkler overspray along the garden's east boundary or south boundary.

Insects and diseases: Good soil drainage is essential. Asparagus plants die during winter if the soil becomes waterlogged.

In Oregon I had to contend with asparagus beetles; they can strip the ferns bare. I've not (yet) encountered them on Tasmania although searching the net suggests they do exist here. Any insect taking more than ten percent of the foliage should be controlled with pyrethrins or spinosad. Neem oil might work. Spray often enough that the leaf loss is small enough that roots still accumulate abundant reserves.

Harvest: In its second year a bed that was started with "two year old" garden centre crowns will produce a few fat spears that you can eat. If a directly seeded row grows well in its first summer then it'll also produce a few fat spears the second spring that you can eat. In the second year take only one spear from each cluster of crowns. I'm sure it'll be incredibly delicious but control yourself; far better to invest—allow the crowns to build food reserves.

In the bed's third spring, spears may be taken until the size of most of them begins to decrease. Probably you'll enjoy three to four weeks of harvesting. In their fourth spring beds provide fat spears for six weeks, even eight weeks. I suggest using this harvesting method—take only fat spears (allow thin ones to grow on) and entirely stop harvesting when most of the spears stop being at least the diameter of your ring finger or when the flavour gets too strong which happens as warmer weather arrives, or else stop harvesting when you're weary of eating asparagus after having already had too much of it (if that be possible) and the garden is now producing an abundance of other vegetables.

Harvest this way: when a spear stands about 300 mm tall, grasp it about 100 mm below the tip and pull it sideways and downwards until the shaft snaps wherever it will. The stalk will be woody below the point it snaps; above that point it'll be tender. Harvest promptly. In one more day the tip starts morphing into a fern.

Saving seed: Asparagus is wind pollinated and needs considerable isolation if genetically pure seed is to be produced, but genetic purity may not matter. Genetic diversity widens the harvest period whilst any grossly off- type or non-productive crowns may be destroyed in their first few years. Seed balls resemble small green berries that turn juicy red when ripe. Each one contains a few black seeds. (In the interest of creating a totally all male bed I should mention here that still green berries that detach from the plant have a remarkable ability to ripen the seeds within them.) To end up with strong seeds let the berries get over-ripe, get close to detaching by themselves before you collect them. Crush them in a bowl or small bucket, mix the crushed pulp with water, stir well and the seeds immediately settle to the bottom.

Pour off the pulp, rinse and pour a few times to remove almost all the pulp, then wash the seeds in a sieve and spread them out on newspaper to dry.

Varieties: I never had space, time or enough interest to do asparagus variety trials. I can only comment on the flavour and productivity of the one variety I grow. I also can comment on two other varieties because for a few years Annie and I more than covered the council rates and other fees on the quarter acre block we used for our food garden by producing hundreds of "two year old" crowns for Allen's Nursery, Prospect. The Jersey Knight all male hybrid crowns I've grown make roots twice the length and half again the diameter of open pollinated Mary Washington. I also have grown crowns from UC157F_2. These crowns were about two thirds the size of Jersey Knight. I assume overall productivity would resemble the vigour and size of the crowns. My beds were started by direct seeding UC157F_2. The spears are entirely delicious and most of the crowns make very fat spears. What I most like about UC157 is that half the crowns put up spears in September and somewhat less than half put up their first spears in early October and a few don't put up any until later in October.

Dry gardening: I am speculating here. A new bed started from either seed or crowns takes irrigation the first year. But it won't take much because all you have to water is a strip 300 mm wide. After that year asparagus should survive without any irrigation in naturally moisture-retentive deep open soil and should produce adequately *if fertilised early each spring, if the bed is kept well weeded and thinly mulched and if there's plenty of unoccupied weed free bare soil to either side of the bed to help supply moisture.*

Sweet Corn

(Zea mays)

Corn's genetic program commands the plant to grow ever taller until *its biocomputer has measured the accumulation of sufficient heat to trigger seed making.* Then tassels and cobs develop. The tassels on top releases pollen which tends more to fall than to blow away; the plumes of silks emerging from cobs catch pollen. There is one silk for every seed in the cob. Reproduction doesn't start because the plant has grown for a certain number of days or has formed a genetically predetermined number of leaves. Agronomists use a measure called the heat unit (HU) to predict when a corn variety will start making seeds. The average annual accumulation of heat units varies by location and is calculated approximately this way: starting from the last usual spring frost add up the number of hours during each 24-hour period that the temperature is above 10°C and multiply that number of hours by the ever changing number of degrees the temperature is above 10°. Then add up every day's total until the first usual frost at summers end.

The quickest maturing sweet corn variety I know of was bred to grow on the Canadian prairies. It needs 1,340 HU. Most varieties that we can buy need 1,600-1,800 HU. A few late varieties require 1,800 to 2,000 HU. Varieties intended for growing in hot places (and often considered "early-maturing" there) can require over 3,000 HU. Where summer is hot-hot, like Brisbane, 3,000 HU may accumulate in 50 summer days. The warmest microclimate in Tasmania doesn't accumulate 3,000 HU over the entire summer. Try growing a heat loving Queensland variety in Tasmania and by the end of March there'll be a 4 metre tall plant just starting to put up tassels.

I tried that once in Oregon just to see it happen. I used a variety called Truckers Favorite White from a reputable seed seller in steamy South Carolina—a state with a summer weather like the hot season at the Sunshine Coast, Qld. The catalogue said Truckers took 67 days to make ripe corn. My plants were 4.5 metres tall 130 days after sowing and were just beginning to form tassels. Then I got frost.

Culture: Any silk that does not catch a grain of pollen will not form a seed, leaving an empty space in the ear. Corn arranged in single long rows may form ears with empty spots. So corn should be sown in blocks that are at least two rows wide and at least two metres long and better, three rows wide and three metres long. That way all the silks receive pollen. When I grow corn I temporarily join two 1,200 mm wide raised beds by digging up and fertilizing the 600 mm wide path between them.

Rain or sprinkler irrigation happening at the same time pollen is falling may cause empty spaces in the ears so avoid overhead watering when pollen is dropping. (Corn pollen has a pleasant odour and the particles are large enough to be visible.)

Corn seed does not germinate when the soil temperature is below 15°C. Best to delay sowing until the soil is a few degrees warmer than 15°. Corn seedlings are killed by frost. They take 7 to 10 days to germinate so the first sowing could be made a few days before the last anticipated frost date. However, an early as possible sowing too often germinates poorly and grows very slowly at first. I get better results and harvest only a few days later by sowing a week after the tomatoes are put out.

Corn is a medium-demand crop; prepare the bed for a low-demand crop and plan to side-dress. Corn is a grass, like wheat; it can be highly productive in soils that are low in organic matter if it gets enough nutrients. Corn responds to compost but if you have to skimp on spreading organic matter then the corn patch is a good spot to miss.

Sowing method number one is best for large areas: place seeds in furrows about 25 mm deep, the parallel furrows 750 mm apart; drop one seed every 100 mm. A few weeks after germination, thin so there is one seedling every 300 mm. Method two produces plenty for us two oldies: Cut a thin stick exactly 30 cm long. Use it to measure in-the-row spacing. Cut another stick 75 cm long. Use that one to measure space between rows. Stretch a string to mark the first row. On positions 30 cm apart along the string, sow two seeds by pinching them tightly between thumb and index finger and then jabbing the seeds 2 cm to 3 cm into just-loosened soil, mimicking the jab planter Nineteenth Century American subsistence farmers used. After one row has been sown, move the string sideways 75 cm and repeat.

Moderately side dress the entire between row space about one week after germination. Thin to one plant per position by the time the plants are 20 cm tall. Should both seeds fail to germinate at a position then allow two plants to grow on at the next position in the row or directly across in the next row. The extra plant fills the gap. Keep the weeds thoroughly hoed until the corn has formed a dense leaf canopy that effectively suppresses weeds. Then keep your feet out of the patch until it's time to harvest.

Garden planning: Hybrid varieties get ripe uniformly. Over 10 days all the ears on a hybrid variety will go from barely ripe enough to eat to overdone and getting starchy. When I was living in the United States I'd simultaneously sow three or four different hybrid varieties, each one required different amounts of HU so that one sowing could be harvested over five- to six-weeks. But Australia Quarantine severely—immorally in my opinion—prevents everyone from importing corn seeds except a seedcorn producing business. Consequently Australian garden seed companies offer very few varieties. So I make several sowings with the best variety I can buy. The first sowing goes in one week after there will be no further frost danger; the last sowing no later than mid December. In the South make the final sowing by November 30.

I usually grow salad greens or winter brassicas on the bed after the first corn sowing has been harvested. After the last patch has been harvested I start a winter green manure. I also could overwinter Spring Hero cabbages, broad beans, onions or garlic after the last corn harvest. Corn leaves nothing in the soil that antagonizes any species.

Insects and diseases: Earworms are close relatives of the cabbage grub. I have only seen a few in Tassie. Earworms can be reduced to a tolerable level with Dipel sprayed directly on the silks: the first spray about a week after the tassels drop pollen (which happens before the grubs eat their way into the ear); best to spray once more about 10 days later. In North America the earworm is a major pest, gardeners there mix Dipel in mineral oil and apply it to the silks with a brush.

Harvest: Indications of ripeness differ by variety. Some varieties signal they're ready when the ear wrappers start browning off; and/or the ears may lean away from the stalk when ready for picking. And ripe ears always plump up.

Before starting to harvest I always peek into the ends of a few ears because indisputably, yellow varieties are ripe enough to eat when the seeds are no longer pale yellow.

Saving seed (and growing corn as grain): The heavy pollen doesn't blow far; two hundred metres of isolation will prevent most crossing if the seed patch is upwind of nearby patches that are releasing pollen. Considering Tasmania's variable winds, this strategy seems doubtful. Commercial seed fields get 1.5 km isolation. The colour and flavour of each seed is set by the genes of the parent plant *and* by genes from the pollen that fertilized the seed. Practically speaking what that means is that if multicoloured field corn grows near yellow sweet corn and both drop pollen at the same time, then every ear in the yellow corn patch will form more than a few kernels with different colours, textures and flavours.

A well bred open pollinated sweet corn variety should produce about two thirds of what a hybrid makes and could taste terrific. Unfortunately, most of the traditional OP varieties have greatly degenerated. When thinning a row of OP corn keep the plants with the thickest stalks that also grow tall, remove slow growing plants and those with thin stalks.

The best way I know to make selections that improve an open-pollinated sweet corn variety is first to provide abundant interplant spacing. This encourages tillering (the formation of secondary stalks that often make smaller ears). If many of the plants in your variety will form tillers then you can eat the big ear on the main stalk and still make seeds. As you harvest each main ear immediately remove the wrappers. If it looks like a desirable ear (and you can taste it raw which is a delicious treat), then seeds may be saved from small ears on tillers. This approach also selects for tillering, which I consider to be a useful trait that, for commercial considerations, has been selected against in modern varieties. However, if very few plants tiller, or none, this strategy is unworkable.

Corn seeds will not serve as the fundamental food of a self sufficient Tasmanian household because even early-maturing varieties rarely achieve seed that sufficiently dries in the field before rains or heavy dews arrive. So when the weather worsens pull the plants, roots and all, hang them upside down in small bundles and allow them to finish drying under cover, best inside a shed; be sure to give them lots of air circulation. To avoid inbreeding depression of vigour save seed from at least 50 plants.

Varieties: Hybrid sweet corn varieties that were in use before the 1980s usually provided a flavoursome treat. Many hybrids developed since then taste to me like watery sugar with a faint corny afterhint. Because there still are some Americans whose sense of taste has not become completely depraved there still are many excellent hybrid varieties being used.

These days there is much interest in developing productive open pollinated varieties. Johnny's, Territorial, and Adaptive offer them. All these OP varieties provide excellent flavour. Unfortunately, AQIS (or whatever its politically correct name is these days) makes bringing corn seed here impossible for a gardener to do legally—and equally impossible for a small seed business. In my opinion, AQIS's justification for this restriction has always been a deception that profits a few at the expense of everyone else. So what's new about that!

True Gold (SH, BIRD) is an OP that makes good sized ears with the corny-corn flavour I prefer. Amish Butter (SH) is an OP that makes corn meal and also is good eating as sweet corn.

Hybrid sweet corn varieties can provide excellent flavour and produce a greater yield which is why they replaced traditional open pollinated sorts and why traditional OP varieties like Golden Bantam were allowed to degenerate past the point of reconstruction. Southern Harvest provides good hybrids. Yeats' Sun-n-Snow is also good. Fothergill's has several. Bicolour hybrids can make very pleasurable eating.

Early maturing varieties can either make fairly large ears with shallow bland-tasting kernels or else they can make small ears with decent flavour. Here's why: corn stores up sugar in the stalk as it grows taller. Then it switches to reproductive mode and quickly uses up the stored sugar while forming seed. To experience this please chew on the sugary pith of a corn stalk shortly before tasselling starts. Taste another one few weeks later when the ears are filling with seeds; this stalk will not be even slightly sweet. Most early hybrid varieties are bred for commercial use. The shops want large attractive-looking ears and the farmer wants a variety that finishes early when the price is higher. But there ain't no free lunch, not even in the garden. Large size combined with early maturity can only be achieved when the ear mainly forms shallow kernels filled with sugary water.

Dry-gardening: Make 400 mm diameter hills on a 1,200 x 1,200 grid, each hill gets a full cup of COF deeply dug into it. Best do this mid-August so the nutrients work their way down where the soil retains moisture during summer. Sow four seeds in each hill. Gradually thin each hill to the one best plant. This is more or less how native Americans did it. Open pollinated varieties that are given such wide interplant spacing may tiller aggressively (form many ear-bearing stalks); the corn patch may get fuller than you'd expect. Do a web search for "three sisters garden."

Horseradish

(Armoracia rusticana)

Unsupervised horseradish quickly becomes a horribly invasive weed that makes roots so thin and so twisted, that it is not convenient to use them. By "horribly" I mean that in garden soil it can spread five metres in one year. Any fragment of horseradish root is capable of waiting months before putting up leaves and then trying to take over the entire universe. But with forethought you can grow easy-cleaning easy-peeling roots and *keep the plant from spreading.*

Culture: Start your patch with a piece of root. Almost any piece will do in a pinch but a crown or part of a crown is best. Anyone afflicted by horseradish growing in their vegie plot will have hundreds of root pieces with leaves already emerging they'll be delighted for you to take away. Your goals for the first year are to (1) grow some long, fairly straight root pieces; and (2) keep the wildly spreading plant under control.

This is of extreme importance: forcibly confine the plant by surrounding the horseradish patch with regularly mowed lawn extending at least two metres on all sides. Better, three metres.

It need not be a large patch; one bed 1,500 mm by 1,500 mm will produce all the horseradish root a big family could ever use. Concerning containment: if the plant puts up any seed stalks, cut them off before any seed forms.

Horseradish is a low demand crop. The bed should be deeply dug and loosened by working in a thicker than usual layer of compost and the usual dose of COF. Repeat that once a year.

Shallowly plant *only one* crown or root piece in the bed's centre about 25 mm below the surface. Do this in spring. Keep the bed weed free all summer. Irrigate enough to keep it growing.

In April, patiently dig the bed, meticulously search out and remove *every bit* of horseradish root. Dig in such a way that long pieces will come out intact, not having been cut by the spade. The goal is to obtain a few fairly straight pieces with the diameter of a pencil that are at least 300 mm long and better, 450 mm long.

After unearthing a long root piece take the end that grew from the centre and trim it off square. At the further end clip the root at a 45 degree angle. That way, next spring there'll be no doubt about which end grows the top and which end grows the root system. You'll almost certainly end up with several long pieces. Tie them in a loose bundle with all the square cuts at one end and the angle-cuts on the other. Bury that bundle in the horseradish bed under 50 mm of soil. Let the bundle rest over the winter.

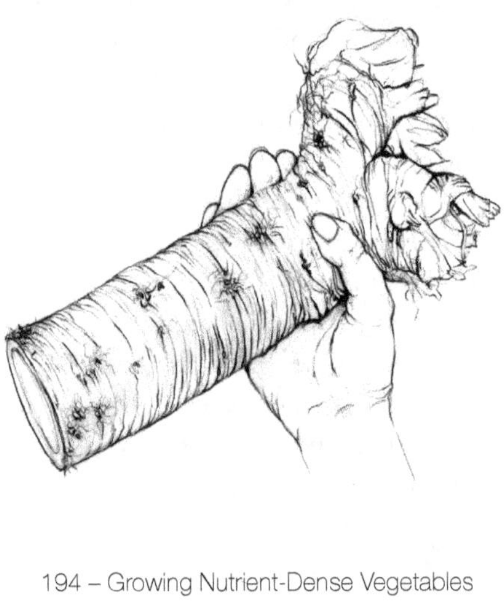

Civilized horseradish roots:
Now you're ready to produce long clean straight easy to wash, very fat horseradish roots.

August. Dig up the bundle of root pieces. Spread compost and COF and dig it in; dig the invading grass back. If you turn up any more horseradish root fragments, remove and send them to the tip, *not to the compost heap.*

If your bed is, as I suggested, 1,500 x 1,500, grow only two big roots. Two will provide plenty. Make two furrows 25 mm deep, parallel, centred in the bed, with about 500 mm between them. Horizontally place one root in each furrow, making note of which end was cut off square. Cover them with soil.

A great many leaves will soon emerge along the entire length of each root piece. Then comes step (1): gently uncover the root starting with the end you cut off square. Make sure 25 mm at the end you cut off at 45 degrees is undisturbed; that's where feeder roots will be allowed to develop. You'll discover many fine roots emerging from the entire length. Starting at the square-cut end, gently lift the flexible root just enough to slide a finger underneath it and break off all feeder roots except those coming from the last 25 mm of the angle-cut end. *Do not disturb that 25 mm section.* And break off all leaves except the cluster at the square-cut end. All the leaves the plant will be allowed to make will emerge from this spot. Now put it back in the furrow and pull an inch of soil over the root piece.

Step (2): There probably will be dozens of little horseradish plants emerging from bits of overlooked root. Treat these as the nastiest weeds imaginable. If you repeatedly cut them off or tease the root segment out before it can store more food they *will* use up their food reserve and die. Eventually.

Then once a month, November, December, January, February and March, repeat step 1. The root will get fatter; you will have to scrape more soil over it to make sure it stays well covered until the next manicure. Repeat step (2) every time you see a horseradish weed.

By April the root should be 50 mm in diameter. Dig it up. All the leaves will be clustered at the square-cut end. Cut and/or break them off. Wash the root and let it dry. Put the clean dry root into a plastic bag; keep that in the fridge to be used at your convenience. It usually keeps for many months.

Painstakingly dig the bed after harvest; extract a few long thin roots to hold over to establish next year's crop. Destroy every other bit of root.

I warn you: if the barrier of infertile, compacted soil around the patch is too narrow—if the plant escapes to a cultivated fertile bed—you'll never again want to grow horseradish. I first tried this method inside the garden fence. It took me several years of persistent hoeing as far away as eight metres to finally eliminate the plant.

Globe Artichoke

(Cynara scolymus)

Globe artichoke is a nearly spineless thistle that makes edible flowers that, like thistle, quickly forms and releases seeds attached to white fuzz that floats in the breeze. If the flowers are harvested young before any internal fuzz develops then the vegetable is far better tasting.

After flowering in spring the main plant forms many secondary plantlets around its base that soon will crowd the bed, making next year's flowers small. So the old plant is dug out and a few secondaries are replanted, best in another spot. They'll bloom next spring.

Culture: Globe artichoke is sufficiently frost hardy to survive Tasmanian winter anywhere that a lemon tree barely can. Globe artichoke seeds always produce a diversity. Some plants form sharp spines on the flowers that make handling them unpleasant. Some plants make better tasting bigger flowers with more edible material in them. Rather than starting a dozen plants from seed in order to (hopefully) find one highly desirable plant from which to propagate more plants for a great many years to come I suggest finding a gardener with a proven good plant and request a few secondaries.

The main stem dies after flowering; secondary growth takes over. However, now there will be five, or eight small plants growing in close competition. If all of them are allowed to develop then the following spring's artichokes will be far more numerous but much smaller. The total weight harvested may be less, not more. And the proportion of inedible flower material to useable food will be greater.

So every year the old plant should be dug up after Christmas, the secondaries (suckers) are separated, leaving some root attached if possible. Then two suckers are planted close together in each new position. I think starting new plants every summer is essential. I think moving to a position that hasn't grown artichokes before is better.

It may seem hopeless to establish a secondary during summer's heat, especially when most of them have few or no roots. But it isn't hopeless because the suckers store heaps of moisture. If the base is buried 30-50 mm deep, if all but the smallest few leaves are removed to reduce moisture loss and if it is watered every other day for a few weeks, it'll probably take root. Even if it seems to completely die back most of them will come good and grow.

It helps enormously to provide temporary shade until they take root. A plastic patio chair over them would do. When I gardened on a bush property I pushed the stems of a dozen bracken ferns into the soil close around the secondary so that fern leaves formed a temporary awning. The ferns soon withered but even then they made partial shade. In each position I always start two secondaries that are a few inches apart; if both get established I dig one (now it has roots on it) and put it elsewhere or kill it.

A secondary can grow itself into quite a large plant by the following spring if given fertile soil. So make their positions at least 1,000 mm x 1,000 mm; 1,200 mm x 1,200 mm is better. If you crowd them the flowers will be smaller next spring. This is a medium demand crop. I suggest side-dressing early in March to increase winter growth and again in August to encourage larger flowers. The first (king) flower is by far the biggest, followed by secondary and tertiary flowers that get ever smaller. Then the harvest is finished; the original plant dies back. If the plant is not dug and divided its secondaries take over the position.

Garden Planning: Two or three plants should provide enough for most people. The plants should be a metre tall and equally broad by mid-spring.

Insects and Diseases: I have never experienced any problems.

Harvest: Cut the flowers with an inch of stem attached when they're about three quarters developed, well before the petals start spreading apart. Leave a flower too long on the bush and it develops internal fuzz. Artichoke hearts from mostly sized up, still-fuzzless flowers are utterly delicious.

Saving Seed: Entirely possible. Simply do not cut the flower until the seeds and the white cottony fuzz they are attached to are ready to fly. It is best to sow the seeds as soon as they have been released and winter the seedlings over. Provide lots of nutrients. Next spring you'll watch a highly variable bunch of plants produce a highly variable lot of flowers so start at least a dozen positions. The game will be won when you discover one great plant.

Varieties: There are two "varieties" commonly on offer as seeds—a green one and a purple one. Be cautious about buying a garden centre seedling; it may be a rooted secondary from a productive plant (good) or it may have been started from seed, in which case the odds are far greater than 10:1 against it being an excellent plant.

Okra

(Hibiscus esculentus)

My first vegie garden was in the steamy San Fernando Valley, a suburb of Los Angeles. There I grew 1,500-mm-tall okra bushes. Each branching bush yielded a few pods almost every day over several months. The pods were so tender and sweet when eaten raw that they rarely made it into the kitchen. Because of that, frozen or canned okra disgusts me now. Okra on a supermarket produce counter? Way too old! Okra that gets airfreighted to Tsing Wah, an Asian market in Launceston, has proven to be delicious. Sometimes.

I made a great many unsuccessful attempts to grow okra in Oregon and more such attempts in Tasmania. I can state with fair certainty that growing okra outside of a *polytunnel or greenhouse* is not practical in Tasmania. I have tried warming the okra bed with black plastic; I have trialled every available variety including so called early hybrids. I have direct seeded okra; I have raised seedlings and transplanted them. My best Tasmanian outdoor result happened in an unusually hot summer when a few weak, stressed-looking plants about 60 cm tall yielded a few miniscule pods.

Additional Reading

I think understanding "why-to" is far more important than knowing how-to because desire precedes action. A careful reading of the books listed below indisputably shows how soil fertility determines human health as much or more than making healthy food choices does. I'd like the whole world to be healthier so I have put every title in this list online for free download at http://www.soilandhealth.org

Albrecht, William. *Soil Fertility and Animal Health.* Webster City, Iowa: Fred Hahne Printing Co., 1958. The book explains how the regional pattern of available soil minerals varies more by climate than by the rocks the soil derived from and that climate mostly determines if the land produces nutrient-dense protein-rich food or if it mainly produces less nutritious carbohydrate foods and fibres. Animals (and by implication, humans) breed well and live long—or not that well and not so long—according to which type of soil they eat from. Albrecht published hundreds of scientific papers, journal articles and even a many years-long series of health magazine articles. This, his only book, encapsulates all his major messages. A reprint is currently in print, sold as "The Albrecht Papers, Vol. 2" by Acres, USA.

Dale, Tom and Vernon Gill Carter. *Topsoil and Civilization.* Norman, Oklahoma: University of Oklahoma Press, 1955. A survey of world history that explains how every previous civilization fell because they degraded their agricultural resource base. The book asks, quite pointedly, how long ours is going to endure.

Elliot, Robert. *The Clifton Park System of Farming.* London: Faber & Faber, 1943. Originally published in 1898 as *Agricultural Changes.* Elliot developed long rotations by sowing arable fields to deep-rooting grasses, clovers and broad leaf weeds. The paddock would be returned to cropping after four to eight years. When cropping lowered soil organic matter levels too far, the field would be restored by again growing grass/clover/herbal mixtures.

Howard, Albert. *Farming and Gardening For Health or Disease.* London: Faber and Faber, 1945 (also called *The Soil and Health* when it was published by Rodale Press in the USA). Howard explains that soil fertility determines human and animal health. Howard's disciples incorrectly believed soil fertility is only accurately measurable by its organic matter content. Albert Howard was the founder of the organic farming and gardening movement.

Howard, Albert and Yeshwant D. Wad. *The Waste Products of Agriculture: Their Utilisation As Humus.* London: Oxford University Press, 1931. This is Howard's most important scientific publication, detailing the method for making superlative compost he developed at Indore Research Farm.

Jenny, Hans. *Factors of Soil Formation: A System of Quantitative Pedology.* New York: Dover, 1994. Originally published in 1941. One of the most important books about soil ever written. Reading Jenny is essential to understanding agricultural soils. This is a scientific text that can be understood without maths, however, a well grasped secondary school science education and a touch of geology makes this book fully comprehensible. Dover Press publishes an inexpensive paperback reprint.

King, F.C. *Farmers of Forty Centuries: or Traditional Agriculture in China, Korea and Japan.* 1911. A classic of holistic agricultural literature. King was a masterful observer of farming. This is, if nothing else, a great travel book.

Krasilnikov, N.S. *Soil Microorganisms and Higher Plants.* Academy of Sciences of the USSR: Moscow, 1958. Translated in Israel by Dr. Y. Halperin. Printed in the USA by the Government Printing Office. In its era this book was the ultimate study of the microbial process in soil as it relates to agriculture. Industrial production of agricultural inputs was limited in the Soviet Union of the 30s, 40s and 50s. Soviet agronomic research could not focus upon the use of chemicals spread voluminously because chemical fertilizers and pesticides could not have been produced in large enough quantity. So Krasil'nikov observed soil microbiology and found ways to improve plant growth with special composts and microbial ferments of the sort that could be made by the farmer in an old barrel. All these "primitive" solutions are based on understanding complex interactions between soil microbes and crop species.

Parnes, Robert. *Fertile Soil, A Grower's Guide To Organic and Inorganic Fertilizers.* Davis, California: Ag Access, 1990. This is a scarce but useful book and is very expensive when you finally turn up a used copy.

Price, Weston, D.D.S. *Nutrition and Physical Degeneration.* New York: Paul B. Hoeber, Inc., 1939. Dr. Price was a highly respected dental researcher who focused on prevention rather than on treatment. In the 1930s Price visited many extremely isolated communities where *everyone* enjoyed extraordinary good health, long life and virtual immunity to disease. Tooth decay was non-existent. Over several years Price journeyed to remote parts of Scotland and Switzerland, Canada, Alaska, Peru, Africa, Down Under, etc. where he observed extraordinarily healthy—and extremely remote—communities that did not—because they could not—partake of the industrial food system. Contains remarkable photographs that plainly reveal the differences between healthy bodies and physically degenerated bodies. These photographs testify far better than words ever could. No one who closely examines Price's photos will ever view the health and appearance of their friends, their neighbours or their own face in the mirror in the same way.

Smith, J. Russell. *Tree Crops: A Permanent Agriculture.* New York: Harcourt & Brace, 1929. Any plowed field sloping more than three percent (3 metres fall in 100 metres of run) will lose its topsoil within a few centuries (sometimes a lot quicker). That much soil loss undermines the resource base that allows civilization to exist. Tree crops on sloping land prevent soil loss and thus lead to the possibility of a permanent civilization. Smith shows us photos of places and people mostly eating food from trees and considers the potential for tree cropping in North America.

Tiedjens, Victor. *More Food From Soil Science: The Natural Chemistry of Lime in Agriculture.* New York: Exposition Press, 1965. Tiedjens is right up there with Albrecht on the list of those who most advanced the growing of nutrient-dense food.

Tiedjens, Victor. *Olena Farm, USA: An Agricultural Success Story.* New York: Exposition Press, 1969. Tiedjens chronicles how he restored an exhausted Ohio farm mainly by the use of agricultural lime.

Weaver, John. *Root Development of Vegetable Crops.* New York: McGraw Hill, 1927. A classic study filled with species-by-species illustrations, each one worth a thousand words. Fully understanding what's seen above the soil line takes an appreciation what the plant is trying to accomplish below ground. The drawings in Chapter 9 of the book you are reading now were reproduced from Weaver.

Widstoe, John A. *Dry Farming.* New York: MacMillan, 1911. By reading between the lines of this book one can see how lack of ethics and greed led farmers to ignore Widstoe's warnings, making the American Great Plains dust bowl inevitable. This book greatly helped enable me to understand dry gardening.

Wrench, G.T. , *The Wheel of Health.* London. C.W. Daniel Company, Ltd., 1939. This is Dr. Wrench's exploration of the Hunza, a mountain people in what is now northern Pakistan. The Hunza were renowned for longevity and vigour. This book should form the foundation of inquiry into healthy living. It should be required reading to graduate from every high school. In *The Wheel of Health* you will encounter two other renowned health explorers: Sir Robert McCarrison and Sir Albert Howard. You will also have the opportunity to spend time with Dr. Wrench, who was an individualist possessed of the most admirable intelligence.

Conversions

For use by readers more familiar with US or UK measurements.
All conversions are close enough for practical purposes.

Temperature

Celsius	Fahrenheit	Context
0°C	32°F	Freezing point
5°C	41°F	Cool soil, early spring
10°C	50°F	Minimum for most seed germination
15°C	59°F	Good growing conditions
20°C	68°F	Ideal for most vegetables
25°C	77°F	Warm season crops
30°C	86°F	Hot — stress for cool-climate crops

Area

Metric	US and UK	Context
1 m^2	10 sq ft	Small bed area
10 m^2	100 sq ft	Typical garden bed (1 deciare)
100 m^2	1,000 sq ft	Larger garden plot
1,000 m^2	¼ acre	Large garden / small holding

Weight

Metric	US and UK	Context
25 g	1 oz	Small fertiliser quantities
100 g	3.5 oz	Fertiliser per bed
250 g	9 oz	COF quantities
500 g	1 lb 2 oz	COF quantities
1 kg	2.2 lbs	Bulk fertiliser
5 kg	11 lbs	Bag quantities
25 kg	55 lbs	Bulk bag quantities

Distance & Depth

Metric	US and UK	Context
1 cm	⅜ inch	Very shallow seed depth (fine seeds)
2 cm	¾ inch	Shallow seed depth
5 cm	2 inches	Transplant depth
10 cm	4 inches	Spacing, small plants
20 cm	8 inches	Spacing, medium plants
30 cm	12 inches (1 foot)	Row spacing
50 cm	20 inches	Wide row spacing
1 metre	39 inches (~3 feet)	Bed width

Volume

Metric	US	UK	Context
5 ml	1 teaspoon	1 teaspoon	Trace element dosing
20ml	1⅓ tablespoons	1⅓ tablespoons	AU = 20ml, UK/US = 15 ml
250 ml	1 cup (8 fl oz)	scant ½ pint	Small liquid quantities
500 ml	1 pint (16 fl oz)	scant 1 pint	Liquid fertiliser
1 litre	1 quart (approx)	1¾ pints	Watering, liquid feed
10 litres	2.6 gallons	2.2 gallons	Watering can capacity
20 litres	5.3 gallons	4.4 gallons	COF mixing quantity

Cool Climates

This book uses "cool-climate" to describe regions with mild winters and summers that rarely turn brutally hot — the temperature range in which most cool-season vegetables thrive without bolting, scorching, or stalling. It includes:

- Coastal Victoria
- The Great Southern coast of Western Australia (Albany, Denmark)
- Tasmania (Lutruwita)
- Cascadia — the maritime Pacific coast west of the Cascade Range, from northern California through western Oregon and Washington to the Lower Mainland and southern coast of British Columbia
- The South Island of New Zealand (Te Waipounamu)
- Chile, south of Santiago
- Southern England (especially the southwest) and Wales
- Ireland
- Holland, the cooler parts of Belgium, Brittany, and Normandy
- Coastal northern Spain
- Western coastal Norway

Most of these share the same underlying climate: mild, wet winters and cool-to-mild summers with no real dry season. A handful — coastal Victoria, the WA Great Southern, Cascadia, and Chile south of Santiago — are technically a different type: dry summers rather than wet, even though they're just as mild. Cascadia in particular sees 100 or more rainless days during the period of greatest heat.

If you garden in one of these dry-summer regions, the temperatures in this book should suit you, but you'll need to irrigate through summer in a way that gardeners in the wetter regions above generally don't.

If your region isn't listed here, try this test: do your summers regularly climb past the high 20s°C (mid-80s°F) for extended stretches, and do your winters reliably drop below freezing for weeks at a time? If neither is true, you're likely gardening in cool-climate territory, whatever your local name for it.

The principles in this book travel further than the regions above. Building fertile soil, growing nutrient-dense vegetables, working with rather than against your conditions — none of that is specific to a cool climate. What won't transfer directly is timing: planting dates and season length are tied to local conditions, so gardeners elsewhere should adapt the calendar in this book to their own, rather than follow it directly.

Steve closes his Preface by hoping this guide might inspire similar books for other climates. Until one exists for yours, the thinking behind this one still applies.

About the Author

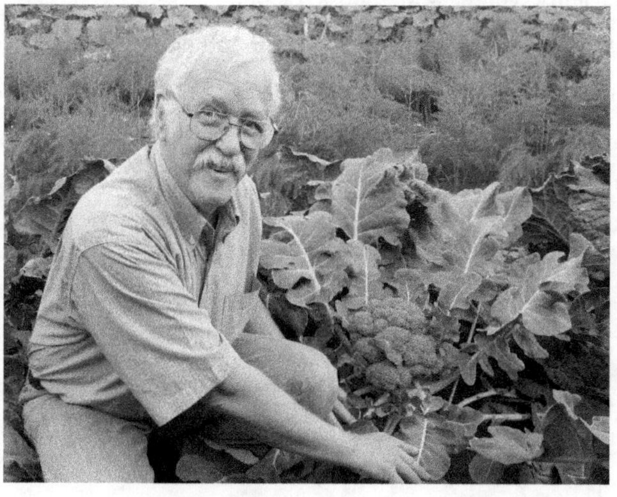

Steve Solomon has been growing most of his own food for over fifty years — first in Oregon, where he founded Territorial Seed Company and wrote *Growing Vegetables West of the Cascades*, the classic food gardening manual for western Oregon and Washington. Then in Tasmania, moving to the island in 1998. This book sprang from that second chapter, with roughly half his growing life spent in each place, across two of the world's finest cool-temperate growing regions.

To found Territorial Seed Company and conduct its extensive variety trials, Steve reached far beyond what organic gardeners typically need to know — coming to understand agriculture as spoken by qualified plant breeders and agronomists. His most recent book, *The Intelligent Gardener*, shows how to create balanced, fully remineralised soil using laboratory soil test results.

Steve is also the founder of the Soil and Health Library (soilandhealth.org), a free online archive of rare and out-of-print books on organic farming, nutrition and self-sufficiency — a resource used by researchers and growers around the world.

Steve believes that growing nutrient-dense food is one of the most powerful things a person can do for their own health — and that most people, with the right knowledge, can do it. This book is that knowledge.

About the Publisher

Melliodora Publishing was started by Su Dennett and her partner David Holmgren, co-originator of permaculture, to produce books and other media to support people in their permaculture journey, while bypassing the traditional gatekeepers of the publishing industry. We aim to minimise adverse environmental impacts of the whole book creation, including printing, logistics and marketing chain, while providing a fair share return to authors, illustrators, editors and other creative contributors to the publishing process. At all times we are guided by permaculture ethics and principles.

MELLIODORA
PUBLISHING

For more see **melliodora.com**

For more on permaculture see **permacultureprinciples.com**

For more on David Holmgren see **holmgren.com.au**;
for his take on possible climate change futures see **futurescenarios.org**;
and for his practical strategies for a resilient future see **retrosuburbia.com**

www.ingramcontent.com/pod-product-compliance
Lightning Source LLC
LaVergne TN
LVHW080050210926
848481LV00011B/3318
9780645606577